T0305803

Global Regulations of Medicinal, Pharmaceutical, and Food Products

Medicine regulation demands the application of sound medical, scientific, and technical knowledge and skills, and operates within a legal framework. Regulatory functions involve interactions with various stakeholders (e.g., manufacturers, traders, consumers, health professionals, researchers, and governments) whose economic, social, and political motives may differ, making implementation of regulation both politically and technically challenging. This book discusses regulatory landscape globally and the current global regulatory scenario of medicinal products and food products comprehensively.

Features:

- Discusses how recent developments of medicinal and food products have opened up innovative solutions for many of the current challenges societies face presently.
- Explores the manifold variations between the regulatory bodies in different countries that have not previously been collected to this extent.
- Presents details on the substantial progress in analytical methodologies for labeling applications and the creation of appropriate test criteria for pharmaceuticals and their safety analysis.
- Reviews how more worldwide collaboration and cooperation in the regulatory area is still required.

Global Regulations of Medicinal, Pharmaceutical, and Food Products

Edited by Faraat Ali and Leo M.L. Nollet

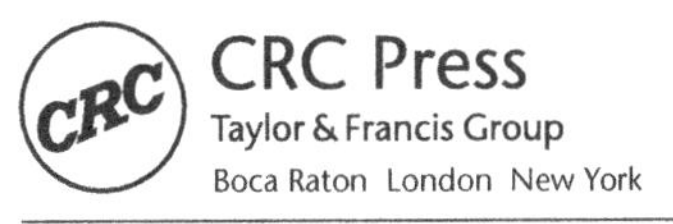

CRC Press is an imprint of the
Taylor & Francis Group, an **informa** business

Designed Cover image: Shutterstock

First edition published 2025
by CRC Press
2385 Executive Center Drive, Suite 320, Boca Raton, FL 33431

and by CRC Press
4 Park Square, Milton Park, Abingdon, Oxon, OX14 4RN

CRC Press is an imprint of Taylor & Francis Group, LLC

Library of Congress Cataloging-in-Publication Data
Names: Ali, Faraat, editor. | Nollet, Leo M. L., 1948– editor.
Title: Global regulations of medicinal, pharmaceutical, and food products / edited by Faraat Ali, Manager, Department of Inspection and Enforcement, Pharmaceutical Development Laboratory Services, BoMRA, Botswana; Leo M. L. Nollet, University College Ghent, Belgium.
Description: First Edition. | Boca Raton : CRC Press, 2024. | Includes bibliographical references and index. |
Identifiers: LCCN 2023057884 (print) | LCCN 2023057885 (ebook) | ISBN 9781032283623 (hardback) | ISBN 9781032283692 (paperback) | ISBN 9781003296492 (ebook)
Subjects: LCSH: Medical laws and legislation. | Drugs—Law and legislation. | Pharmacy—Law and legislation. | Food law and legislation.
Classification: LCC K3601 .G57 2024 (print) | LCC K3601 (ebook) | DDC 344.04/232—dc23/eng/20240316
LC record available at https://lccn.loc.gov/2023057884
LC ebook record available at https://lccn.loc.gov/2023057885

ISBN: 978-1-032-28362-3 (hbk)
ISBN: 978-1-032-28369-2 (pbk)
ISBN: 978-1-003-29649-2 (ebk)

DOI: 10.1201/9781003296492

Typeset in Times Lt Std
by Apex CoVantage, LLC

Contents

Preface

The use of poor quality, substandard, and falsified medicines can result in therapeutic failure, resistance to medicines, and sometimes death. It also undermines confidence in health technology systems, health professionals, pharmaceutical manufacturers, and distributors. Money spent on ineffective, unsafe, and poor quality medicines is wasted—whether by patients/consumers or insurance schemes/governments. Governments have the responsibility to protect their citizens in the areas where the citizens themselves are not able to do so. Thus, governments of different countries need to establish strong national regulatory authorities (NRAs) to ensure that the manufacture, trade, and use of medicines are regulated effectively. In broad terms the mission of NRAs is to protect and promote public health. Medicines regulation demands the application of sound scientific (including but not limited to medical, pharmaceutical, biological, and chemical) knowledge and specific technical skills, and operates within a legal and regulatory framework. The basic elements of effective drug regulation have been laid down in several World Health Organization guidance documents. Medicines regulation incorporates several mutually reinforcing activities, all aimed at promoting and protecting public health. These activities vary from country to country in scope and implementation. What makes medicines regulation effective? Regulatory functions involve interactions with various stakeholders (e.g., manufacturers, traders, consumers, health professionals, researchers, and governments) whose economic, social, and political motives may differ, making implementation of regulation both politically and technically challenging. Medicines regulation has an administrative part, but far more important is the scientific basis for it. All medicines must meet three criteria: be of good quality, safety, and efficacy. The judgments about medicines quality, safety and efficacy should be based on solid and regulatory convergence science.

The specific factors for NRA include a clear mission statement; adequate medicines legislation and regulation; appropriate organizational structure and facilities; clearly defined NRA roles and responsibilities; adequate and sustainable financial resources, including resources to retain and develop staff; appropriate tools, such as standards, guidelines, and procedures, international collaboration, convergence, regulatory practice and reliance with other NRAs and health authorities.

The same arguments apply for food. Food safety standards are a set of requirements that foods and food manufacturers must meet to produce and serve safe food products for human consumption. Food safety standards are interpreted differently in each country. All food companies must follow food safety standards for the protection of public health. Laws that lay out food safety standards are always complex, and most acts and food regulations affecting the food industry are no exception. These standards are essential elements of all food companies to protect public health from food safety risks while serving quality foods. Some standards and food safety requirements are designed to address food safety issues before they even occur.

Different countries have different interpretations of what is safe for their constituents. The differences may be based on lifestyle, tradition, quality of food ingredients, and scientific knowledge. Higher bodies, such as the Codex Alimentarius Commission, may be consulted to make decisions.

Standards for food safety are established based on scientific evidence and risk assessment. Their aim is to prevent the occurrence of different foodborne illnesses. They are applied throughout the entire food supply chain to ensure that raw materials and finished products are processed safely.

Recent development of medicinal and food products has opened up a world of possibilities for innovative solutions to most of the current challenges societies face presently. On the other hand, product development evolves quicker than the regulatory landscape and frameworks. This is because of the complexity of specific pharmaceuticals and food products, the unavailability of an internationally standardized regulatory framework, and worldwide regulatory landscape differences. In the last two decades, scientific institutions and regulatory agencies have put in a lot of effort to meet these issues. However, there has been substantial progress in analytical methodologies for labeling applications and the creation of appropriate test criteria for pharmaceuticals and their safety analysis.

More worldwide collaboration and cooperation in the regulatory area is still required. The growing presence of pharmaceutical products in almost every sphere of science, especially in nano-pharmaceutical and personal care areas, has again proved the vital significance of unregulated products in today's world. However, it has also led to concerns regarding their associated safety, efficacy, and toxicity issues among the public and scientific communities. Here comes the role of the regulators to ensure the maintenance of regulatory concerns of medicinal and food products, hence maintaining the confidence and trust of the public. However, because of the complicated nature of the recently developed medicinal and food products, they pose challenges for the regulators to form necessary legislation, guidelines, and rules.

This book focuses on and comprehensively discusses the regulatory landscape globally including registration, evaluation, marketing authorization, testing, characterization, recent regulation, challenges, safety assessments, regulatory standards documents, and the current global regulatory scenario of medicinal products and food products.

This book has two sections. The first section, "Global Regulatory Perspectives of Medicinal and Pharmaceutical Products," consists of 14 chapters that discuss the challenges, safety aspects, and regulations of medicinal and pharmaceutical products in different countries and continents. An overview of regulatory matters is also provided. In the second section, Global Regulatory Perspectives of Food Products," these same items are discussed in five chapters in terms of food products.

The editors of this book would like to thank all contributors for their excellent work and their time spent in preparing their chapters.

Thank you very much to my coeditor, Faraat Ali, for his enthusiasm while working on this project.

Leo M.L. Nollet

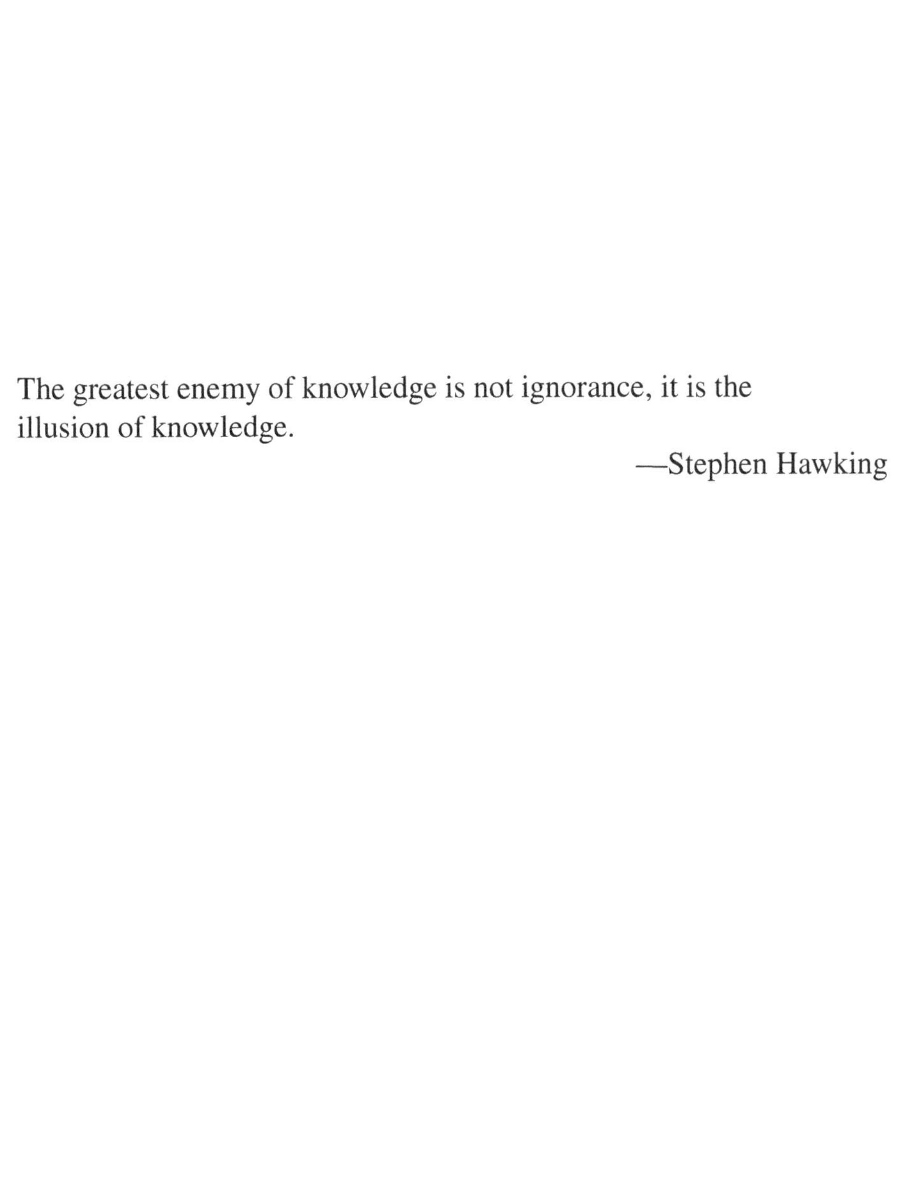

The greatest enemy of knowledge is not ignorance, it is the illusion of knowledge.

—Stephen Hawking

About the Editors

Faraat Ali presently working as Manager of Department of Inspection and Enforcement, Pharmaceutical Development Laboratory Services (Formerly National Drug Quality Control Laboratory), Botswana Medicines Regulatory Authority (BoMRA), Gaborone, Botswana. Mr Ali is a Graduate Pharmaceutical Scientist and completed Master of Pharmacy in Pharmaceutical and Medicinal Chemistry from Uttar Pradesh Technical University, India; Post Graduate Diploma in Drug Regulatory Affairs (PGDDRA) from Jamia Hamdard, India; and Post Graduate Diploma in Management (PGDM) from WITS Business School, University of Witwatersrand, South Africa. He has over 9 years of rich and varied experience in analytical research and development, regulatory system strengthening (RSS), regulatory and scientific affairs, drug and formulation development and public health, working in various positions in top ranking pharmaceutical industries (including Teva API India Ltd, Akums Drugs and Pharmaceuticals Ltd.) and standard drug regulatory setting in India (specifically the Indian Pharmacopoeia Commission (IPC), Ministry of Health and Family Welfare, Government of India). He initiated his career as a research trainee in Teva API India Limited, Gajraula, India. He has published more than 60 scientific publications/book chapter in various national and international journals to his credit. Ali is a member of World Health Organization-National Control Laboratory (WHO-NCL) Network for Biologicals & Vaccines, American Chemical Society, Regulatory Affairs Professional Society (RAPS), American Association of Pharmaceutical Scientists (AAPS) and life member of IPGA.

Leo M.L. Nollet earned an MS (1973) and PhD (1978) in biology from the Katholieke Universiteit Leuven, Belgium. He is an editor and associate editor of numerous books. He edited for M. Dekker, New York—now CRC Press of Taylor & Francis Publishing Group—the first, second, and third editions of *Food Analysis by HPLC* and *Handbook of Food Analysis*. The last edition is a two-volume book. Dr. Nollet also edited the *Handbook of Water Analysis* (first, second, and third editions) and *Chromatographic Analysis of the Environment* (third and fourth editions with CRC Press). With F. Toldrá, he coedited two books published in 2006, 2007, and 2017: *Advanced Technologies for Meat Processing* (CRC Press) and *Advances in Food Diagnostics*. With M. Poschl, he coedited the book *Radionuclide Concentrations in Foods and the Environment*, also published in 2006 (CRC Press). Dr. Nollet has also coedited with Y. H. Hui and other colleagues on several books: *Handbook of Food Product Manufacturing* (2007), *Handbook of Food Science, Technology, and Engineering* (CRC Press, 2005), *Food Biochemistry and Food Processing* (first and second editions; 2006 and 2012), and the *Handbook of Fruits and Vegetable Flavors* (2010). In addition, he edited *Handbook of Meat, Poultry, and Seafood Quality* (first and second editions; 2007 and 2012). From 2008 to 2011, he published five volumes on animal product-related books with F. Toldrá: *Handbook of Muscle Foods Analysis*, *Handbook of Processed Meats and Poultry Analysis*, *Handbook of Seafood and Seafood Products Analysis*, *Handbook of Dairy Foods Analysis* (second edition in 2021), and *Handbook of Analysis of Edible Animal By-Products*. Also, in 2011, with F. Toldrá, he coedited two volumes for CRC Press: *Safety Analysis of Foods of Animal Origin* and *Sensory Analysis of Foods of Animal Origin*. In 2012, they published the *Handbook of Analysis of Active Compounds in Functional Foods*. In a coedition with Hamir Rathore, *Handbook of Pesticides: Methods of Pesticides Residues Analysis* was marketed in 2009; *Pesticides: Evaluation of Environmental Pollution* in 2012; *Biopesticides Handbook* in 2015; and *Green Pesticides Handbook: Essential Oils for Pest Control* in 2017. Other finished book projects include *Food Allergens: Analysis, Instrumentation, and Methods* (with A. van Hengel; CRC Press, 2011) and *Analysis of Endocrine Compounds in Food* (2011). Dr. Nollet's recent projects include *Proteomics in Foods* with F. Toldrá (2013) and *Transformation Products of Emerging Contaminants in the Environment: Analysis, Processes, Occurrence, Effects, and Risks* with D. Lambropoulou (2014). In the series Food Analysis & Properties, he edited (with C. Ruiz-Capillas) *Flow Injection Analysis of Food Additives* (CRC Press, 2015) and *Marine Microorganisms: Extraction and Analysis of Bioactive Compounds* (CRC Press, 2016). With A.S. Franca, he coedited *Spectroscopic Methods in Food Analysis* (CRC Press, 2017), and with Horacio Heinzen and Amadeo R. Fernandez-Alba he coedited *Multiresidue Methods for the Analysis of Pesticide Residues in Food* (CRC Press, 2017). Further volumes in the series Food Analysis & Properties are *Phenolic Compounds in Food: Characterization and Analysis* (with Janet Alejandra Gutierrez-Uribe, 2018), *Testing and Analysis of GMO-containing Foods and Feed* (with Salah E. O. Mahgoub, 2018), *Fingerprinting Techniques in Food Authentication and Traceability* (with K. S. Siddiqi, 2018), *Hyperspectral Imaging Analysis and Applications for Food Quality* (with N.C. Basantia, Leo M.L. Nollet, Mohammed Kamruzzaman, 2018), *Ambient Mass Spectroscopy Techniques in Food and the Environment* (with Basil K. Munjanja, 2019), *Food Aroma Evolution: During Food Processing, Cooking, and Aging* (with M. Bordiga, 2019), *Mass Spectrometry Imaging in Food Analysis* (2020), *Proteomics in Food Authentication* (with S. Ötleş, 2020), *Analysis of Nanoplastics and Microplastics in Food* (with K.S. Siddiqi, 2020), *Chiral Organic Pollutants, Monitoring and Characterization in Food and the Environment* (with Edmond Sanganyado and Basil K. Munjanja, 2020), *Sequencing Technologies in Microbial Food Safety and Quality* (with Devarajan Thangardurai, Saher Islam, Jeyabalan Sangeetha, 2021), *Nanoemulsions in Food Technology: Development, Characterization, and Applications* (with Javed Ahmad, 2021), *Mass Spectrometry in Food Analysis* (with Robert Winkler, 2022), *Bioactive Peptides from Food: Sources, Analysis, and Functions* (with Semih Ötles, 2022), and *Nutriomics: Well-being through Nutrition* (with Devarajan Thangadurai, Saher IslamJuliana Bunmi Adetunji, 2022).

Contributors

Usama Ahmad
Department of Pharmacy
Integral University
Lucknow, UP, India

Shaima Ahmadeen
Quality Evaluation of Biological Products Saudi Food and Drug Authority (SFDA) Riyadh
KSA

Jitin Ahuja
Department of Consumer Affairs Ministry of Consumer Affairs
New Delhi, India

Md. Akbar
Faculty of Pharmacy
Al-Kareem University
Katihar, Bihar, India

Tausif Alam
School of Pharmaceutical Sciences Lingaya's Vidyapeeth
Faridabad, Haryana, India

Faraat Ali
Department of Inspection and Enforcement
Laboratory Services Botswana Medicines Regulatory Authority Gaborone, Botswana

Hasan Ali
Department of Pharmacy Meerut
Institute of Technology Meerut
Uttar Pradesh, India

Vazahat Ali
MJP Rohilkhand University
Bareilly, Uttar Pradesh, India

Varisha Anjum
Department of Food and Biotechnology School of Medical Sciences
South Ural State University
Chelyabinsk, Russia

Irfan Ansari
School of Pharmaceutical Sciences Lingaya's Vidyapeeth
Faridabad, Haryana, India

Vishal Dixit
School of Pharmaceutical Sciences Lingaya's Vidyapeeth
Faridabad, Haryana, India

Ramesh K. Goyal
Department of Pharmacology School of Pharmacy
Delhi Pharmaceutical Sciences and Research University
Pushp Vihar, New Delhi, India

Parveen Kumar Goyal
Department of Pharmacy Panipat Institute of Engineering and Technology
Panipat, Haryana, India

Anam Ilyas
Medicinal Chemistry and Molecular Modelling Lab Department of Pharmaceutical Chemistry School of Pharmaceutical Education and Research Jamia
Hamdard, New Delhi, India

Babar Iqbal
Formulation and Development Unicure India Ltd. Noida
Uttar Pradesh, India

Anas Islam
Department of Pharmacy Integral University
Lucknow, Uttar Pradesh, India

Gaurav Pratap Singh Jadaun
Indian Pharmacopoeia Commission Ministry of Health & Family Welfare Government of India
Ghaziabad, Uttar Pradesh, India

Pritya Jha
Department of Pharmacy Banasthali Vidyapeeth
Banasthali, Rajasthan, India

Vivekanandan Kalaiselvan
Indian Pharmacopoeia Commission Ministry of Health & Family Welfare Government of India
Ghaziabad, Uttar Pradesh, India

Nishith Keserwani
Indian Pharmacopoeia Commission National Coordination Centre Pharmacovigilance Programme of India
Ghaziabad, Uttar Pradesh, India

Rishi Kumar
Indian Pharmacopoeia Commission National Coordination Centre Pharmacovigilance Programme of India
Ghaziabad, Uttar Pradesh, India

Rutendo J. Kuwana
Incidents and Substandard/Falsified Medical Products Team Regulation and Safety of Medicines Unit World Health Organization
Geneva, Switzerland

Kumari Neha
Department of Pharmaceutical Chemistry Delhi Institute of Pharmaceutical Sciences and Research DPSR University
New Delhi, India

Leo M.L. Nollet
University College Ghent Ghent
Belgium

Irina Potoroko
Department of Food and Biotechnology School of Medical Sciences South Ural State University
Chelyabinsk, Russia

Doaa Rady
Egyptian Drug Authority Cairo
Egypt

Evans Sagwa
US Pharmacopeial Convention PQM Kenya

Vishesh Sahu
Amity Institute of Pharmacy Amity University
Noida, Uttar Pradesh, India

Colin Shamhuyarira
Kairos University Sioux Falls
South Dakota

Arvind Kumar Sharma
Department of Pharmacology School of Pharmacy Delhi Pharmaceutical Sciences and Research University
New Delhi, India

Khushboo Sharma
School of Pharmaceutical Sciences Lingaya's Vidyapeeth
Faridabad, Haryana, India

Neeraj Kant Sharma
Department of Pharmacy Meerut Institute of Technology Meerut
Uttar Pradesh, India

Tarani Prakash Shrivastava
Department of Pharmacology School of Pharmacy Delhi Pharmaceutical Sciences and Research University
New Delhi, India

Meghna Amrita Singh
Department of Pharmaceutics School of Pharmacy Delhi Pharmaceutical Sciences and Research University
New Delhi, India

Neelam Singh
Department of Pharmacy ITS College of Pharmacy
Ghaziabad, Uttar Pradesh, India

Sandeep Kumar Singh
Department of Pharmaceutical Sciences Birla Institute of Technology
Ranchi, Jharkhand, India

Manisha Trivedi
Indian Pharmacopoeia Commission Ministry of Health & Family Welfare Government of India
Ghaziabad, Uttar Pradesh, India

Yayra Timothy Tuani
Department of Chemistry and Biochemistry University of Maryland College Park
Maryland

Sharad K. Wakode
Department of Pharmaceutical Chemistry Delhi Institute of Pharmaceutical Sciences and Research DPSR University
New Delhi, India

Section 1

Global Regulatory Perspectives of Medicinal and Pharmaceutical Products

1 Introduction, Challenges, and Overview of Regulatory Affairs

Faraat Ali, Kumari Neha, Anam Ilyas, and Hasan Ali

1.1 INTRODUCTION

Every industry must complete a first experimental exercise in pharmaceutical product design to generate acceptable and sustainable goods. The process of implementing concepts in a structured manner results in a product that meets quality standards. Pharmaceutical items are manufactured and constructed under a number of compendial constraints and are subject to the rules of various country constitutions that have been formed after a great deal of testing. Nearly all nations have their own regulatory bodies that are responsible for enforcing laws, rules, and standards for medication improvement, registration, licensing, producing goods, categorizing, and marketing of pharmaceutical goods. In addition to national regulatory bodies, certain international associations are also promoting drug safety through the development of guidelines for product approval, distribution, manufacturing, price control, marketing, advertising, and intellectual property rights protection (Franco, 2013). Table 1.1 provides a complete list of regulatory bodies from various nations for fast and easy reference. Drug regulation promotes a number of activities to ensure the safety, effectiveness, and quality of drugs (Wirthumer-Hoche and Bloechl-Daum, 2016). The pharmaceutical corporation must set up a regulatory affairs department that actively participates in all phases of drug development, from clinical research to marketing and post-marketing surveillance, to comply with regulatory standards. It serves as a liaison between the drug regulatory organizations and the pharmaceutical sector (De Frutos, 2013).

The pharmaceutical sector is constantly up against competitors from around the world and must operate under pressure to provide products on schedule, under budget, and according to standards. These three crucial requirements, which are governed by rules and laws, determine whether a product is successful or unsuccessful (Gabe et al., 2015). Before scheduling a new medication, the pharmaceutical business must take the legal and regulatory requirements into account. Therefore, understanding legal and regulatory frameworks from the outset of drug discovery helps researchers integrate their findings and create a research roadmap (Dimasi et al., 2016). After the phases of medication research and discovery are completed, commercial production follows

DOI: 10.1201/9781003296492-2

TABLE 1.1
Regulatory Bodies and Their Functions

ICH	*International Council for Harmonisation of Technical Requirements for Pharmaceuticals for Human Use*: Issues guidelines defining quality, safety, efficacy, and related aspects for developing and registering new medicinal products in Europe, Japan, and the United States.
CDSCO	*Central Drugs Standard Control Organization, Ministry of Health & Family Welfare, Government of India*: Provides drug regulatory requirements in India.
EMA	*European Medicines Agency*: Decentralised body of the European Union headquartered in London prescribes guidelines for inspections and general reporting and all aspects of human and veterinary medicines.
FDA	*US Food and Drug Administration*: Issues regulations, guidelines, notifications, news, and other communications.
MHRA	*Medicines and Healthcare Products Regulatory Agency*: Responsible for ensuring efficacy and safety of medicines and medical devices in the United Kingdom; produces news, warnings, information, and publications.
PMDA	*Japanese Pharmaceutical and Medical Devices Agency*: An Independent Administrative Institution responsible for ensuring the safety, efficacy, and quality of pharmaceuticals and medical devices in Japan.
Health Canada	The federal department responsible for health-related issues in Canada; issues advisories, warnings, recalls, reports, publications, activities, legislation, and guidelines.

established guidelines that are periodically reviewed by the regulatory body in the country where the goods are intended for sale. However, scientists must ensure that a developed or state-of-the-art medication satisfies all regulatory standards before moving forward with commercial manufacture (Pezzola and Sweet, 2016) because there will be a significant loss of time, money, and the reputation of the company if the product fails during processing. As a result, all pharmaceutical enterprises are concerned about regulatory matters because the introduction of novel and inventive medicines will determine the fate of their businesses (Glick et al., 2014). Drug approval is a laborious procedure, and production facilities, documentation, and experimental expertise all work together to make it successful. Therefore, working in tandem with regulatory bodies becomes the duty of regulatory affairs experts (Djulbegovic et al., 2014).

Because obtaining regulatory clearance is directly tied to an organization's income, industries periodically look for ways to expedite the process, which can result in regulatory fraud. As a recent example, a multinational corporation was fined $3 billion for paying bribes to doctors to boost the sales of its medicines. Under these conditions, the regulatory body should uphold its moral principles and be resolute in its standards. For this reason, regulatory authorities must closely monitor every facet of medication research, discovery, and marketing. However, regulatory agencies also confront significant challenges in the form of the acceleration of drug development, and they are pressing for more effort and intensity in this area. Regulatory bodies occasionally make situational choices as well, like in the case of the Ebola virus, which has a 50% to 90% fatality rate. The US Food and Drug Administration (FDA) has provided an Ebola vaccine with "animal efficacy rules," which allow for limited flexibility throughout the trial phase and restrict vaccine registration to the use of animal models. Therefore, after vaccination, human interaction with the pathogens is not necessary (Donnelly, 2016). The rules put in place by different organizations are making the process of developing new pharmaceuticals more complicated, but they are also providing a blueprint for how researchers might create safe and efficient medications. Therefore, regulatory bodies play a crucial role in the pharmaceutical sector by aiding in the comprehension of how different laws impact the various aspects of drug research (Spindler and Schmechel, 2016). Moreover, the regulatory landscape for traditional goods, such as tablets, capsules, and immediate-release and extended-release medications, is stable. For the majority of nanotechnology-based medications, however, the development criteria and restrictions remain vague (Lalu et al., 2017; Maheshwari et al., 2015; Sharma et al., 2015; Tekade et al., 2017).

Pharmaceutical regulations are defined as a blend of legal and administrative measures that governments take to ensure the safety, quality, and efficacy of medicines, as well as the relevance and accuracy of product information. Regulations include a variety of documents such as guidelines, approvals, processes, and policies that have different legal bases and authority. Regulations play a significant role in endorsing the safety and efficacy of the approved drugs throughout the world. They control the pricing and quality of drugs. Regulations are required for newly innovated and existing products to recover declining health status. Each country has its own guidelines used for novelty, testing, and marketing of manufacturing drugs, and also for post-marketing studies.

1.1.1 Function of RA

As one of the most heavily regulated sectors in the world, the pharmaceutical business is made up of many distinct laws. Drug regulatory organizations' primary concerns include ensuring the efficacy, safety, and quality of drugs. These days, regulatory bodies are essential to every facet of medication research, including manufacturing, distribution, import, storage, and sales (Gabe et al., 2015).

The primary responsibilities of international regulatory affairs agencies are as follows:

- Assisting with product development, manufacturing, registration, and marketing. Upon an organization's registration application, the regulatory agency initiates verbal and written correspondence with the applicant, advising them on enhanced clinical procedures and documentation that reduce the likelihood of numerous errors. The applicant is encouraged to design a product that is widely accepted by offering global regulatory policy and strategic regulatory controls for product development, manufacture, and registration.
- Developing and maintaining a dependable relationship with regulatory authorities through effective verbal and written communication during response to queries arising during the filing of new drug applications, investigational new drug applications, and abbreviated new drug applications. Groundwork, maintenance, and scheduled appraisal of standard operating procedures, batch manufacturing records, dossiers, temperature control documents, and other documents ensure product quality.

- Creating appropriate labels and pamphlets, such as those with patient information and an overview of the product's features.
- Ensuring that all necessary information is provided on the product, such as the manufacturing date, expiration date, and ingredients. The regulatory agency must establish standard formats for the creation of appropriate labels for each developed drug.
- Completing record data of a company's product and maintaining the records of therapeutic products in accordance with current regulations and guidelines.
- Keeping track of and compiling data on any product's adverse drug responses and assisting the research and development division in addressing them. For instance, the pharmacovigilance division's data gathering efforts may be used to mitigate adverse drug responses, and regulatory bodies play a leading role in data collection.
- Compiling information on new products for physicians and other medical professionals to use safely and effectively, as well as to keep track of records and reports about post-marketing surveillance of new products. Preparing pamphlets and other marketing materials for both new and current medications is also helpful.
- Providing ongoing training to related staff members about record-keeping, reporting, pilot plant operations, research, and development. It should be highlighted that this record aids the company in standard operating procedures compliance and regular manufacturing, which makes audits and inspections easier (Singh et al., 2015).

Health authorities have established laws that must be followed by all pharmaceutical enterprises. These rules guarantee public health and safety in addition to high product quality. Therefore, to function effectively and stay one step ahead of the regulatory landscape, regulatory agencies must be well-versed in both local and global regulatory scenarios. To this end, the agencies require a highly skilled workforce to enforce standard standards. These days, organizations are also striving for global harmonization for more comprehensive regulations, which helps innovators create pharmaceutical items that are acceptable around the world. Product development ought to adhere to best practices for regulations and regulatory standards. Businesses must also complete a series of tasks such as product development and marketing. An organization should have several expert teams working toward a common goal, each with clearly defined tasks and duties, to ensure the efficient adoption and operation of laws. The chemical production and control team, product development, regulatory submissions team, policy and regulatory intelligence team, and promotion and advertising team are all included in the drug regulatory affairs division (Ciociola et al., 2014).

1.1.1.1 Chemistry, Manufacturing, and Control (CMC)

This creative team is concentrated on adhering to modern good laboratory and clinical procedures, as well as information technologies, clinical facilities, good manufacturing practices, validation, audit compliance, and regulatory laboratory inspections. Although the CMC by itself is insufficient to control product quality and manufacturing, the CMC team bears responsibility for validating that the product being marketed is equivalent to the product that has been found safe and effective in various studies, ensuring that the manufacturing process is consistent in producing a product of approved quality, and ensuring that the drug product retains its quality throughout its storage period.

1.1.1.2 Policy and Regulatory Intelligence Team

This group is essential to the creation of products, their production, and registration regulations. Every business engages in regulatory intelligence to varying degrees, with opportunities arising from variations in resources, location, and enterprise size that are acknowledged to facilitate regulatory compliance. This team keeps an eye out for changing trends in the global regulatory landscape and creates policies that align with regulatory agency guidelines. They also look into standards and precedents to provide intelligence and anticipate input, enabling strong, proactive regulatory strategies. The group gathers, tracks, and evaluates regulatory data from various internal and external sources before sharing filtered information with commentary from relevant company staff and expert explanation through various channels, including portfolio strategy and day-to-day operations.

1.1.1.3 Advertising Team

To guarantee that the communication materials for promotion and advertising are both feasible and compliant, the marketing and product development teams collaborate closely with the promotion and advertising team. According to Bostrom (2009), it serves as the main point of contact for promotional and advertising materials with the regulatory bodies.

1.1.1.4 Regulatory Submissions Team

This group is in charge of putting together, submitting, and disseminating regulatory submissions to the international regulatory organizations. Submissions should be user- and reviewer-friendly, accessible, and comprehensive; this is possible thanks to new electronic technology. The strategic focus on using electronic technologies is to gather the dossier from technically proficient groups and submit it electronically in compliance with international standards, allowing for the timely and thorough submission of dossiers to international regulatory bodies (Seimetz, 2017).

1.1.1.5 Product Labeling Team

This team provides strategic guidance for the production of label content and is positioned fundamentally alongside the product development, regulatory, and other technical teams. The team in charge of product labeling is also in charge of creating packaging and container labels, literature and label package inserts, and updating product-related information. This team ensures conformity with the regulatory agency's specific format by coordinating with other relevant technical teams to get the label content reviewed for accuracy. Additionally, it strives to fulfill the deadlines set forth for submitting the label data (Sangshetti et al., 2017).

1.2 GLOBAL REGULATORY BODIES

A substantial amount of highly specific in vitro and nonhuman animal testing (which together make up a drug's nonclinical development program) and clinical research must be completed completely before submitting an appeal by a sponsor to a regulatory agency for a new medicine to be registered for human use in the agency's jurisdiction. Regulatory governance covers the manufacturing process and all facets of clinical research and nonclinical drug development. It is imperative that development projects adhere to regulatory requirements; this cannot be overstated (Davit et al., 2013). From a regulatory standpoint, all experimentation techniques and results should be correctly documented. Regulatory agencies frequently consider that a research experimental procedure and its outcomes are not adequately recorded, indicating that the experiment has not been carried out. Regulatory bodies often encourage sponsors to seek their advice before beginning a full fledged drug development program. As a result, there is an increased level of mutual understanding between the sponsor and the regulatory bodies on the program's overarching objectives, vision, and mission.

The main technical standards for the registration of medications intended for human use are established by the International Council for Harmonisation (ICH). For example, the development of new guidelines (and revisions of existing ones) must involve the active participation of non-ICH regions and other harmonization initiatives like the Southern African Development Community (SADC), Gulf Cooperation Countries (GCC), Asia-Pacific Economic Cooperation (APEC), Association of Southeast Asian Nations (ASEAN), and the Pan American Network for Drug Regulatory Harmonization (PANDRH). Other regulatory bodies are given in Figure 1.1. ICH was founded in 1990 with a number of objectives, one of which is to promote the adoption and use of a few common standards within the framework of the drug development process. A coordinated development method is highly beneficial to enable the prompt introduction of new medication alternatives for populations living in various locations, as sponsors frequently seek to commercialize novel drugs in several nations.

To specify the needs for different parts of drug development programs, nonclinical research, CMC, and clinical trials, ICH multiparty harmonized guidelines were created. Notably, there are several multidisciplinary guidelines, such as those that describe the timing of nonclinical studies in relation to clinical trials and the joint technical document submission structure, in addition to the safety, quality, and efficacy guideline categories, which cover nonclinical, CMC, and clinical topics, respectively. These recommendations, which direct biopharmaceutical research and development operations in their various countries, have been authorized by individual regulatory bodies, who additionally normally give regional guidance on certain themes.

Furthermore, sponsors "translate" the recommendations into customized standard operating procedures (SOPs) for their particular company. In some complex situations, a collection of several SOPs could be necessary to support an overall ICH guideline. New drug development needs cooperation from a wide range of parties, including regulatory bodies. The future of the pharmaceutical industry should move toward a more collaborative framework in which regulatory bodies will aim for a greater degree of convergence. Major players in the drug development process include payers, regulatory bodies, and sponsors. They approach the process with

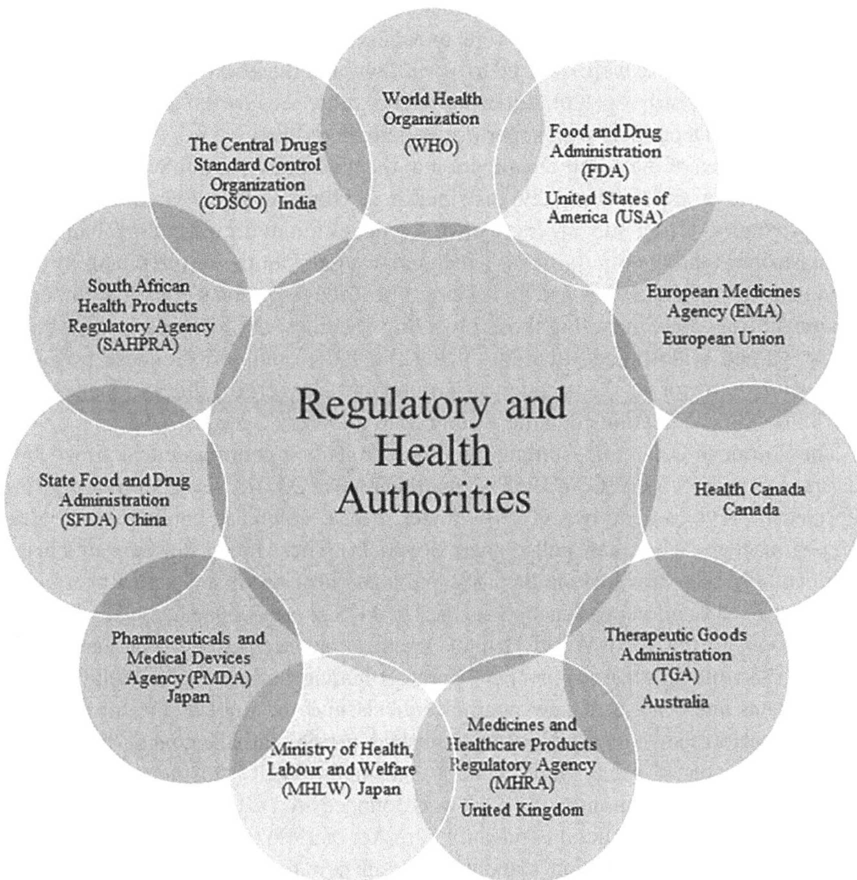

FIGURE 1.1 Regulatory Bodies of Several Countries.

the goal of achieving reimbursement targets while simultaneously advancing the global goal of providing the public with safe, effective, and inexpensive medications (Grignolo, 2013). By using mechanisms such as pre-investigational new drugs and end of phase 2 meetings and distinct protocol assessment in the United States, clinical trial consultations in Japan, and requests for scientific advice and protocol assistance in the EU, sponsors and regulatory agencies are already working together. Maintaining support for collaborative and creative methods requires effective communication between regulatory bodies in various locations (Kramer et al., 2012).

1.3 HISTORICAL DEVELOPMENT

Medications have been used since the development of humankind, and they are not a by-product of everyday usage or consumption. It takes certain knowledge and skill to produce, distribute, and dispense medications. Every culture had its own medical system; interestingly, back then, a medical practitioner had to be self-regulatory. Therefore, regulatory authorities were unnecessary. For instance, in India, those with medical expertise were referred to as *vaidyas*, and these individuals were highly esteemed and morally upright, adhering to the guidelines for creating and recommending pharmaceuticals with superior medicinal qualities.

Since the idea of the commercialization of the medical system first emerged, laws governing the production, use, and distribution of pharmaceutical goods have developed gradually. Using subpar, ineffective, or contaminated medications can result in catastrophic therapeutic failures, which can range from the development of drug resistance to instances that are so severe as to take a person's life. A number of significant tragedies, including those involving vaccines, thalidomide, and sulfanilamide, gained widespread attention during the 1950s and 1960s. These tragedies were a major factor in the creation of stricter laws governing the production and distribution of medications in a more controlled manner (Lezotre, 2013).

The European Economic Commission released its first pharmaceutical directive in Europe, number 65/65/EEC, in 1965. Council Directive 2001/83/EEC harmonized and superseded previous directives in 2001 (Sauer, 2015). Reference books for biological and pharmaceutical items are called pharmacopoeias. These books first appeared in the 16th century; examples include the 1581 publication of the first Spanish pharmacopoeia, the 1618 London pharmacopoeia, the 1820 US pharmacopoeia, the 1864 British pharmacopoeia, the 1951 World Health Organization International Pharmacopoeia, and the 1955 Indian pharmacopoeia. To protect human health and end delays in the development and release of new pharmaceuticals into the market, the International Council for Harmonisation (ICH) was established in 1990 with the goal of establishing quality, effectiveness, safety, and regulatory standards (WHO Document, 2013). The US Pharmacopoeia Committee (USPC) was founded in 1820. The FDA was established as a result of the Federal Food and Drugs Act of 1906 (the Wiley Act). The 1938 Food, Drug, and Cosmetic Act mandated that all new medications need premarketing approval and must be accompanied by documentation of scientific investigation before approval (Gad, 2016). As medical knowledge grows daily, new and innovative technology and treatments are being introduced into the healthcare system. Regulatory bodies must operate with more responsibility and without interruption than innovators to deliver optimal outcomes in a controlled manner for a safe medical system free from risks. Regulatory bodies and organizations need to take a lesson from the numerous instances of uncontrolled pharmaceuticals that we have witnessed in the past. Regulatory bodies are developing future policies and rules by drawing on their extensive historical experience. Although regulatory agencies may learn to eliminate the likelihood of errors and also gain insight into how and why laws are essential for the establishments, organizations can also benefit from historical data and certain case studies when developing and adhering to regulations. Every rule is being created with the pharmaceutical industry and public health experience in mind.

1.4 REGULATORY CHALLENGES

The pharmaceutical sector is heavily regulated. Regulations are always being tightened to guarantee the safety, effectiveness, and high pharmaceutical quality of the medicines that are supplied. Time is becoming a more significant component in enabling patients to receive cutting-edge medical treatments more quickly and live better lives. General challenges faced by countries are given in Figure 1.2. Under the EU's Advanced Therapy Medicinal Products (ATMP) regulatory system, patients can receive medications more quickly in cases when their medical needs are not being satisfied. This is made possible via the adaptive pathway, rapid approval, conditional approval, and hospital exemption. In the United States and Europe, breakthrough designation, personalized medicine, and customized medicine are in vogue. To speed the licensing of important novel medications, Japan established the *sakigake* priority review system, which grants priority assessments, consultations, and assessments. Treatments for illnesses will be completely changed by regenerative medicine, which is advancing with techniques like stem cell treatment. For example, with cell therapy, treating age-related macular degeneration (AMD) has become nearly standard practice. Other ailments, such as diabetes, hepatitis, and arthritis, are getting worse. Dialysis will no longer be

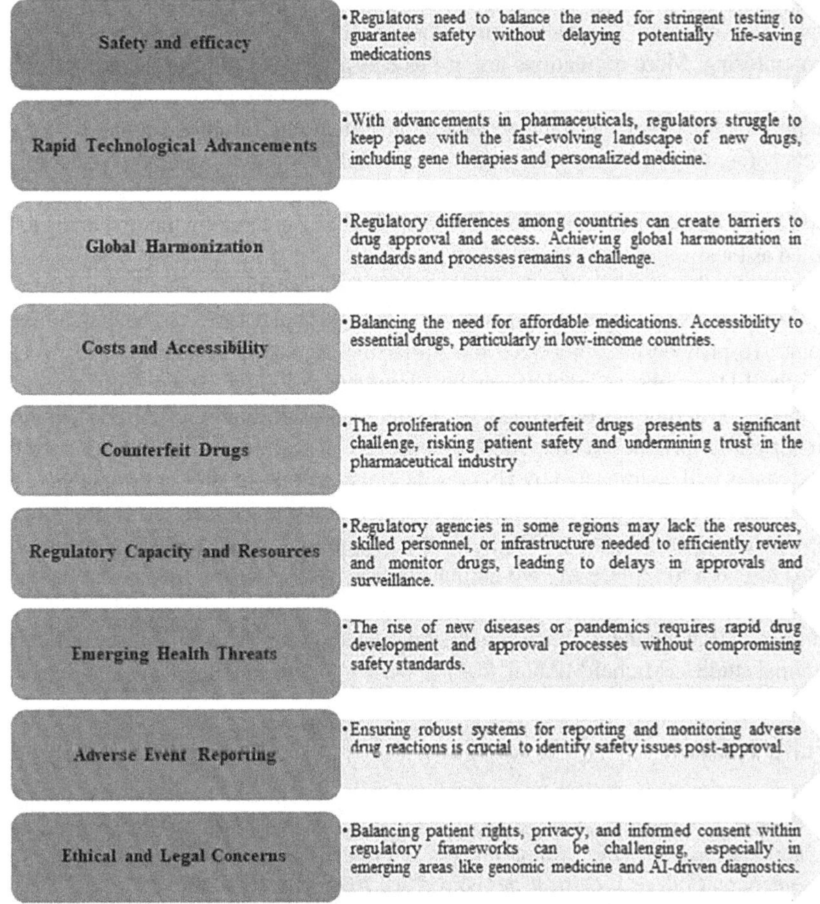

FIGURE 1.2 General Challenges Faced by Countries.

necessary if kidney regeneration is possible. Multi-regional clinical trials (MRCT) are now being conducted in accordance with ICH guideline E 17.

With this approach, the ethnic variables that should be considered while developing new drugs for the appropriate medication classes will become clearer. Along with the new ICH guideline E 17 on basic principles on planning and constructing MRCTs, a modification of the ICH E 5 guideline on ethnic considerations is being considered. The ICH E 17 guideline entered the consultation phase (step 3) after reaching step 2b. Regulatory authorities that oversee drug safety in Japan, the risk evaluation and mitigation system in the United States, EudraVigilance in Europe, and pharmacovigilance in Europe are increasingly focusing on these areas. Additionally, an increasing number of these agencies are emphasizing the need for ICSRs, Adverse Drug Events (ADEs), and Adverse Drug Reactions (ADRs) reporting. The Pharmacovigilance Risk Assessment Committee in the EU is (re-)evaluating the safety of marketed pharmaceuticals and is involved in the safety evaluation of new medications before to approval. Periodic safety update reports are evolving into periodic risk-benefit evaluation reports. The results of post-approval efficacy studies and safety studies are increasingly factored into regulatory decision-making. The EU's pharmaceutical safety is being strengthened by further monitoring. More regulations are in place as a result of the European Medicines Directive. By January 1, 2018, among other criteria, a 2D bar code on every pack will be required. Other obstacles include the establishment of a European center to inspect packets before dispensing to patients and the identification of medicinal products. The United States is now following Europe in the approval of biosimilars, which have been around for more than a decade. Monoclonal antibodies were among the first items to be certified as biosimilars.

Traceability is made possible by the addition of a four-letter rule to the International Nonproprietary Names (INN) that sets the biosimilar apart from the reference listed biologic. To provide the authorized biosimilar the regulatory status of "interchangeable," the FDA seeks an application for "interchangeability." What will happen to the market for additional biosimilars of a reference listed biologic (RLB) if the first interchangeable product of that RLB is approved? The future of medications in the United States will be impacted by US presidential elections, talks over drug prices, and whether the Affordable Care Act will be repealed and replaced. In the United States, compounding pharmacies are subject to new regulations. In addition to encouraging in vitro research to replace in vivo animal studies and permitting the extrapolation of indications for the same mode of action, Europe is loosening its approval policies for biosimilars, allowing the global reference product and introducing the three principles for animal studies (Michel Mikhail, 2017).

REFERENCES

Ciociola, A.A., Cohen, L.B., Kulkarni, P., Kefalas, C., Buchman, A., Burke, C., Cain, T., Connor, J., Ehrenpreis, E.D., Fang, J. and Fass, R., 2014. How drugs are developed and approved by the FDA: Current process and future directions. *Official Journal of the American College of Gastroenterology ACG*, *109*(5), pp. 620–623.

Davit, B., Braddy, A.C., Conner, D.P. and Yu, L.X., 2013. International guidelines for bioequivalence of systemically available orally administered generic drug products: A survey of similarities and differences. *The AAPS Journal*, *15*, pp. 974–990.

de Frutos, M.A., Ornaghi, C. and Siotis, G., 2013. Competition in the pharmaceutical industry: How do quality differences shape advertising strategies? *Journal of Health Economics*, *32*(1), pp. 268–285.

DiMasi, J.A., Grabowski, H.G. and Hansen, R.W., 2016. Innovation in the pharmaceutical industry: New estimates of R&D costs. *Journal of Health Economics*, *47*, pp. 20–33.

Djulbegovic, B., Hozo, I. and Ioannidis, J.P., 2014. Improving the drug development process: More not less randomized trials. *JAMA*, *311*[3], pp. 355–356.

Franco, P., 2013. Orphan drugs: The regulatory environment. *Drug Discovery Today*, *18*(3–4), pp. 163–172.

Gabe, J., Williams, S., Martin, P. and Coveney, C., 2015. Pharmaceuticals and society: Power, promises and prospects. *Social Science & Medicine*, *131*, pp. 193–198.

Gad, S.C., 2016. *Drug safety evaluation*. John Wiley & Sons.

Glick, H.A., Doshi, J.A., Sonnad, S.S. and Polsky, D., 2014. *Economic evaluation in clinical trials*. Oxford University Press.

Grignolo, A., 2013. Collaboration and convergence: Bringing new medicines to global markets in the 21st century. *Therapeutic Innovation & Regulatory Science*, *47*[1], pp. 8–15.

Kramer, D.B., Xu, S. and Kesselheim, A.S., 2012. How does medical device regulation perform in the United States and the European union? *A Systematic Review*.

Lalu, L., Tambe, V., Pradhan, D., Nayak, K., Bagchi, S., Maheshwari, R., Kalia, K. and Tekade, R.K., 2017. Novel nanosystems for the treatment of ocular inflammation: Current paradigms and future research directions. *Journal of Controlled Release*, *268*, pp. 19–39.

Lezotre, P.L., 2013. *International cooperation, convergence and harmonization of pharmaceutical regulations: A global perspective*. Academic Press.

Maheshwari, R., Tekade, M., A Sharma, P. and Kumar Tekade, R., 2015. Nanocarriers assisted siRNA gene therapy for the management of cardiovascular disorders. *Current Pharmaceutical Design*, *21*(30), pp. 4427–4440.

Mikhail, M., 2017. Global regulatory challenges and current hot topics in the regulatory world. In *Pharmaceutical regulatory affairs and IPR*. Pharm Regul Aff, 6:2 (Suppl).

Pezzola, A. and Sweet, C.M., 2016. Global pharmaceutical regulation: The challenge of integration for developing states. *Globalization and Health*, *12*, pp. 1–18.

Sangshetti, J.N., Deshpande, M., Zaheer, Z., Shinde, D.B. and Arote, R., 2017. Quality by design approach: Regulatory need. *Arabian Journal of Chemistry*, *10*, pp. S3412–S3425.

Seimetz, D., 2017. The key to successful drug approval: An effective regulatory strategy. In *Life science venturing: Herausforderung—spezifika—prozess* (pp. 139–165). Springer Fachmedien Wiesbaden.

Sharma, R., Agrawal, U., Mody, N. and Vyas, S.P., 2015. Polymer nanotechnology based approaches in mucosal vaccine delivery: Challenges and opportunities. *Biotechnology Advances*, *33*(1), pp. 64–79.

Singh, V.K., Romaine, P.L. and Seed, T.M., 2015. Medical countermeasures for radiation exposure and related injuries: Characterization of medicines, FDA-approval status and inclusion into the strategic national stockpile. *Health Physics*, *108*(6), p. 607.

Spindler, G. and Schmechel, P., 2016. Personal data and encryption in the European general data protection regulation. *Journal Intellectual Property Information Technology & Electric Commerce Law*, *7*, p. 163.

Tekade, R.K., Maheshwari, R., Soni, N., Tekade, M. and Chougule, M.B., 2017. Nanotechnology for the development of nanomedicine. In *Nanotechnology-based approaches for targeting and delivery of drugs and genes* (pp. 3–61). Academic Press.

Wirthumer-Hoche, C. and Bloechl-Daum, B., 2016. Current issues in drug regulation. In *Clinical pharmacology: Current topics and case studies* (pp. 19–31). Cham: Springer.

2 Safety Perspectives of Medicinal Products

Rishi Kumar, Nishith Keserwani, and Parveen Kumar Goyal

2.1 INTRODUCTION

Medicinal products are being regulated by drug regulatory authorities of respective countries throughout the world. Quality, safety, and efficacy of medicinal products are the three important parameters that need stringent rules and regulations for patient safety. The safety of medical products is established by various facets of the preclinical study of the molecule(s), and pre-formulation studies are also necessary to establish the products scientifically safe for consumption for therapeutic use. Clinical trials (CTs) play an important role in establishing the safety of medicinal products.

This chapter focuses on the rules and regulations of the post-marketing surveillance of medical products in various countries. In the last two decades, the legislation about pharmacovigilance has improved significantly. As described by the World Health Organization (WHO), pharmacovigilance is the science and activities of detection, assessment, understanding, and prevention of adverse drug reactions and any other drug-related problems [1].

2.2 SAFETY OF MEDICINAL PRODUCTS

Any medicinal products may cause serious adverse events if they are used without the supervision of healthcare professionals. The safety of medicinal products is of paramount importance to ensure that they provide benefits without causing harm to patients. To achieve this, regulatory agencies around the world require rigorous testing and evaluation of medicinal products before they are approved for use.

The safety evaluation of medicinal products typically includes:

1. *Preclinical studies*: These are laboratory studies done on animals or in vitro to assess the safety and potential toxicity of a new drug. This stage is important to determine whether the drug should proceed to CT.
2. *Clinical trials*: These are studies conducted on humans to evaluate the safety, efficacy, and dosage of a new drug. CTs are typically done in three phases, with each phase involving a larger number of participants.

 DOI: 10.1201/9781003296492-3

3. *Post-marketing surveillance*: Once a drug is approved for use, regulatory agencies require continuous monitoring of its safety through pharmacovigilance. This involves monitoring the adverse drug reactions, unexpected side effects, and interactions with other drugs.

In addition to these evaluations, regulatory agencies also require pharmaceutical companies to comply with good manufacturing practices (GMP) to ensure the safety and quality of the drug during manufacturing and distribution [2].

2.3 PRECLINICAL STUDIES OF MEDICINAL PRODUCTS

Preclinical studies are laboratory tests that are conducted on animals or in vitro to evaluate the safety and potential toxicity of a new drug before it is tested on humans in CT. These studies are an essential component of drug development and are used to determine whether a drug is safe enough to proceed to CT.

Preclinical studies typically include the following:

1. *Pharmacodynamics*: These studies evaluate how a drug affects the body, including its mechanism of action, therapeutic dose range, and potential side effects.
2. *Pharmacokinetics*: These studies evaluate how the body affects the drug, including absorption, distribution, metabolism, and excretion.
3. *Toxicology*: These studies evaluate the safety of the drug, including its potential to cause toxicity and adverse effects in animals.
4. *Formulation development*: These studies evaluate the optimal formulation and delivery method for the drug.

Preclinical studies are conducted as per the regulatory guidelines and standards, such as the International Council for Harmonisation (ICH) guidelines. These guidelines provide an outline for the design and conduct of preclinical studies, ensuring that they are conducted in a scientifically sound and ethical manner.

The preclinical studies are used to evaluate whether a drug is safe and effective enough to proceed to CT in humans. If a drug passes preclinical testing, it may be granted permission to move to the next stage of development, which involves testing in humans in CT [3].

2.4 CLINICAL TRIALS OF MEDICINAL PRODUCTS

CT are studies conducted on human volunteers to evaluate the safety, efficacy, and dosage of a new medicinal product. These studies are conducted in several phases, and each phase involves a progressively larger number of participants.

The different phases of CT are as follows:

1. *Phase 0*: Phase 0 CTs, also known as exploratory Investigational New Drug studies, are a relatively new type of CTs that involves the administration

of sub-therapeutic doses of a drug to a small group of healthy volunteers (usually less than 15) to determine its pharmacokinetics and pharmacodynamics. Phase 0 trials are usually conducted early in the drug development process to help pharmaceutical companies in determining whether a drug is worth pursuing further. These trials are designed to provide initial safety and pharmacokinetic data on the drug, with the goal of minimizing the risks to patients in subsequent CTs.

The main objectives of Phase 0 trials include:

- Establishing the pharmacokinetics and pharmacodynamics of the drug in humans.
- Assessing the safety of the drug at sub-therapeutic doses.
- Identifying suitable biomarkers that can be used to evaluate the drug's effectiveness.

Phase 0 trials are conducted under the same regulatory oversight as other CTs and are subject to the same ethical considerations. However, because the doses administered are below therapeutic levels, the risks to participants are generally lower than in other types of CTs. If the results of a Phase 0 trial are positive, the drug may proceed to Phase 1 trials, which involve the administration of higher doses of the drug to a larger group of healthy volunteers to evaluate its safety and tolerability.

2. *Phase 1*: This is the first stage of CT and involves a small group of healthy volunteers (usually less than 100). The primary objective of this phase is to evaluate the safety and tolerability of the new drug entity, as well as its pharmacokinetics and pharmacodynamics.
3. *Phase 2*: This phase involves a larger group of patients (usually a few hundred) who have the disease to be treated or the condition that the drug is intended to treat. The primary objective of this phase is to evaluate the efficacy of the drug and to determine the optimal dose range.
4. *Phase 3*: This phase involves a much larger group of patients (usually several thousand) and is designed to confirm the safety and efficacy of the drug in a larger population. This phase is also used to assess the drug's effectiveness compared with standard treatments or placebos.
5. *Phase 4*: This phase involves the post-marketing surveillance of the drug and involves ongoing monitoring of the drug's therapeutic safety in a larger patient population.

The results of CTs are used by regulatory agencies to evaluate the safety and efficacy of the drug and to determine whether it should be approved for use by the general population [4].

2.5 HISTORY OF PHARMACOVIGILANCE

The word *pharmacovigilance* (composed of two words: *pharmakon*, a Greek word meaning "medicinal substance," and *vigilia*, a Latin word meaning "to keep watch") simply means to keep monitoring any medicinal product in clinical use for adverse reactions. The history of pharmacovigilance is about 175 years old; on January 29, 1848, a young girl named Hannah Greener living in the northern region of England met an unfortunate death due to the administration of chloroform as an anesthetic drug during the removal of infected toenail. At that time, Sir James Simpson, a medical professional, had recently introduced chloroform as a safe and potent anesthetic in clinical practice. It was hypothesized that she might have succumbed to a fatal arrhythmia or pulmonary aspiration. To comprehend the circumstances of Hannah's demise, an investigation was conducted; however, the efforts made couldn't find the exact cause of her death and it remained unknown. Nevertheless, this event opened a new chapter for monitoring any medicinal product in clinical use, which later on evolved as pharmacovigilance [5]. In India, pharmacovigilance came into view in 1986 for monitoring formal adverse drug reactions.

2.6 CASE STUDIES IN PHARMACOVIGILANCE

The use of excipients in the production of pharmaceuticals needs to be taken care of while using: some chemicals may cause serious adverse events in human beings if not controlled specifically; for example the solvent, diethylene glycol, has been the cause of concern across the world. The first case of diethylene glycol toxicity was observed in 1937; This was also known as the sulfanilamide tragedy, which caused the death of 100 children in the United States. The thalidomide tragedy has drastically changed the perception of the people in terms of drug regulation and safety perspective. This drug led to the occurrence of 10,000 serious events among children, many of the children who were born with phocomelia, that is, children born with a bone deformity. This tragedy led to the foundation of the Program for International Drug Monitoring by the WHO in 1968. After this tragedy, regulatory authorities of many countries started taking pharmacovigilance seriously, and it is continuously evolving. The recent case of cough syrup deaths in Gambia is a recent example of deaths due to diethylene glycol–contaminated solvent used in the preparation of the cough syrup. The above examples have made it a point that there is a strong need for an effective pharmacovigilance system for the safety of medicinal products.

2.7 ROLE OF WORLD HEALTH ORGANIZATION IN THE SAFETY OF MEDICINAL PRODUCTS

After the thalidomide tragedy in 1961, during the 16th World Health Assembly in 1963, resolution number 16.36 was passed, which states that "a systematic collection of information on serious adverse drug reactions during the development and particularly after medicines have been made available for public use." Subsequently the WHO started the Programme for International Drug Monitoring (PIDM) in 1968.

Initially, the PIDM was started with ten countries; at present, the program has 155 full member countries and 21 associated members, which they shall be full members in due time [6].

2.8 UPPSALA MONITORING CENTRE, SWEDEN

The Uppsala Monitoring Centre (UMC) is the WHO Collaborating Centre for International Drug Monitoring. It is worthy to praise the efforts of the UMC in establishing strong and effective networks of member countries for pharmacovigilance. It has provided various information technology tools like VigiBase, VigiFlow, VigiLyze, and VigiAccess, which help member countries in the collection, collation, and analysis of Individual Case Safety Reports (ICSRs). In addition, all the safety information related to medical products can be compared and shared with other member countries. In a nutshell, the UMC provides a common platform for assessing the safety of medicinal products that can be used by all member countries in the best possible way for patient safety [7].

2.9 PHARMACOVIGILANCE REGULATIONS, US FOOD AND DRUG ADMINISTRATION (FDA)

Adverse event(s) reporting is a vital and indispensable requirement imposed by the FDA, ensuring that pharmaceutical companies, healthcare professionals, and consumers promptly report any adverse event(s) or suspected adverse reaction(s) associated with the approved drug(s), encompassing both serious and non-serious occurrences. Recognizing the significance of this process, the FDA has established the MedWatch program, which serves as a dedicated platform, facilitating the reporting of such events. Furthermore, the FDA diligently conducts post-marketing safety monitoring to proactively identify the potential safety concerns that might have eluded detection during the rigorous CT phase(s). This ongoing surveillance is achieved through the use of various systems, including the FDA Adverse Event Reporting System (FAERS) and the Sentinel Initiative—a nationwide electronic system specially designed to monitor the safety of medical products regulated by the FDA [8].

To further safeguard public health, the FDA possesses the authority to enforce Risk Evaluation and Mitigation Strategies (REMS) for certain drugs that are known to possess inherent safety risks. REMS entails a comprehensive set of strategies implemented by manufacturers to ensure the safe use of these products. These strategies may encompass crucial elements such as medication guides, communication plans aimed to enhance awareness among healthcare professionals and patients, or restricted distribution programs that ensure the product is only accessible to individuals for whom the benefits outweigh the potential risks [9].

In its commitment to ensuring the utmost safety of approved drugs, the FDA continually reviews safety information and actively engages with manufacturers, directing them to update drug labels promptly with any new safety information that may arise. Additionally, the FDA may issue safety communications for targeting healthcare professionals and the general public, effectively disseminating essential safety concerns and promoting informed decision-making in the use of medications.

Recognizing that safety concerns extend beyond national boundaries, the FDA actively engages in collaboration with regulatory agencies and organizations both domestically and internationally. This collaborative approach fosters the exchange of safety information and promotes global pharmacovigilance efforts, ultimately benefiting patients worldwide. Through these multifaceted efforts, the FDA remains steadfast in its mission to protect public health and ensure the safe use of approved drugs.

2.10 CENTRAL DRUGS STANDARD CONTROL ORGANIZATION (CDSCO), INDIA

The National Regulatory Authority of India, known as CDSCO, is involved in the regulation of pharmacovigilance, done through the Pharmacovigilance Programme of India (PvPI), a programme supported by the Government of India. The structure of the PvPI is unique in the world and is explained in Figure 2.1.

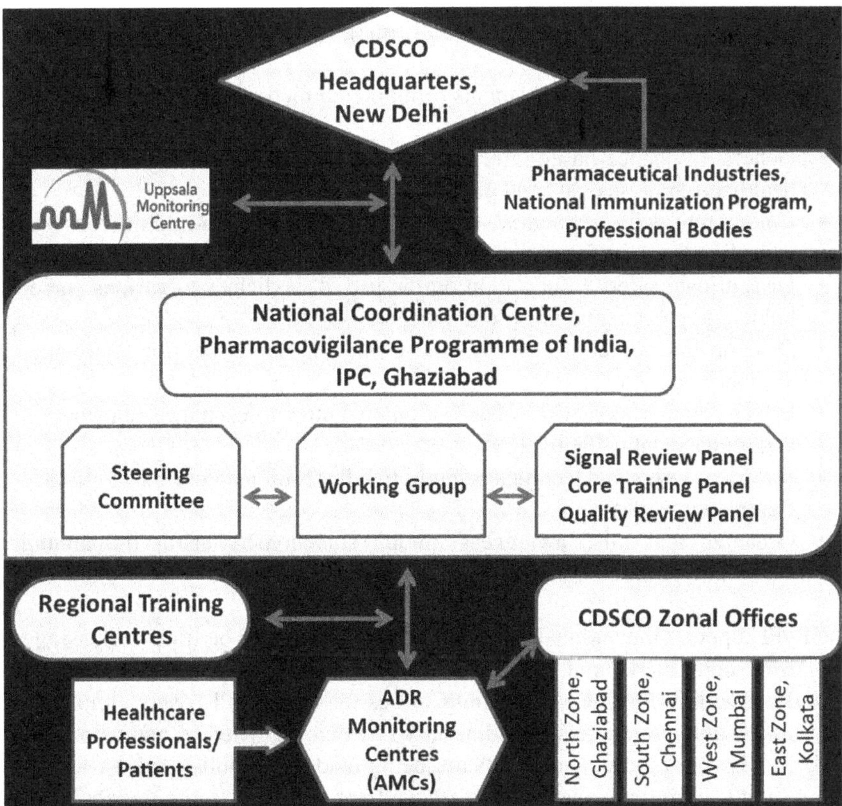

FIGURE 2.1 Structure of the Pharmacovigilance Programme of India.

The PvPI is a significant drug safety monitoring initiative by the Government of India. It plays a pivotal role in collecting and analyzing adverse events related to drugs. Monitoring of adverse drug reactions (ADR) is imperative as it significantly contributes to global morbidity and mortality. Initially launched in July 2010 by the Ministry of Health & Family Welfare (MoHFW) and the All India Institute of Medical Sciences (AIIMS), New Delhi served as the National Coordination Centre (NCC) for PvPI. However, a subsequent order dated April 15, 2011, from the MoHFW led to the transfer of PvPI from AIIMS, New Delhi to the Indian Pharmacopoeia Commission (IPC), Ghaziabad. Since then, IPC has been entrusted with the responsibility of being the NCC for PvPI. Furthermore, the Materiovigilance Programme of India and the Haemovigilance Programme of India also fall under the ambit of PvPI. The mission of PvPI is to safeguard the health of the Indian population by ensuring that the benefits of using medicine outweigh the associated risks. The vision is to enhance patient safety and the welfare of the Indian population by monitoring the safety of medicines and reducing the risks associated with their use.

The objectives of the PvPI are as follows:

- Establish a nationwide system to ensure patient safety through comprehensive drug safety monitoring.
- Identify and analyze new signals and emerging risks from reported adverse events.
- Conduct benefit-risk assessments of marketed medications to inform regulatory authorities.
- Generate evidence-based information on the safety of medicines to support healthcare professionals and patients.
- Collaborate with regulatory agencies in the decision-making process regarding the use of medications.
- Disseminate safety information on the use of medicines to various stakeholders to prevent and minimize risks.
- Develop into a recognized National Centre of Excellence for Pharmacovigilance activities.
- Foster collaboration with other National Centres to exchange information and manage data effectively.
- Provide training and technical support to other National Pharmacovigilance Centres worldwide.
- Organize and raise awareness among stakeholders about the annual National Pharmacovigilance Week (September 17–23).

The PvPI supports the national drug regulatory authority to be timely releasing signals, drug safety alerts, and package insert leaflet changes, if any. At present PvPI is working with 842 ADR Monitoring Centres in India. PvPI covers almost all 28 states and 7 union territories of India; only one union territory remains to have an ADR Monitoring Centre, and efforts are being made to establish at least one ADR Monitoring Centre there. Various tools have been provided to the stakeholders for seamless reporting of ADRs to PvPI, such as the ADR PvPI mobile app, available on the Google Play store for Android mobile users; the ADR Reporting Form; the ADR Reporting Helpline (1-800-180-3024); and the Consumer ADR Reporting Form [10].

2.11 NATIONAL MEDICAL PRODUCTS ADMINISTRATION (NMPA), CHINA

ADR reporting in China involves the active participation of healthcare professionals, pharmaceutical manufacturers, and the general public, who are encouraged to report ADRs to the National Medical Products Administration (NMPA). Reporting channels include the National Adverse Drug Reaction Monitoring System (NADRMS) and an online reporting platform. The NMPA may require the submission of risk management plans (RMPs) as part of the registration process for certain drugs, outlining strategies and measures to identify, characterize, and minimize the associated risks. Post-marketing surveillance is conducted by the NMPA to monitor the safety and effectiveness of drugs on the market, involving routine inspections, audits, and the collection and analysis of safety data. The NMPA employs various methods for signal detection and evaluation, thoroughly assessing the potential safety signals from ADR reports and other data sources to determine the need for regulatory actions, such as labeling updates or restrictions. Safety communications are issued by the NMPA to healthcare professionals and the public to disseminate important drug safety information, and the authority exists to request pharmaceutical companies to update drug labels with new safety information [11].

2.12 EUROPEAN MEDICAL AGENCY (EMA), EUROPE

European pharmacovigilance practices encompass a range of key elements and databases managed by the European Medicines Agency (EMA). One such database is the EudraVigilance platform, a centralized repository that gathers and stores information on suspected adverse reactions reported within the European Union (EU) and European Economic Area (EEA). This system streamlines the collection, analysis, and monitoring of safety data on medicinal products. ADR reporting mandates that marketing authorization holders, healthcare professionals, and patients report suspected adverse drug reactions to the national competent authorities of EU member states, who then submit these reports to the EMA via the EudraVigilance platform. The EMA uses advanced methodologies and data analysis techniques to detect potential safety signals from the reported adverse reactions and various data sources, which serve as a foundation for further evaluation and potential regulatory action. Conducting comprehensive benefit-risk assessments throughout the life cycle of medicinal products is another critical task undertaken by the EMA, which entails evaluating the balance between a drug's benefits and risks. These assessments may lead to the implementation of additional risk minimization measures, such as updated product information, changes in prescribing or administration practices, or the initiation of further studies. Marketing authorization holders are required to develop and submit RMPs to the EMA, outlining strategies to identify, characterize, prevent, or mitigate the risks associated with their medicinal products. These plans are subject to periodic review and updating as new safety information emerges. The EMA actively issues safety communications to healthcare professionals and the public to disseminate essential drug safety information, collaborating with marketing authorization holders to ensure timely updates to product information, including summaries of product characteristics (SmPCs) and patient information leaflets. Moreover, the EMA engages in extensive collaboration and international cooperation, working closely with national competent authorities within the EU and EEA and forging partnerships on a global scale to share safety information and promote harmonized pharmacovigilance practices [12].

The pharmacovigilance regulations in Europe are continually evolving to adapt to scientific advancements and emerging safety concerns. The EMA plays a pivotal role in ensuring the ongoing monitoring and safety of medicinal products in the European region.

2.13 THERAPEUTIC GOODS ADMINISTRATION (TGA), AUSTRALIA

Adverse event reporting is a crucial component of the Therapeutic Goods Administration (TGA) in Australia, which relies on active participation from healthcare professionals, consumers, and pharmaceutical companies to report adverse events associated with therapeutic products. These reports can be conveniently submitted through the online Adverse Event Management System or the Yellow Card Scheme. The TGA maintains the Database of Adverse Event Notifications, a comprehensive repository that collects and stores adverse event reports. To identify potential safety signals and facilitate further investigation, the TGA employs advanced signal detection methods using the reported data. RMPs play a vital role in the approval process, as pharmaceutical companies may be required to develop these plans for high-risk products. RMPs provide strategies for identifying, characterizing, preventing, or minimizing risks associated with the use of therapeutic products. Safety communication is paramount, and the TGA issues advisories and alerts to healthcare professionals and the public, disseminating essential safety information about therapeutic products. TGA collaborates with pharmaceutical companies to ensure the timely updates of product information and consumer medicine information with the latest safety data. The TGA conducts post-market monitoring activities, encompassing surveillance programs, audits, and inspections of pharmaceutical manufacturers to ensure compliance with safety standards and regulatory requirements, thereby ensuring ongoing safety and efficacy of therapeutic products.

The TGA actively participates in international collaborations and exchanges related to pharmacovigilance. It collaborates with regulatory authorities from other countries and regions to share safety information and contribute to global pharmacovigilance efforts [13].

2.14 PHARMACEUTICAL AND MEDICAL DEVICE AGENCY (PMDA), JAPAN

Pharmacovigilance in Japan is overseen by the Pharmaceuticals and Medical Devices Agency (PMDA). The PMDA plays a crucial role in monitoring the safety of pharmaceuticals and medical devices in Japan. The Adverse Drug Reactions Reporting System (ADRS) is the primary mechanism through which healthcare professionals, patients, and pharmaceutical companies report ADRs. The PMDA conducts post-marketing surveillance and employs advanced signal detection methods to identify potential safety signals from reported ADRs and other data sources. RMPs may be required for high-risk products to outline strategies to identify, prevent, and minimize risks. The PMDA also collaborates internationally, sharing safety information and contributing to global pharmacovigilance efforts. Overall, the PMDA's pharmacovigilance system ensures the ongoing monitoring and safety of pharmaceuticals and medical devices in Japan [14].

2.15 MEDICINE AND HEALTHCARE PRODUCTS REGULATORY AGENCY (MHRA), UNITED KINGDOM

The United Kingdom is a pioneer in the field of pharmacovigilance. The pharmacovigilance system in the United Kingdom is being managed by the Medicine and Healthcare Products Regulatory Agency (MHRA), which launched the Yellow Card system to collect data related to ADRs in the UK population; later, the ADR reporting form was adopted in other countries.

The Yellow Card system, which was launched in 1964, is an important tool for monitoring the safety of medicines in the United Kingdom. Healthcare professionals, patients, and consumers are encouraged to report suspected adverse reactions to the MHRA through the Yellow Card system. The system collects valuable data on ADRs, including information about the medicine involved, the nature of the adverse reaction, and the patient's demography.

The data collected through Yellow Cards is further used to identify various safety signals related to the use of medicines. The pharmacovigilance system of the United Kingdom is considered to be advanced [15].

2.16 HEALTH CANADA, CANADA

Pharmacovigilance in Canada is overseen by Health Canada, the country's regulatory authority for health products. Health Canada has implemented a robust system for monitoring and ensuring the safety of medicines and medical devices in the Canadian market. The Canada Vigilance Program serves as the national system for collecting and analyzing ADR reports. Healthcare professionals, consumers, and pharmaceutical companies are encouraged to report ADRs to Health Canada through the Canada Vigilance Online Adverse Reaction Reporting System. Health Canada conducts signal detection and risk assessment activities to identify potential safety signals and takes appropriate regulatory actions whenever necessary to protect public health. They also collaborate with international partners and regulatory agencies to share safety information and contribute to global pharmacovigilance efforts [16].

2.17 CHALLENGES

There are many challenges being faced by regulators for pharmacovigilance, including the following:

1. Lack of interest of healthcare professionals in pharmacovigilance activities.
2. Overcrowded hospitals due to a large physician-to-patient ratio in developing and low- and middle-income countries.

3. Lack of awareness.
4. Lack of tools for ADR reporting and perception of ADR reporting for pharmacovigilance.
5. Stringent pharmacovigilance regulation for the safety of medicinal products.

The International Council for Harmonisation of Technical Requirements for Pharmaceuticals for Human Use (ICH) guidelines related to pharmacovigilance are:

1. ICH E2A: Clinical Safety Data Management: Definitions and Standards for Expedited Reporting.
2. ICH E2B(R3): Electronic Transmission of Individual Case Safety Reports (ICSRs): Implementation Guide—Data Elements and Message Specification.
3. ICH E2C(R2): Periodic Benefit-Risk Evaluation Report (PBRER).
4. ICH E2D: Post-Approval Safety Data Management: Definitions and Standards for Expedited Reporting.
5. ICH E2E: Pharmacovigilance Planning.
6. ICH E2F: Development Safety Update Report (DSUR).
7. ICH E2F(R1): DSUR—Questions and Answers.
8. ICH E2F(R2): DSUR—Data Elements for Transmission of Individual Case Safety Reports.
9. ICH E4: Dose-Response Information to Support Drug Registration.
10. ICH E6(R2): Good Clinical Practice: Integrated Addendum to ICH E6(R1).
11. ICH E19: Optimization of Safety Data Collection.

These guidelines have been adopted by various countries for making effective pharmacovigilance systems in their respective territories. They will also help in the cross-border strengthening of the pharmacovigilance system. Various other tools like the Identification of Medicinal Products are products in development that shall be launched by WHO for easy and fast identification of medicinal products and shall subsequently help to trace products from manufacturer to end user.

2.18 DRUG SAFETY ALERTS BY VARIOUS DRUG REGULATORY AUTHORITIES IN 2023

The authors referred to various online resources of several regulatory bodies, studied drug safety alerts, and identified various drug alerts issued by such authorities. Some significant safety alerts recently issued by FDA, CDSCO, TGA, MHRA, and Health Canada are mentioned in Tables 2.1–2.5.

In India, the National Pharmacovigilance Centre aims to raise awareness among healthcare professionals and patients/consumers by issuing drug safety alerts. This initiative encourages individuals to vigilantly observe the potential occurrence of ADRs associated with the use of suspected drugs mentioned in the preceding tables. In the event of encountering such reactions, individuals are strongly urged to submit reports to the NCC PvPI, IPC. This can be done by completing the Suspected

Adverse Drug Reactions Reporting Form/Medicines Side Effect Reporting Form for consumers, available at www.ipc.gov.in. Alternatively, reports can also be submitted using the ADR PvPI Android mobile app or by contacting the PvPI Helpline at 1-800-180-3024.

Tables 2.1–2.5 clearly indicate that various regulatory authorities issue drug safety alerts for patient safety in their respective regulatory territories. These alerts may also be reviewed by countries' regulatory authorities to cross-check whether the same product is being sold in their country. There will be a significant improvement in patient safety if the pharmacovigilance systems of different countries are harmonized and the necessary information is shared among all respective authorities using a synchronized platform.

TABLE 2.1
Drug Safety Alerts Issued by the FDA, United States

Sr. No.	Date of Issue	Drug Safety Alert
1.	May 23, 2023	FDA issues final guidance on adjusting for covariates in randomized CTs
2.	May 17, 2023	FDA issues two draft guidance documents for industry to support the approval of pediatric drug products
3.	May 11, 2023	FDA requires updates to clarify labeling of prescription stimulants used to treat attention deficit hyperactivity disorder and other conditions
4.	April 28, 2023	FDA issues final nicotine replacement therapy drug products guidance
5.	April 13, 2023	FDA announces new safety label changes for opioid pain medicines
6.	April 4, 2023	FDA authorizes Gohibic (vilobelimab) injection for the treatment of COVID-19
7.	March 29, 2023	FDA launches the Lupus Treatment Consortium in partnership with the Lupus Research Alliance

TABLE 2.2
Drug Safety Alerts Issued by CDSCO, India

Sr. No.	Date of Issue	Suspected Drugs	Adverse Drug Reactions
1.	June 22, 2023	Teneligliptin	Bullous pemphigoid
2.	May 31, 2023	Levosulpride	Restless legs syndrome
3.	May 31, 2023	Ceftriaxone	Electrocardiogram QT prolonged
4.	April 24, 2023	Ziprasidone	Drug reaction with eosinophilia and systemic symptoms
5.	March 29, 2023	Sulfasalazine	Visual impairment
6.	March 29, 2023	Olmesartan	Muscle spasm and taste disorder
7.	March 29, 2023	Nebivolol	Hyperkalemia
8.	March 29, 2023	Metoprolol	Hyponatremia
9.	February 20, 2023	Amikacin	Blurred vision
10.	February 20, 2023	Cephalosporins	Purpura
11.	January 31, 2023	Amphotericin B	Hearing disorders and tachycardia

TABLE 2.3
Drug Safety Alerts Issued by TGA, Australia

Sr. No.	Date of Issue	Drug Safety Alert
1.	June 8, 2023	Australia tablets pose a serious risk to your health and should not be taken
2.	June 8, 2023	Big Penis USA tablets pose a serious risk to your health and should not be taken
3.	June 8, 2023	Germany Niubian tablets pose a serious risk to your health and should not be taken
4.	June 8, 2023	Multani Kaminividravana Rasa (Kamini) tablets: the TGA has recently tested the contents of Kamini and found ingredients that pose a serious risk if ingested
5.	June 8, 2023	USA Black Gold tablets pose a serious risk to your health and should not be taken
6.	June 1, 2023	Risk of kidney damage with oral anticoagulants: a warning about serious kidney damage has been added to the prescribing information for all oral anticoagulants in Australia
7.	May 31, 2023	EVE Allyl-isopropyl-acetyl-urea tablets: the TGA is warning consumers against taking EVE branded products that contain allyl-isopropyl-acetyl-urea (apronal) as they pose a significant health risk and are prohibited from sale, supply, or use in Australia
8.	May 25, 2023	Counterfeit semaglutide vials: the TGA has detected fake semaglutide, also known as Ozempic, being illegally imported into Australia
9.	May 11, 2023	New safety warning for medicines used in arthritis and other inflammatory conditions: a safety warning has been added to a class of medicines called Janus kinase inhibitors used for chronic inflammatory conditions
10.	January 5, 2023	Nitrosamine impurities in medicines: information for sponsors and manufacturers

TABLE 2.4
Drug Safety Alerts Issued by MHRA, United Kingdom

S. No.	Date of Issue	Drug Safety Alert
1.	June 27, 2023	Calcium chloride, calcium gluconate: potential risk of underdosing with calcium gluconate in severe hyperkalemia
2.	June 27, 2023	Adrenaline auto-injectors (AAIs): new guidance and resources for safe use
3.	May 25, 2023	Febuxostat: updated advice for the treatment of patients with a history of major cardiovascular disease
4.	April 26, 2023	Nitrofurantoin: reminder of the risks of pulmonary and hepatic adverse drug reactions
5.	March 23, 2023	Terlipressin: new recommendations to reduce risks of respiratory failure and septic shock in patients with type-1 hepatorenal syndrome
6.	January 25, 2023	Xaqua (metolazone) 5 mg tablets: exercise caution when switching patients between metolazone preparations

TABLE 2.5
Drug Safety Alerts Issued by Health Canada, Canada

S. No.	Date of Issue	Drug Safety Alert
1	July 7, 2023	Rhinaris nasal mist: one lot was recalled because of the risk of microbial growth which may lead to infection
2	June 1, 2023	Nature's Bounty Kids Multivitamin Gummies were recalled because of missing label information that could create a choking hazard for children under 4 years old
3	March 16, 2023	Robikids and Solmux are unauthorized children's syrups for thinning mucus and may pose serious health risks
4	February 7, 2023	Amitriptyline antidepressant drugs were recalled because of a nitrosamine impurity
5	January 17, 2023	Evusheld (tixagevimab and cilgavimab for injection): risk of prophylaxis or treatment failure due to antiviral resistance to specific SARS-CoV-2 subvariants

2.19 CONCLUSION

Pharmacovigilance, since its inception in response to drug disasters especially the thalidomide tragedy, has come a long way and is currently integrated with cutting-edge technologies to ensure the safe use of medicinal products. To achieve and strengthen the safety aspects of medicinal products in every country, all need to contribute to international collaborations and adopt either already established guidelines by several regulatory authorities or create their own regulatory guidelines so that international harmonization for safe, effective, and rational use of medicinal products can be achieved.

REFERENCES

[1] R. Kumar, P. Kumar, V. Kalaiselvan, I. Kaur, and G. N. Singh, "Best practices for improving the quality of Individual case safety reports in pharmacovigilance," *Ther. Innov. Regul. Sci.*, vol. 50, no. 4, pp. 464–471, July 2016, https://doi.org/10.1177/2168479016634766.

[2] S. G. Suke, P. Kosta, and H. Negi, "Role of pharmacovigilance in India: An overview," *Online J. Public Health Inform.*, vol. 7, no. 2, p. 223, June 2015, https://doi.org/10.5210/OJPHI.V7I2.5595.

[3] H. Langhof, W. W. L. Chin, S. Wieschowski, C. Federico, J. Kimmelman, and D. Strech, "Preclinical efficacy in therapeutic area guidelines from the U.S. food and drug administration and the European medicines agency: A cross-sectional study," *Br. J. Pharm.*, vol. 175, no. 22, pp. 4229–4238, Nov. 2018, https://doi.org/10.1111/BPH.14485.

[4] J. K. Aronson, "What is a clinical trial?," *Br. J. Clin. Pharm.*, vol. 58, no. 1, p. 1, July 2004, https://doi.org/10.1111/J.1365-2125.2004.02184.X.

[5] G. Fornasier, S. Francescon, R. Leone, and P. Baldo, "An historical overview over Pharmacovigilance," *Int. J. Clin. Pharm.*, vol. 40, no. 4, p. 744, Aug. 2018, https://doi.org/10.1007/S11096-018-0657-1.

[6] "Guidelines for the regulatory assessment of medicinal products for use in self-medication." Published by WHO, 2000.

[7] S. Olsson, "The role of the WHO programme on international Drug monitoring in coordinating worldwide drug safety efforts," *Drug Saf.*, vol. 19, no. 1, pp. 1–10, 1998, https://doi.org/10.2165/00002018-199819010-00001.

[8] R. E. Gliklich, N. A. Dreyer, and M. B. Leavy, "Adverse event detection, processing, and reporting," 2014, [Online], www.ncbi.nlm.nih.gov/books/NBK208615/ (accessed July 12, 2023).

[9] N. J. Kachuck, "Registries, research, and regrets: Is the FDA's post-marketing REMS process not adequately protecting patients?," *Ther. Adv. Neurol. Disord.*, vol. 4, no. 6, p. 339, 2011, https://doi.org/10.1177/1756285611424461.

[10] "About us—Indian pharmacopoeia commission," www.ipc.gov.in/mandates/pvpi/pharmacovigilance-skill-development-programme.html (accessed July 12, 2023).

[11] H. Song, X. Pei, Z. Liu, C. Shen, J. Sun, Y. Liu, L. Zhou, F. Sun, and X. Xiao, "Pharmacovigilance in China: Evolution and future challenges," *Br. J. Clin. Pharm.*, vol. 89, no. 2, pp. 510–522, Feb. 2023, https://doi.org/10.1111/BCP.15277.

[12] M. Banovac, G. Candore, J. Slattery, F. Houyez, D. Haerry, G. Genov, and P. Arlett, "Patient reporting in the EU: Analysis of EudraVigilance data," *Drug Saf.*, vol. 40, no. 7, pp. 629–645, July 2017, https://doi.org/10.1007/S40264-017-0534-1/FIGURES/13.

[13] J. H. Martin, and C. Lucas, "Reporting adverse drug events to the therapeutic goods administration," *Aust. Prescr.*, vol. 44, no. 1, p. 2, Feb. 2021, https://doi.org/10.18773/AUSTPRESCR.2020.077.

[14] K. Mori, M. Watanabe, N. Horiuchi, A. Tamura, and H. Kutsumi, "The role of the pharmaceuticals and medical devices agency and healthcare professionals in post-marketing safety," *Clin. J. Gastroenterol.*, vol. 7, no. 2, pp. 103–107, 2014, https://doi.org/10.1007/S12328-014-0474-6.

[15] A. U. Rehman, S. N. Khalid, R. Zakar, U. Hani, M. Zakria Zakar, and F. Fischer, "Patients' perception of the pharmacovigilance system: A pre-diagnostic and post-interventional cross-sectional survey," *Front. Pharm.*, vol. 13, p. 936124, Nov. 2022, https://doi.org/10.3389/FPHAR.2022.936124/BIBTEX.

[16] N. Raj, S. Fernandes, N. R. Charyulu, A. Dubey, R. G. S., and S. Hebbar, "Post-market surveillance: A review on key aspects and measures on the effective functioning in the context of the United Kingdom and Canada," *Ther. Adv. Drug Saf.*, vol. 10, p. 204209861986541, Jan. 2019, https://doi.org/10.1177/2042098619865413.

3 Regulations in the United States

Kumari Neha, Faraat Ali, Rutendo J. Kuwana, and Sharad K. Wakode

3.1 INTRODUCTION

Pharmaceutical regulations are defined as blend of lawful, managerial procedures that administrations take to guarantee the protection, excellence, and efficiency of drugs, in addition to the significance and exactness of product information. The term *regulation* refers to a wide range of papers with various legal justifications and authorities, including instructions, authorizations, procedures, legislation, and so on [1]. It plays a significant part in endorsing the harmlessness and effectiveness of approved medicines worldwide. It regulates the pricing and quality of drugs. Regulations are required for newly innovated and existing products to recover declining health status. Each country has its own guidelines used for novelty, testing, and marketing of manufacturing drugs, and for post-marketing studies. Laws are the guidelines created by a body that analyzes legislation to make them more easily put into practice. Compared to legislation, they might be enacted relatively swiftly and easily. For instance, the US Food, Drug, and Cosmetic Act of 1938 is governed by the US Food and Drug Administration (FDA). Regulations often grow considerably bigger than the scope of the underlying statute. The regulation of medications in the United States is a complex and multifaceted system that is designed to certify the safety and efficacy of medicinal products [2]. This system comprises numerous federal and state agencies, laws, regulations, and policies that work together to oversee the expansion, analysis, approval, and selling of drugs. This chapter will provide an outline of the drug guideline system in the United States, including the organization accountable for medication regulation, the drug approval process, and the ongoing monitoring and oversight of drugs once they are on the market. The regulatory framework for medications in the United States is shaped by a number of factors, including legal, political, and economic considerations. In many cases, the federal government plays a central role in developing and enforcing drug regulations, although state and local governments also have significant regulatory authority [3].

One of the of the organizations working under the roof of the Department of Health and Human Services (HHS), the FDA, validates the quality, effectiveness, and purity of meals, both human and animal medications, biological substances,

DOI: 10.1201/9781003296492-4

and medical equipment [4]. There are 11 operational divisions within HHS, including three human services organizations and eight US Public Health Service organizations. These examinations supervise a range of medical and social services and carry out vital research for the country [5]. As seen in Figure 3.1, the FDA is made up of five separate offices that oversee various operations. It is the responsibility of the FDA to promote and protect public health. Clinical trials (CTs) and the acceptance of new drug applications (NDAs) are the two steps in the FDA's drug approval process. Only after the proposal of an investigational new drug (IND) application does the FDA approval procedure begin [6]. The Center for Drug Evaluation and Research (CDER) carries out health campaigns to find safe and beneficial medications to enhance health. It harmonizes prescription and over-the-counter (OTC) medications, combining biological treatments and generic pharmaceuticals [7].

The OTC Monograph System or the NDA Protocol establishes OTC medications [8]. The primary difference among both processes is that the NDA procedure requires official FDA preapproval (Figure 3.2), whereas the monograph-based approach does not require official filing or acceptance. The pharmaceutical item must fully adhere to the labelling standards outlined in Title 21 of the Code of Federal Regulations along with the monograph [9].

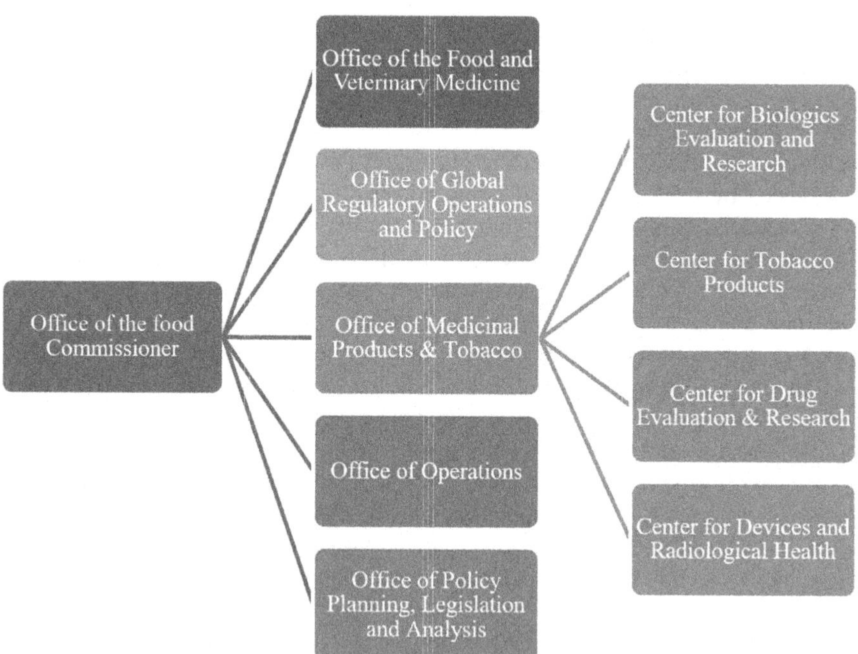

FIGURE 3.1 Organizational Chart of the FDA.

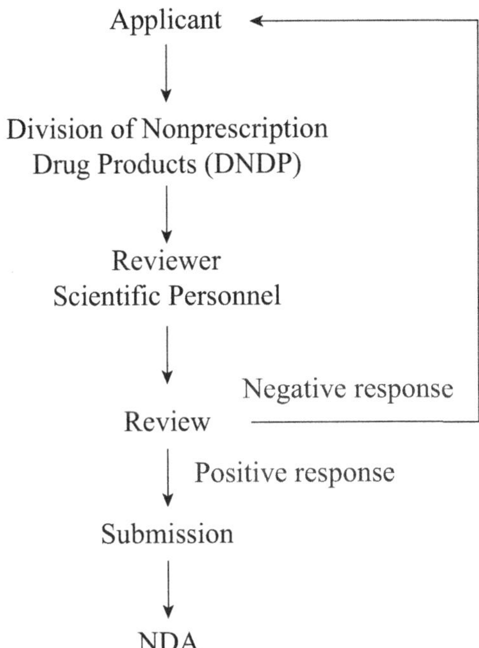

FIGURE 3.2 Development of OTC Drugs by the NDA Process.

3.2 HISTORY OF DRUG REGULATION IN THE UNITED STATES

The antiquity of medicine regulation in the United States can be outlined back to the early 20th century, when concerns about the protection and efficiency of medicines led to the development of the first medication laws. These laws aimed to protect the public from fraudulent and dangerous drugs by requiring manufacturers to disclose the contents of their products and the claims made for them. Since the 1906 Pure Food and Drugs Act was employed by President Theodore Roosevelt, FDA drug regulation has undergone significant evolution [10].

Over time, the scope of drug regulation expanded to encompass a varied choice of issues, counting the approval and marketing of new drugs, the protection and efficacy of existing medicines, and the prevention of drug abuse and addiction. In many cases, drug regulatory policies have been developed in response to crises or public outcry, such as the thalidomide scandal of the 1960s, the AIDS epidemic of the 1980s and 1990s, and the opioid epidemic of the 2010s [11].

3.3 LEGAL FRAMEWORK FOR DRUG REGULATION

The instruction for drugs in the United States is primarily the responsibility of the FDA, which is a federal agency within the Department of Health and Human

Services [12]. The FDA is answerable for ensuring the safety and effectiveness of all drugs sold in the United States, as well as regulating the production, dispersal, and labeling of these medicines [13]. CDER, the Center for Food Safety and Applied Nutrition (CFSAN), and the Center for Biologics Evaluation and Research (CBER) are the three centers where the FDA principally allocates its research for the production of drugs, biologics, devices, combination products, and foods.

In addition to the FDA, several other federal agencies play a role in drug regulation. The National Institutes of Health (NIH) is responsible for funding investigation into the safety and effectiveness of drugs, whereas the Centers for Disease Control and Prevention (CDC) monitors the safety of drugs once they are on the market [14]. The Drug Enforcement Administration (DEA) controls the creation, circulation, and supply of sensitive materials, such as opioids, whereas the Department of Justice (DOJ) imposes federal drug rules and protocols.

At the state level, the regulation of drugs is primarily the responsibility of state pharmacy boards and health divisions. These agencies are answerable for regulating the dispensing of drugs by pharmacies and other healthcare providers, as well as overseeing the licensing and training of pharmacists [15].

3.4 DRUG APPROVAL PROCESS

The process for authorizing new medications in the United States is lengthy and complex, and is designed to guarantee that medications are reliable and efficient before they are sold to the public. The drug approval process is overseen by the FDA, which has the authority for medication approval or rejection depending on safety concerns and effectiveness [16].

The drug approval process typically begins with preclinical testing, which involves laboratory and animal research to determine the suitability and safety of a medication. If the preclinical testing is successful, the drug developer can then apply for an IND proposal with the FDA, which allows them to begin testing the drug in humans (Figure 3.3).

The next phase of the pharmaceutical authorization procedure is CTs, which are normally carried out in three stages. A small number of young volunteers takes part in phase I studies, which are intended for assessing the drug's effectiveness and dosing. A greater number of participants participates in the second stage of trials with the disease or condition being targeted by the drug; these CTs are designed to determine the medicine's efficacy and any negative effects it may cause. The stage three trials, which involve an even greater number of recipients, are intended to verify the medication's efficacy and assess its safety [17].

If the medicine performs successfully in these clinical studies, the pharmaceutical manufacturer can submit a proposal to the FDA for approval. The FDA reviews the data from the CTs and decides as to whether the medicine is suitable and secure for consumption in the general population. The medicine may be offered for sale to consumers if FDA approves it.

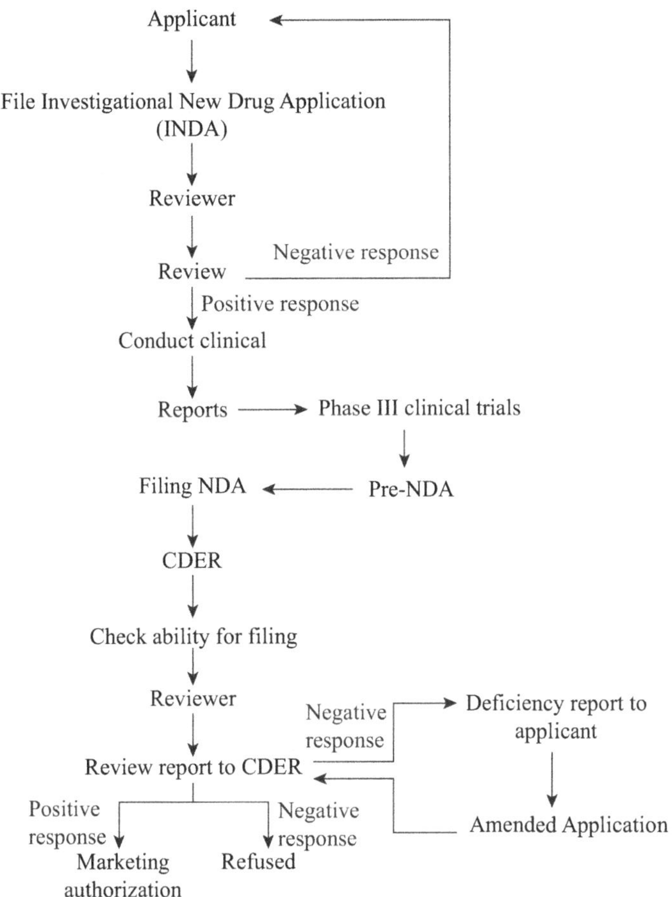

FIGURE 3.3 FDA Approval Process of a Drug.

3.5 POST-MARKET OVERSIGHT

In the United States, post-market surveillance is a critical component of drug regulation. Once a medicine has been accepted for use by the FDA, it enters the post-market phase, during which the efficacy and safety of the medication are continually monitored. CDER is accountable for monitoring the safety of drugs in the post-market phase. CDER uses a variety of tools and programs to collect and analyze statistics regarding the efficacy and quality of medications, including adverse event reporting, digital health record facts, and post-market scientific studies [18].

One important tool for post-market oversight is the FDA Adverse Event Reporting System (FAERS), which is maintained by the FDA. FAERS collects reports of adverse events, such as side effects or other unexpected reactions, from healthcare providers, patients, and drug manufacturers. The data collected in FAERS is used to identify potential safety issues with drugs and to inform regulatory decisions. Another important program used in post-market surveillance is the FDA's Sentinel Initiative, which uses electronic health record data to monitor the reliability of medications and other medical products [19]. Sentinel allows the FDA to rapidly identify potential safety issues and to conduct post-market studies to further investigate these issues. In addition to these programs, the FDA may necessitate post-market clinical lessons to further evaluate the safeties and reliability of drugs. These reports may be required as a condition of approval or may be initiated in response to safety concerns identified in the post-market phase [20].

Overall, post-market surveillance plays a critical role in ensuring the ongoing protection and efficiency of medications in the United States. By continually monitoring drugs in the post-market phase, the FDA can recognize and address latent secure issues and certify that patients are receiving safe and effective treatments.

3.6 DRUG REGULATION IN THE UNITED STATES

The FDA is in charge of regulating drug formulation in the United States. Thus the agency ensures that drugs are secure and reliable for their proposed use and that they are manufactured to high quality standards. The FDA requires that all new drug formulations undergo rigorous testing before they can be approved for use. This testing includes preclinical studies to assess the secure and reliability of the medicine, as well as CTs to determine the optimal dosage and to assess any potential side effects. Manufacturers are required to provide scientific proof for the safety of new drugs as to their intended use before placing on the market.

Once a drug formulation has been approved, the FDA continues to regulate it through post-market surveillance. This includes monitoring adverse events and conducting additional studies if safety concerns arise. The FDA also regulates drug formulations in terms of their labeling and packaging. Drug labels must provide accurate information about the drug's uses, dosage, side effects, and potential interactions with other drugs. Drug packaging must also be designed to prevent contamination and to ensure that the drug remains stable during storage and transportation. Drug formulations are also direct to strict manufacturing protocols, recognized as good manufacturing practices (GMPs). These regulations require that drug manufacturers maintain a high level of quality control in their production processes and that they meet specific standards for cleanliness, equipment maintenance, and documentation.

Overall, drug formulation guidelines in the United States are aimed at ensuring that medicines are innocuous and active for their proposed use, and that they are manufactured to the highest quality standards. This helps to defend the health and well-being of patients who rely on these drugs for their medical care.

CDER has initiatives to help with the new approach methodologies (NAMs) qualification process for drug development tools. The goal of NAMs is to demonstrate that a technique may be applied repeatedly to a specific governing context of use deprived of needing the submission of authentication information for the respective application [21]. As an example, it is a victory for the FDA and for patients with US asthma and chronic obstructive pulmonary disease that approved generic dry powder inhalers (DPIs) have now entered the market. Numerous generic DPIs have been approved thanks to the FDA supporting exploration and converting existing considerate of DPI achievement into a suitable bioequivalence pathway conveyed via product-specific guidelines. FDA is dedicated to easing regulatory burdens and advancing scientific knowledge for complicated drug-device amalgamation products like DPIs [22].

3.7 COMMON TECHNICAL DOCUMENT (CTD)

With the most depth at the base and higher-level summaries, the Common Technical Document (CTD) has five parts and is organized hierarchically. Since the previous reform of the vaccine prequalification method, the CTD format has seen a considerable increase in usage worldwide. Several nations that import previously approved pharmaceuticals demand the submission of a CTD format dossier for registrations of its goods. The majority of producers have generated a dossier in CTD format that they have used to register the product in one or more countries. The information found in Module 1 is not found in Modules 2, 3, 4, or 5, yet it is necessary to evaluate the product for prequalification purposes. In accordance with Figure 3.4, Modules 2, 3, 4, and 5 share the common format and substance of dossiers presented to various authorities:

Module 2: Common Technical Document Summaries (in accordance with ICH recommendations M4Q, M4S, and M4E).
Module 3: Quality (as per ICH M4Q).
Module 4: Nonclinical Study Reports (as per ICH M4S).
Module 5: Clinical Study Reports (as per ICH M4E).

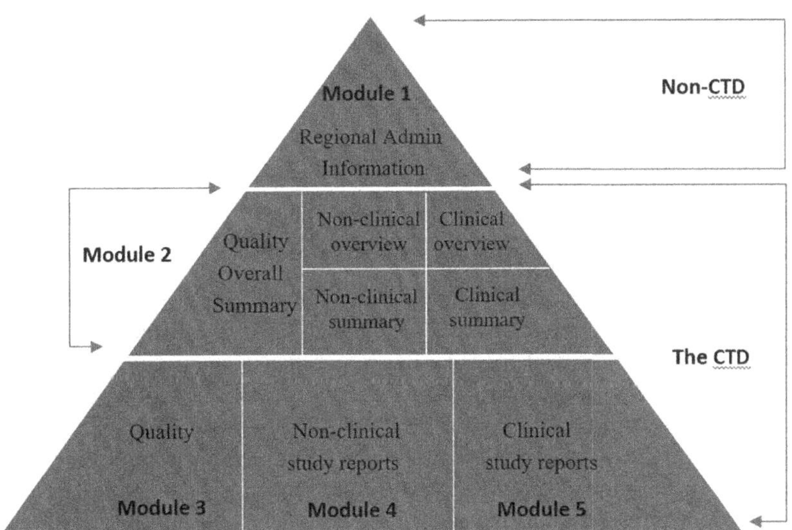

FIGURE 3.4 Common Technical Document Organization.

3.8 FOOD ADDITIVES AMENDMENT

The FDA sets standards for what constitutes food that is adulterated, mislabeled, or hazardous. An FDA amendment was passed to distinguish between additives to food items that are generally recognized as safe (GRAS) and those that might modify food attributes and need marketing permission. A product's manufacturer must demonstrate its safety for human consumption before receiving marketing permission.

3.9 CURRENT CHALLENGES IN US DRUG REGULATIONS

There are several current challenges facing drug regulation in the United States:

- *Opioid epidemic*: The United States is currently facing an opioid epidemic, which has been fueled by the over-prescription of prescription painkillers. The challenge for drug regulators is to balance the need for pain relief with the risks of addiction and overdose.
- *Rising drug prices*: The cost of prescription drugs in the United States has been rising at an alarming rate, making it difficult for many patients to afford necessary medications. Regulators are struggling to find ways to balance the need for innovation and investment in drug development with the need for affordable medications [23].
- *Regulatory capture*: There are concerns that drug companies have too much influence over the regulatory process, leading to a lack of oversight and accountability. Regulators need to ensure that they are independent and transparent in their decision-making [24].
- *FDA favors procedure*: The FDA sanction procedure for new drugs can be lengthy and expensive, leading to delays in getting new treatments to patients. Regulators are exploring ways to streamline the process while still ensuring the well-being and efficacy of new drugs.
- *Drug shortages*: There have been shortages of some critical drugs in recent years, which can have serious consequences for patients. Regulators are working to identify the causes of these shortages and develop solutions to prevent them from happening in the future [25].

3.10 LIMITATIONS ON DRUG REGULATIONS

One limitation of drug regulation in the United States is the potential for regulatory capture, where the interests of the drug industry may influence the regulatory process. The pharmaceutical industry has a significant amount of political influence, and there have been concerns that this can lead to a lack of regulatory oversight. Another limitation is the complex and lengthy process of drug approval by the FDA, which can delay access to new treatments for patients. The approval process is designed to ensure safety and efficacy, but it can also be costly and time-consuming, which may limit innovation and investment in drug development [26].

Additionally, the high cost of prescription drugs is a significant limitation of drug regulation in the United States. The cost of drugs can be prohibitively expensive for some patients, which can result in poor health outcomes and reduced access to necessary treatments. Finally, the regulatory system in the United States can vary between states, which can lead to inconsistencies and confusion for patients and healthcare providers. This lack of uniformity can create challenges for drug manufacturers who must navigate multiple regulatory systems.

3.11 CONCLUSION

In conclusion, drug regulation in the United States is a multifaceted and rigorous method that includes multiple phases of testing, review, and monitoring. The FDA is in charge of managing the regulation of drugs, and it uses a science-based approach to assess the safeness and persuasiveness of novel remedies. The FDA's medicine evaluation process is designed to ensure that new drugs are harmless and active before they are accepted for usage by patients. This process includes preclinical testing, CTs, and a thorough review of the data by the FDA's expert reviewers.

Once a drug is approved for use, the FDA continues to monitor its safety and effectiveness through post-market surveillance. This includes tools such as adverse event reporting, electronic health record data, and post-market clinical studies. Overall, drug directive in the United States is aimed at protecting the community well-being by assuring that medications are innocuous and active before they are marketed to patients. Although the regulatory process can be lengthy and costly, it is an essential component of the healthcare system, and it helps to ensure that patients receive safe and effective treatments.

REFERENCES

[1] Lezotre, P.L. (2013). *International Cooperation, Convergence and Harmonization of Pharmaceutical Regulations: A Global Perspective.* Academic Press. https://doi.org/10.1016/B978-0-12-800053-3.00001-X.

[2] Regulatory Authorities for Drug Safety National Academies of Sciences, Engineering, and Medicine. (2007). *The Future of Drug Safety: Promoting and Protecting the Health of the Public.* The National Academies Press. https://doi.org/10.17226/117

[3] *Laws, Regulations, Policies and Procedures for Drug Applications | FDA.* www.fda.gov/drugs/development-approval-process-drugs/laws-regulations-policies-and-procedures-drug-applications

[4] McGuire, S. (2011). US department of agriculture and US department of health and human services, dietary guidelines for Americans, 2010. Washington, DC: US government printing office, January 2011. *Advances in Nutrition*, *2*(3), 293–294.

[5] National Center for Health Statistics (US), & National Center for Health Services Research. (1994). *Health, United States.* US Department of Health, Education, and Welfare, Public Health Service, Health Resources Administration, National Center for Health Statistics.

[6] Jawahar, N., & Lakshmi, V.T. (2017). Regulatory requirements for the drug approval process in US, Europe and India. *Journal of Pharmaceutical Sciences and Research*, *9*(10), 1943–1952.

[7] Narang, S. (2018). Pharmaceutical regulations in the United States: An overview. *Pharmaceutical Medicine and Translational Clinical Research*, 157–174.

[8] Engel, L.W., & Straus, S.E. (2002). Development of therapeutics: Opportunities within complementary and alternative medicine. *Nature Reviews Drug Discovery*, *1*(3), 229–237.

[9] Bobka, M.S. (1993). The 21CFR online database: Food and drug administration regulations full-text. *Medical Reference Services Quarterly*, *12*(1), 7–15.

[10] *The History of Drug Regulation | FDA*. www.fda.gov/about-fda/histories-fda-regulated-products/history-drug-regulation

[11] Klantschnig, G., & Dele-Adedeji, I. (2021). Opioid of the people: The moral economy of tramadol in Lagos. *Politique Africaine*, *16*(3), 85–105.

[12] Rägo, L., & Santoso, B. (2008). Drug regulation: History, present and future. *Drug Benefits and Risks: International Textbook of Clinical Pharmacology*, *2*, 65–77.

[13] Johnson, R. (2012). *The Federal Food Safety System: A Primer*. Congressional Research Service.

[14] Smith, M.B., Haney, E., McDonagh, M., Pappas, M., Daeges, M., Wasson, N., Fu, R., & Nelson, H.D. (2015). Treatment of myalgic encephalomyelitis/chronic fatigue syndrome: A systematic review for a national institutes of health pathways to prevention workshop. *Annals of Internal Medicine*, *162*(12), 841–850.

[15] Mankar, S.D., Gholap, V.D., Zende, T.P., & Dighe, R.S. (2014). Drug regulatory agencies in India, USA, Europe and Japan: A review. *International Journal of Institutional Pharmacy and Life Sciences*, *4*(2), 288–300.

[16] Kashyap, U.N., Gupta, V., & Raghunandan, H.V. (2013). Comparison of drug approval process in United States & Europe. *Journal of Pharmaceutical Sciences and Research*, *5*(6), 131.

[17] Van Norman, G.A. (2016). Drugs and devices: Comparison of European and US approval processes. *JACC: Basic to Translational Science*, *1*(5), 399–412.

[18] Downing, N.S., Shah, N.D., Aminawung, J.A., Pease, A.M., Zeitoun, J.D., Krumholz, H.M., & Ross, J.S. (2017). Postmarket safety events among novel therapeutics approved by the US Food and Drug administration between 2001 and 2010. *Jama*, *317*(18), 1854–1863.

[19] Wallach, J.D., Egilman, A.C., Dhruva, S.S., McCarthy, M.E., Miller, J.E., Woloshin, S., Schwartz, L.M., & Ross, J.S. (2018). Postmarket studies required by the US Food and Drug administration for new drugs and biologics approved between 2009 and 2012: Cross sectional analysis. *BMJ*, *361*.

[20] Bhasale, A.L., Sarpatwari, A., De Bruin, M.L., Lexchin, J., Lopert, R., Bahri, P., & Mintzes, B.J. (2021). Postmarket safety communication for protection of public health: A comparison of regulatory policy in Australia, Canada, the European Union, and the United States. *Clinical Pharmacology & Therapeutics*, *109*(6), 1424–1442.

[21] Avila, A.M., Bebenek, I., Mendrick, D.L., Peretz, J., Yao, J., & Brown, P.C. (2023). Gaps and challenges in nonclinical assessments of pharmaceuticals: An FDA/CDER perspective on considerations for development of new approach methodologies. *Regulatory Toxicology and Pharmacology*, *139*, 105345.

[22] Newman, B., Babiskin, A., Bielski, E., Boc, S., Dhapare, S., Fang, L., Feibus, K., Kaviratna, A., Li, B.V., Luke, M.C., Ma, T., & Gaglani, D.K. (2022). Scientific and regulatory activities initiated by the US food and drug administration to foster approvals of generic dry powder Inhalers: Bioequivalence perspective. *Advanced Drug Delivery Reviews*, 114526.

[23] Bewley-Taylor, D.R. (2003). Challenging the UN drug control conventions: Problems and possibilities. *International Journal of Drug Policy*, *14*(2), 171–179.

[24] Shah, R.B., & Khan, M.A. (2009). Nanopharmaceuticals: Challenges and regulatory perspective. *Nanotechnology in Drug Delivery*, 621–646.

[25] Huang, S.M., Abernethy, D.R., Wang, Y., Zhao, P., & Zineh, I. (2013). The utility of modeling and simulation in drug development and regulatory review. *Journal of Pharmaceutical Sciences*, *102*(9), 2912–2923.

[26] Jumelle, C., Gholizadeh, S., Annabi, N., & Dana, R. (2020). Advances and limitations of drug delivery systems formulated as eye drops. *Journal of Controlled Release*, *321*, 1–22.

4 Regulations in the European Union

Anam Ilyas, Faraat Ali, Vishesh Sahu, and Doaa Rady

4.1 INTRODUCTION

Drug regulation plays a crucial role in ensuring the safety, efficacy, and quality of medicines. The primary objective of drug regulation is to protect public health and ensure patient safety. By implementing robust regulatory processes, authorities can evaluate the safety profile of drugs before they are approved for use. This includes assessing potential risks, monitoring adverse reactions, and taking necessary actions to minimize harm to patients [1,2]. Drug regulation ensures that medicines are rigorously evaluated for their intended therapeutic benefits. Regulatory agencies assess clinical trial data and scientific evidence to determine if a drug is effective in treating the targeted condition. This helps to prevent the marketing of ineffective or insufficiently tested drugs, safeguarding patients from potential harm and unnecessary expenses [3]. It establishes quality standards for the manufacturing, packaging, and labelling of medicines. By enforcing good manufacturing practices, regulators ensure that drugs are produced consistently, meeting stringent quality standards. This helps prevent contamination, incorrect dosages, and substandard products, ensuring that patients receive safe and reliable medicines [4]. Regulatory agencies conduct thorough assessments of the risks and benefits associated with medicines. This evaluation considers factors such as the severity of the condition being treated, available alternative treatments, and potential side effects. By conducting a balanced risk-benefit analysis, drug regulation helps healthcare professionals and patients make informed decisions about the use of specific medications. Drug regulation includes robust pharmacovigilance systems to monitor the safety profile of drugs once they are on the market. Adverse drug reactions and unexpected side effects can be reported, collected, and analysed to identify any emerging safety concerns. Regulatory authorities can then take appropriate actions, such as issuing warnings, updating product labelling, or even withdrawing drugs from the market if necessary [5]. A well-regulated pharmaceutical sector enhances public trust and confidence in the healthcare system. When patients know that medicines undergo rigorous evaluation and monitoring, they can have greater confidence in their safety and effectiveness. This trust is essential for patient compliance, healthcare provider confidence, and the overall success of the healthcare system. Drug regulation is critical to protect patients from potentially unsafe or ineffective medicines. It ensures that medicines meet high safety, efficacy, and

DOI: 10.1201/9781003296492-5

quality standards, promoting public health and providing the foundation for effective healthcare delivery [6].

4.1.1 Role of the European Union in Harmonizing Regulations across Member States

The role of the European Union in harmonizing regulations across member states is crucial for several reasons. It aims to establish a single market within its member states where goods, services, and capital can flow freely. Harmonizing regulations across member states is essential to eliminate trade barriers and create a level playing field for businesses. By harmonizing regulations related to drug approval, safety standards, labelling requirements, and clinical trials, the EU facilitates the movement of medicines across borders, ensuring consistent quality, safety, and efficacy standards. Harmonized regulations enable the EU to establish common safety standards for medicines, ensuring that patients across member states receive equally safe and effective treatments [4,7]. By aligning regulations, the EU can strengthen pharmacovigilance systems, enable consistent monitoring of adverse drug reactions, and enhance post-marketing surveillance activities. This coordinated approach helps identify safety issues promptly, take appropriate actions, and protect patients from potential harm. Harmonization of regulations facilitates the timely availability of medicines across the EU, ensuring equitable access for patients in all member states [8,9]. A harmonized regulatory framework streamlines the process for marketing authorization, reducing duplication of efforts and accelerating the introduction of new drugs into the market. This helps avoid delays in patient access to innovative treatments, particularly for rare diseases or conditions with limited therapeutic options. Harmonizing regulations across member states improves the efficiency and effectiveness of the regulatory process. Sharing best practices, standardizing procedures, and aligning assessment criteria minimize duplication of work and reduces regulatory burdens for pharmaceutical companies [10]. Harmonization also fosters regulatory convergence, enabling regulatory authorities to pool resources, exchange information, and collaborate on scientific assessments. This cooperative approach enhances the overall efficiency of the regulatory system, ensuring timely evaluations and robust decision-making. Harmonized regulations contribute to the competitiveness of the EU pharmaceutical industry globally. By establishing consistent standards, the EU facilitates the development and registration of medicines within its borders, making it an attractive market for pharmaceutical companies. A harmonized regulatory framework also simplifies regulatory compliance for manufacturers, especially for those operating across member states. This consistency and efficiency support the growth of the pharmaceutical industry, encourage research and development investments, and foster innovation within the EU [11]. The EU actively collaborates with regulatory authorities from around the world to harmonize regulations at the international level. This collaboration facilitates mutual recognition of regulatory decisions, reducing duplicative evaluations and promoting global access to safe and effective medicines. The EU plays an active role in international forums and initiatives to share expertise, align regulatory standards, and promote convergence among regulatory authorities.

4.2 HISTORICAL BACKGROUND AND DEVELOPMENT OF DRUG REGULATION IN THE EU

The EU has a well-established framework for drug regulation that has evolved over several decades. The development of this regulatory system was driven by the need to ensure the safety, efficacy, and quality of pharmaceutical products available in the EU market [12–14].

A historical background and overview of the development of drug regulation in the EU is provided here.

1. *Early stages*:
   - In the 1960s and 1970s, individual EU member states had their own drug regulatory systems with varying standards and procedures.
   - The thalidomide tragedy in the 1960s, where a drug caused severe birth defects, highlighted the importance of harmonizing drug regulation to protect public health.
2. *Creation of the European Medicines Agency (EMA)*:
   - In 1995, the European Medicines Evaluation Agency (EMEA) was established as a centralized regulatory authority for the evaluation and supervision of medicines in the EU.
   - The EMEA was responsible for coordinating the scientific evaluation of medicines across member states and providing recommendations to the European Commission.
3. *Legal framework*:
   - The main legislation governing pharmaceuticals in the EU is Directive 2001/83/EC, commonly known as the Pharmaceuticals Directive, which establishes the regulatory framework for human medicines.
   - The directive outlines requirements for drug authorization, clinical trials, labelling, pharmacovigilance (monitoring drug safety), and post-approval changes.
4. *Centralized procedure*:
   - The EU operates a centralized procedure for the authorization of certain types of medicines, including biotechnology products, orphan drugs, and medicines for specific diseases.
   - Under the centralized procedure, a single marketing authorization is granted by the European Commission, valid in all EU member states, based on a recommendation from the EMA.
5. *Mutual recognition procedure*:
   - For most medicines, the mutual recognition procedure allows companies to seek authorization in one EU member state, known as the "reference member state," and then have other member states recognize that authorization.
   - The mutual recognition procedure facilitates the free movement of medicines within the EU while ensuring a consistent level of regulatory oversight.
6. *Strengthening regulation*:
   - Over time, the EU has introduced various measures to strengthen drug regulation. This includes the introduction of pharmacovigilance legislation to enhance the monitoring and reporting of adverse drug reactions.

- The EU also established the European Monitoring Centre for Drugs and Drug Addiction (EMCDDA) to address issues related to illicit drugs.

7. *Evolution of regulations*:
   - Drug regulation in the EU continues to evolve to address emerging challenges and advancements in science and technology.

In recent years, there has been a focus on improving patient access to innovative medicines, streamlining clinical trial procedures, and strengthening the evaluation of the benefits and risks of medicines.

4.2.1 Importance of Regulatory Harmonization for Cross-Border Access to Medicines

Regulatory harmonization plays a crucial role in facilitating cross-border access to medicines. Harmonized regulations help to ensure that medicines available across different countries meet consistent standards of safety, efficacy, and quality. It reduces the risk of patients being exposed to substandard or unsafe products. By establishing common requirements for authorization, clinical trials, and post-marketing surveillance, regulatory harmonization enhances patient safety [15]. When regulations are harmonized, pharmaceutical companies can seek authorization for their products in multiple countries simultaneously or through a centralized procedure. This streamlines the process and reduces duplication, allowing medicines to reach the market more efficiently. It also encourages pharmaceutical companies to invest in research and development, knowing that they can access a larger market with a single approval. Harmonized regulations can foster competition by creating a level playing field for pharmaceutical companies. When companies can easily access multiple markets, it encourages competition, which can lead to lower prices for medicines [16]. This benefit is particularly relevant for generic medicines as regulatory harmonization facilitates their timely entry into the market, increasing affordability and accessibility. Regulatory harmonization can create an environment that encourages innovation. When pharmaceutical companies face consistent and transparent regulatory processes, it becomes easier for them to develop and introduce innovative medicines. Harmonized regulations can also provide mechanisms for expedited approval pathways for breakthrough therapies, benefiting patients by accelerating access to potentially life-saving treatments [17]. In regions where regulatory harmonization exists, there is a higher likelihood that medicines approved in one country will be available in others. This reduces disparities in access to essential medicines and improves the availability of a broader range of treatment options for patients. Harmonized regulations remove unnecessary barriers that can impede the importation and distribution of medicines, facilitating their movement across borders. Regulatory harmonization fosters collaboration among regulatory authorities from different countries. This collaboration allows for the sharing of information, expertise, and best practices, leading to more efficient and effective regulatory processes [18]. The exchange of information can help regulators make informed decisions, conduct joint assessments, and align regulatory requirements, benefiting all participating countries.

4.2.2 European Medicines Agency (EMA)

The EMA is a decentralized agency of the EU responsible for the scientific evaluation, supervision, and regulation of medicinal products. It plays a central role in the authorization, monitoring, and regulation of medicinal products within the EU, contributing to the harmonization of regulatory standards and procedures across member states. The EMA is headquartered in Amsterdam and collaborates with regulatory authorities, industry stakeholders, and healthcare professionals to promote access to safe and effective medicines for patients in the European Union [19].

4.2.3 Objectives of EMA

The EMA has several primary objectives that guide its activities and its mandate [20].

1. *Protecting public health*: The EMA's foremost objective is to safeguard public health by ensuring that medicinal products available in the EU are safe, effective, and of high quality. The agency assesses the risks and benefits of medicines to determine their suitability for patient use.
2. *Promoting access to medicines*: The EMA strives to promote timely access to medicines for patients within the EU. By evaluating the safety, efficacy, and quality of medicinal products, the agency contributes to the authorization and availability of new treatments and therapies.
3. *Harmonizing regulatory standards*: The EMA works toward harmonizing regulatory standards and procedures across EU member states. By developing and maintaining guidelines, the agency aims to create a consistent regulatory framework that ensures a high level of oversight for medicines throughout the EU.
4. *Facilitating innovation*: The EMA encourages and facilitates innovation in the pharmaceutical industry. It provides scientific advice and support to companies during the development and authorization process, helping them navigate regulatory requirements and bring innovative medicines to the market.
5. *Ensuring regulatory compliance*: The agency aims to ensure compliance with regulatory requirements and good manufacturing practices in the pharmaceutical industry. Through inspections, regulatory procedures, and guidelines, the EMA promotes adherence to high quality standards and helps maintain the integrity of the EU pharmaceutical market.
6. *Enhancing pharmacovigilance*: The EMA plays a critical role in pharmacovigilance, the monitoring and assessment of the safety of authorized medicines. The agency collects and analyses data on adverse drug reactions and takes appropriate regulatory actions to protect public health, such as updating product information, imposing restrictions, or withdrawing medicines from the market if necessary.
7. *Collaborating with stakeholders*: The EMA actively collaborates with various stakeholders, including regulatory authorities from EU member states,

patient organizations, healthcare professionals, and the pharmaceutical industry. Collaboration aims to foster information sharing, exchange expertise, and incorporate diverse perspectives into regulatory decision-making processes.

By pursuing these objectives, the EMA strives to ensure the availability of safe, effective, and high quality medicines, promote public health, and contribute to the overall well-being of patients within the European Union.

4.2.4 Functions of the EMA [19]

1. *Scientific evaluation*: The EMA coordinates the scientific evaluation of medicinal products for human and veterinary use. It assesses the data on quality, safety, and efficacy provided by pharmaceutical companies during the authorization process.
2. *Regulatory oversight*: The EMA provides regulatory oversight throughout the life cycle of a medicinal product. It grants marketing authorizations for specific types of medicines through centralized procedures and provides recommendations for the approval of medicines in decentralized and mutual recognition procedures.
3. *Pharmacovigilance*: The EMA is responsible for monitoring the safety of authorized medicines through pharmacovigilance activities. It collects and evaluates data on adverse drug reactions, assesses risks, and takes appropriate regulatory actions to protect public health.
4. *Scientific advice*: The EMA offers scientific advice to pharmaceutical companies during the development and evaluation of medicinal products. This advice helps companies align their development plans with regulatory requirements and optimize the quality and efficiency of their data.

4.3 RESPONSIBILITIES OF THE EMA [21]

1. *Regulatory harmonization*: The EMA promotes the harmonization of regulatory standards and procedures across EU member states. It develops guidelines and standards to ensure a consistent approach to the evaluation and regulation of medicines within the EU.
2. *Guidelines and standards*: The EMA develops and maintains a wide range of guidelines covering various aspects of pharmaceutical development, clinical trials, safety monitoring, and regulatory procedures. These guidelines provide guidance and ensure consistency in the evaluation and regulation of medicinal products.
3. *Information dissemination*: The EMA provides public access to information on its activities, including assessment reports of medicinal products, guidelines, safety communications, and transparency initiatives. It aims to foster transparency and engage stakeholders in its decision-making processes.

4.4 STRUCTURE OF THE EMA [21]

1. *Management board*: The management board consists of representatives from EU member states, the European Commission, and the European Parliament. It provides strategic direction, supervises the agency's work, and approves the budget.
2. *Executive director*: The executive director is appointed by the management board and is responsible for the day-to-day operations of the EMA. The executive director leads the agency's staff and ensures the efficient implementation of its tasks.
3. *Scientific committees*: The EMA has several scientific committees composed of experts from EU member states. These committees, such as the Committee for Medicinal Products for Human Use (CHMP) and the Pharmacovigilance Risk Assessment Committee (PRAC), provide scientific advice, evaluate data, and make recommendations on regulatory matters (Figure 4.1).
4. *Working parties*: The EMA has various working parties and expert groups that focus on specific areas, such as biologics, vaccines, paediatrics, and herbal medicines. These groups contribute to the development of guidelines, provide specialized expertise, and support the agency's work in specific therapeutic areas or regulatory topics.

4.4.1 Guidelines of the EMA [22]

The EMA develops and maintains a wide range of guidelines to provide guidance and ensure consistency in the evaluation and regulation of medicinal products within the EU. These guidelines cover various aspects of pharmaceutical development, authorization, safety monitoring, and regulatory procedures. Here are some key categories and examples of guidelines issued by the EMA:

1. *Quality guidelines*: Guidelines on pharmaceutical quality, including requirements for chemical and biological quality control, stability testing, and manufacturing processes.
2. *Nonclinical guidelines*: Guidelines on the nonclinical evaluation of medicinal products, covering areas such as pharmacology, toxicology, and safety testing in animals.
3. *Clinical guidelines*: Guidelines on clinical development and evaluation of medicinal products, including guidelines on specific therapeutic areas, clinical trial design, statistical methods, and ethical considerations.
4. *Safety guidelines*: Pharmacovigilance guidelines on the monitoring, reporting, and assessment of adverse drug reactions, risk management plans, signal detection, and benefit-risk assessment.
5. *Paediatric guidelines*: Guidelines specific to the development and evaluation of medicinal products for use in the paediatric population, aiming to ensure safe and effective treatments for children.

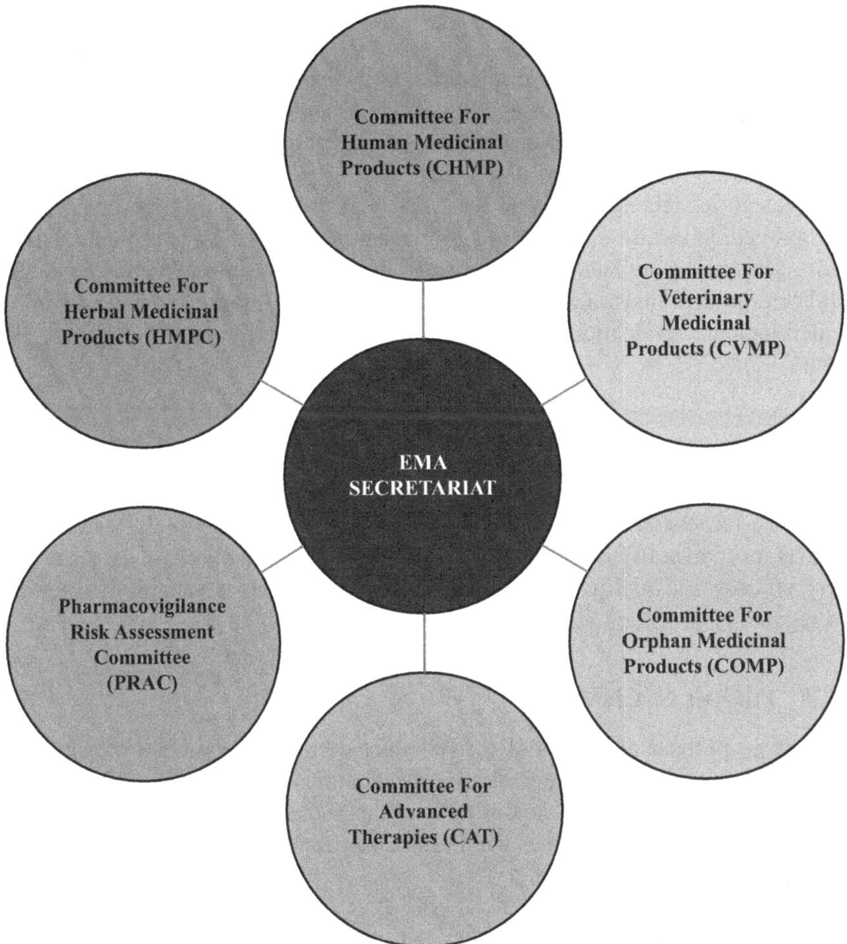

FIGURE 4.1 EMA and its Scientific Committees.

6. *Orphan medicines guidelines*: Guidelines addressing the development and authorization of medicinal products designated as orphan drugs, which are intended for the treatment of rare diseases.
7. *Biosimilars guidelines*: Guidelines on the development, evaluation, and regulation of biosimilar medicinal products, which are highly similar to already authorized biological medicines.
8. *Herbal medicinal products guidelines*: Guidelines on the quality, safety, and efficacy assessment of herbal medicinal products, including traditional herbal medicines and herbal combination products.
9. *Advanced therapy medicinal products (ATMP) guidelines*: Guidelines covering the regulation and development of advanced therapy medicinal

products, such as gene therapies, cell therapies, and tissue-engineered products.

10. *Regulatory and procedural guidelines*: Guidelines on regulatory procedures, such as marketing authorization applications, variations, post-approval changes, labelling, and packaging requirements.

These categories represent a broad overview, and the EMA regularly updates and adds new guidelines to address emerging scientific, regulatory, and public health needs. The guidelines serve as important tools for pharmaceutical companies, healthcare professionals, regulatory authorities, and other stakeholders involved in the development, evaluation, and regulation of medicinal products within the EU (Figure 4.2).

4.4.2 Committee for Medicinal Products for Human Use (CHMP)

The CHMP is one of the scientific committees operating within the EMA. It is responsible for evaluating and providing scientific recommendations on medicinal products for human use in the EU. The CHMP plays a critical role in assessing the safety, efficacy, and quality of medicines, as well as their risk-benefit profiles, to support regulatory decision-making [23].

4.4.3 Purpose of CHMP

The primary purpose of the CHMP is to conduct scientific assessments of medicinal products for human use and provide expert recommendations to the EMA and the European Commission [24]. The CHMP plays a crucial role in ensuring the safety, efficacy, and quality of medicines within the European Union. Here are the key purposes of the CHMP:

1. *Scientific evaluation*: The CHMP conducts comprehensive scientific evaluations of medicinal products, considering data on their quality, safety, and efficacy. This evaluation involves reviewing preclinical and clinical data submitted by pharmaceutical companies during the marketing authorization application process.
2. *Risk-benefit assessment*: The CHMP assesses the risk-benefit profile of medicinal products by carefully weighing the therapeutic benefits they provide against their potential risks. This assessment helps determine whether the benefits of a medicine outweigh the risks and contribute to the overall benefit-risk balance.
3. *Authorization and post-authorization recommendations*: Based on its scientific evaluation, the CHMP provides recommendations to the EMA on the authorization of medicinal products. It advises on the conditions of use, therapeutic indications, dosages, contraindications, warnings, and precautions associated with the medicines. The CHMP also advises on post-authorization obligations, including the need for additional studies or safety monitoring.

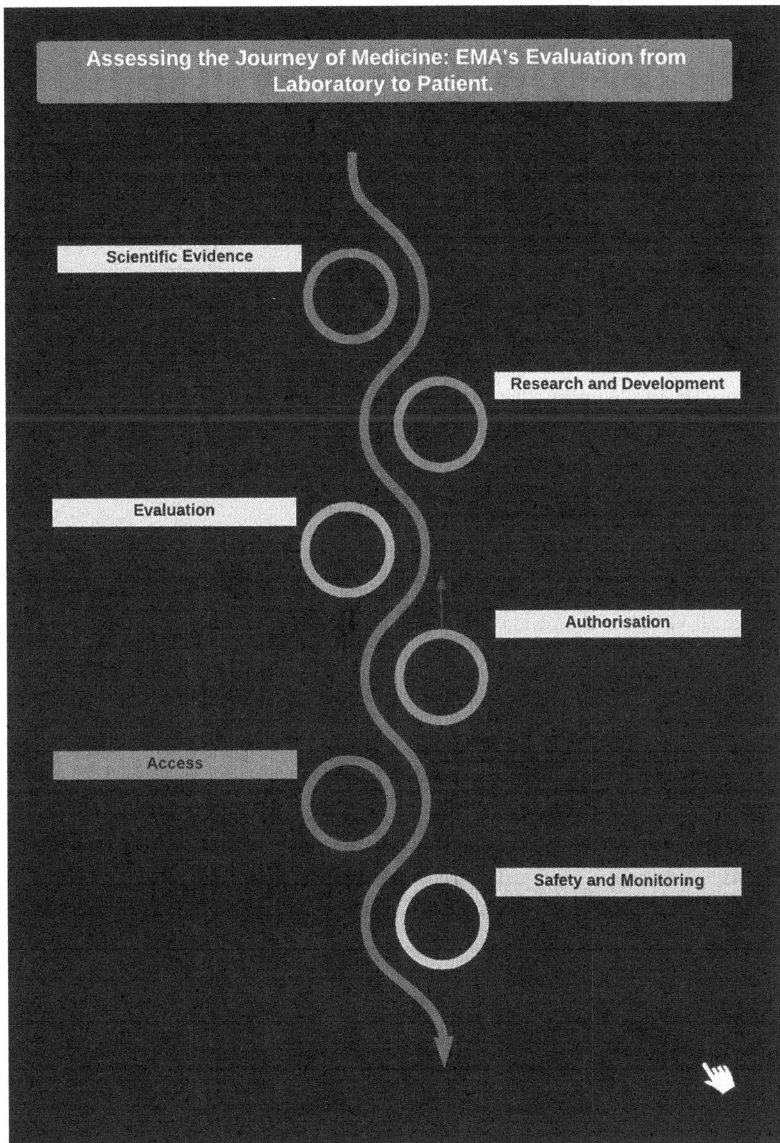

FIGURE 4.2 EMA Evaluation Process Flow.

4. *Harmonization of regulatory standards*: The CHMP plays a key role in promoting the harmonization of regulatory standards and practices across EU member states. It works toward ensuring consistency in the evaluation and regulatory decision-making processes for medicinal products within the EU.

5. *Expert scientific advice*: The CHMP offers expert scientific advice to pharmaceutical companies during the development and evaluation of medicinal products. This advice helps companies align their development plans with regulatory requirements, optimize study designs, and address any scientific or regulatory concerns.
6. *Collaboration and communication*: The CHMP collaborates closely with other EMA committees, national regulatory authorities, and stakeholders to ensure a comprehensive evaluation of medicinal products. It engages in scientific exchanges and dialogue to address any scientific or regulatory challenges and promotes transparency and communication with healthcare professionals, patients, and the public.

By fulfilling these purposes, the CHMP contributes to safeguarding public health by ensuring that only safe, effective, and high quality medicinal products are authorized and available for patients in the European Union.

4.4.4 Composition of CHMP

The CHMP is composed of experts from EU member states who possess specialized knowledge in various scientific disciplines related to medicine [23].

1. *Members*: The CHMP consists of members who are appointed by the European Commission based on their expertise and experience in the evaluation and regulation of medicinal products. The members are nominated by the national competent authorities of EU member states.
2. *Expertise*: The members of the CHMP come from diverse scientific backgrounds, including clinical medicine, pharmacology, toxicology, pharmaceutics, statistics, and other relevant disciplines. This multidisciplinary composition ensures a comprehensive assessment of medicinal products from different perspectives.
3. *Independent experts*: The members of the CHMP act in an independent capacity, serving in their individual expertise rather than representing their respective member states or organizations. They are expected to provide unbiased and objective scientific advice based on their knowledge and experience.
4. *Working groups*: The CHMP may establish working groups consisting of additional experts in specific therapeutic areas or scientific disciplines. These working groups assist the CHMP in conducting in-depth evaluations and providing specialized expertise when needed.
5. *Rotation and term*: The members of the CHMP serve for a designated term, typically 3 years, which can be renewed once. The rotation of members ensures a continuous influx of fresh perspectives and expertise within the committee.
6. *Conflicts of interest*: The members of the CHMP are subject to strict rules and guidelines regarding conflicts of interest. They must declare any potential conflicts and are expected to act in the best interest of

public health and without bias toward any specific stakeholder or interest group.

7. *Support staff*: The CHMP is supported by a secretariat provided by the EMA. The secretariat assists in coordinating the committee's activities, managing administrative tasks, and facilitating communication with stakeholders.

4.4.5 Scientific Evaluation Process

The CHMP follows a rigorous scientific evaluation process to assess the quality, safety, and efficacy of medicinal products within the EU [25].

1. *Marketing authorization application (MAA)*: The evaluation process begins when a pharmaceutical company submits a Marketing Authorization Application for a medicinal product to the EMA. The application includes comprehensive data on the product's quality, safety, and efficacy.
2. *Validation*: The CHMP initially reviews the MAA to ensure it is complete and complies with regulatory requirements. This includes verifying the availability of necessary data and documentation.
3. *Assessment teams*: The CHMP assigns assessment teams consisting of experts with relevant scientific backgrounds to evaluate the medicinal product. The teams analyze the data and conduct a thorough review of the information provided by the pharmaceutical company.
4. *Scientific assessment*: The assessment teams assess various aspects of the medicinal product, including:
   - *Quality*: The evaluation of the product's quality focuses on its manufacturing process, composition, stability, and control of the final product.
   - *Non-clinical evaluation*: This assessment involves reviewing data from preclinical studies, which investigate the product's pharmacology, toxicology, and other relevant non-clinical aspects.
   - *Clinical evaluation*: The clinical evaluation examines data from clinical trials conducted on humans. This includes assessing the trial design, patient population, efficacy outcomes, safety profile, and risk-benefit assessment.
   - *Risk management plan*: The CHMP evaluates the pharmaceutical company's risk management plan, which outlines measures to identify, minimize, and manage potential risks associated with the medicinal product.
5. *Assessment report*: Based on the scientific evaluation, the assessment teams prepare an assessment report summarizing their findings, conclusions, and recommendations. The report includes an evaluation of the product's quality, safety, and efficacy, as well as recommendations for use, dosages, indications, contraindications, and any necessary risk minimization measures.

6. *CHMP meeting*: The assessment report is presented and discussed during a CHMP meeting, where the committee members deliberate on the assessment findings and recommendations. The meeting allows for scientific exchanges, clarifications, and additional discussions if needed.
7. *CHMP opinion*: After the meeting, the CHMP formulates its scientific opinion on the medicinal product. The opinion reflects the committee's assessment of the product's benefit-risk profile and provides recommendations to the European Commission regarding the authorization and conditions of use.
8. *European Commission decision*: The European Commission, considering the CHMP's opinion, makes the final decision on the marketing authorization of the medicinal product within the EU. The Commission may grant authorization, request additional information, or reject the application based on scientific, legal, or ethical considerations.

Throughout the process, the CHMP ensures that the evaluation is based on scientific principles, evidence-based medicine, and a thorough assessment of data provided by the pharmaceutical company. The objective of the CHMP is to safeguard public health by ensuring that authorized medicinal products are of high quality, safe, and effective for patients in the European Union.

4.5 MARKETING AUTHORIZATION PROCESS IN THE EU

The marketing authorization process in the EU is a regulatory procedure that pharmaceutical companies must follow to obtain approval for the marketing and sale of their medicinal products within the EU member states. The EMA plays a central role in coordinating and evaluating applications for marketing authorization in the EU [26–28].

Key steps involved in the marketing authorization process in the EU include the following [29].

1. *Preclinical development*: Pharmaceutical companies conduct extensive laboratory and animal studies to gather data on the safety, quality, and efficacy of medicinal products. These preclinical studies provide the basis for further development.
2. *Clinical trials*: Companies conduct clinical trials on human volunteers to assess the safety and efficacy of the medicinal product. These trials are conducted in multiple phases (Phases I, II, and III) and involve increasing numbers of participants. The data generated from these trials are submitted as part of the marketing authorization application.
3. *MAA*: Once the clinical trials are completed, the pharmaceutical company submits an MAA to the EMA. The application includes comprehensive data on the medicinal product's quality, safety, and efficacy, as well as information on its manufacturing and proposed labelling.
4. *EMA evaluation*: The EMA evaluates the MAA to ensure that the medicinal product meets the necessary quality, safety, and efficacy standards. The

evaluation is carried out by scientific committees, such as the CHMP. The evaluation involves a thorough assessment of the submitted data, including a review of the clinical trial results.

5. *CHMP recommendation*: Based on the evaluation, the CHMP provides a recommendation on whether the medicinal product should be granted marketing authorization. The recommendation considers the balance between the benefits and risks of the product.
6. *European Commission decision*: The European Commission, which has the final decision-making authority, reviews the CHMP recommendation and grants or refuses marketing authorization. The decision is based on the scientific assessment carried out by the EMA and takes into consideration public health and European Union legislation.
7. *Post-authorization*: Once marketing authorization is granted, the pharmaceutical company can market and distribute the medicinal product within the EU member states. However, ongoing pharmacovigilance activities are required to monitor the safety and effectiveness of the product in real-world use.

It is worth noting that there are specific variations and procedures for certain types of medicinal products, such as generic drugs and biosimilars. Additionally, some EU member states may have additional national requirements or procedures for marketing authorization, although the overall process is harmonized across the EU.

4.5.1 Centralized Procedure

The centralized procedure is one of the regulatory pathways available for obtaining marketing authorization for medicinal products in the EU. It is a harmonized and centralized process that allows pharmaceutical companies to apply for marketing authorization that will be valid in all EU member states [30].

4.5.2 Overview of the Centralized Procedure

The centralized procedure is mandatory for certain types of medicinal products, including biotechnology-derived products, orphan drugs, ATMPs, and certain products for the treatment of HIV, cancer, diabetes, neurodegenerative disorders, and autoimmune diseases. It is also available voluntarily for other medicinal products [30]. It is coordinated by the EMA. The EMA conducts a comprehensive scientific evaluation of the medicinal product, involving input from various scientific committees and experts. The pharmaceutical company submits a single MAA to the EMA. The application includes data on the quality, safety, and efficacy of the medicinal product, as well as information on manufacturing, labelling, and packaging. The EMA evaluates the MAA through a robust and standardized process. It involves a thorough assessment of the submitted data, including preclinical and clinical trial results, as well as an evaluation of the benefit-risk balance of the product. The CHMP is the scientific committee responsible for evaluating the medicinal product within the centralized procedure. It reviews the data and provides a scientific opinion on whether the product should be granted marketing authorization. Based on the CHMP's scientific opinion, the European Commission decides on the granting of marketing authorization. The decision applies to all EU member states [31,32].

4.5.3 Benefits of the Centralized Procedure

1. *Single application*: Pharmaceutical companies only need to submit one application for marketing authorization in the EU, avoiding the need for multiple submissions to individual member states.
2. *Harmonized evaluation*: The evaluation of the medicinal product is conducted by the EMA and involves input from various experts and scientific committees. This ensures a consistent and harmonized assessment across all EU member states.
3. *Access to EU market*: Once marketing authorization is granted through the centralized procedure, the pharmaceutical company can market and distribute the medicinal product in all EU member states simultaneously, providing access to a large and unified market.
4. *Streamlined process*: The centralized procedure aims to streamline the regulatory process by reducing duplication of efforts and facilitating a more efficient evaluation and decision-making process.
5. *Scientific expertise*: The involvement of the EMA and the CHMP ensures that the evaluation of the medicinal product is based on the latest scientific knowledge and expertise, leading to robust decisions on the product's quality, safety, and efficacy.
6. *Patient access*: The centralized procedure helps ensure that patients across the EU have timely access to safe and effective medicinal products, particularly those used in the treatment of serious and rare diseases.

4.5.4 Decentralized Procedure (DCP) and Mutual Recognition Procedure (MRP)

The decentralized procedure and mutual recognition procedure are two regulatory pathways for obtaining marketing authorization for medicinal products in the EU. They are alternative processes to the centralized procedure and are used for products that do not fall within the scope of the mandatory centralized procedure or for companies seeking authorization in specific EU member states [32].

4.5.4.1 Decentralized Procedure (DCP)

The DCP is used when a medicinal product is intended to be authorized in multiple EU member states but not through the centralized procedure. It is typically used for products that do not fall under the mandatory centralized procedure, such as generic drugs. The pharmaceutical company selects one EU member state as the reference member state (RMS), which will lead the evaluation process [33]. The RMS is responsible for preparing the assessment report and coordinating the involvement of other member states, known as concerned member states (CMS). The RMS evaluates the medicinal product's quality, safety, and efficacy based on the data provided in the marketing authorization application [27,28]. It prepares an assessment report that includes its evaluation and proposed summary of product characteristics (SmPC), package leaflet, and labelling. The assessment report, along with the application, is then submitted to the CMS for their evaluation [34]. The CMS review the assessment report and decide whether to grant national marketing authorization based on the RMS evaluation. If disagreements arise, a decision is made through the Coordination Group for Mutual Recognition and Decentralised Procedures—Human (CMDh) to resolve them. Each CMS decides independently on whether to grant national marketing authorization based on the evaluation conducted by the RMS and the assessment report. The marketing authorization granted in each CMS is valid only in that specific member state.

4.5.4.2 Mutual Recognition Procedure (MRP)

The MRP is used when a medicinal product is already authorized in one EU member state, the RMS, and the pharmaceutical company seeks authorization in other EU member states. The pharmaceutical company first obtains marketing authorization in the RMS through the centralized procedure or another valid procedure. The pharmaceutical company then applies to the CMS, seeking recognition of the marketing authorization granted by the RMS. The RMS provides the CMS with the assessment report, including the evaluation of the medicinal product's quality, safety, and efficacy, as well as the approved SmPC, package leaflet, and labelling. The CMS evaluates the assessment report provided by the RMS and decides whether to grant national marketing authorization based on the RMS evaluation. If disagreements arise, they are resolved through the CMDh [27]. Each CMS decides independently on whether to grant national marketing authorization based on the evaluation conducted by the RMS. The marketing authorization granted in each CMS is valid only in that specific member state [35].

Both the DCP and MRP aim to facilitate the authorization process for medicinal products across multiple EU member states by leveraging the work already conducted in one member state. These procedures help streamline the regulatory process, reduce duplication of efforts, and promote timely access to safe and effective medicinal products within the EU.

4.5.5 Difference between Centralized and Decentralized Procedures

Centralized Procedures	Decentralized Procedures
Mandatory for specific types of products (e.g., biotechnology-derived products, orphan drugs).	Used for products not covered by mandatory centralized procedure or for specific member states.
Involves a single marketing authorization application (MAA) submitted to the European Medicines Agency (EMA).	Involves selecting a reference member state (RMS) and concerned member states (CMS).

(Continued)

(Continued)

Centralized Procedures	Decentralized Procedures
Evaluation and decision-making are conducted at the EU level.	RMS leads the evaluation and prepares the assessment report.
Scientific evaluation is performed by the EMA's scientific committees, such as the Committee for Medicinal Products for Human Use (CHMP).	CMS review the assessment report and decide on national marketing authorizations.
Marketing authorization is valid in all EU member states simultaneously.	Marketing authorization is granted independently by each member state.
Provides access to the entire EU market.	Facilitates authorization in multiple member states.
The centralized procedure is coordinated by the EMA.	The decentralized procedure requires coordination between RMS and CMS.
The centralized procedure involves a single evaluation at the EU level.	The decentralized procedure involves separate evaluations in each member state.
The centralized procedure provides a single marketing authorization valid in all member states.	The decentralized procedure results in separate national authorizations.

4.6 EUROPEAN DIRECTORATE FOR THE QUALITY OF MEDICINES AND HEALTHCARE (EDQM)

The EDQM is an organization operating under the Council of Europe, dedicated to ensuring the quality, safety, and efficacy of medicines and healthcare products in Europe. The EDQM is responsible for establishing and promoting quality standards, conducting scientific research and analysis, and providing technical expertise and support to member states. It operates through various activities such as the development and maintenance of the European Pharmacopoeia, certification of substances, pharmacovigilance, and international cooperation. The EDQM plays a crucial role in harmonizing regulatory practices, promoting public health, and facilitating the availability of safe and effective medicines across Europe [36].

4.6.1 Role of the EDQM in Setting Quality Standards for Medicines and Healthcare Products

The role of the EDQM in setting quality standards for medicines and healthcare products is essential for ensuring the safety, efficacy, and quality of these products throughout Europe [37].

Key aspects of the EDQM's role in setting quality standards include the following.

1. *European Pharmacopoeia (Ph. Eur.)*: The EDQM is responsible for the development, maintenance, and publication of the European Pharmacopoeia, which is a comprehensive collection of quality standards for medicinal substances and products used in Europe. It includes monographs, general chapters,

and guidelines that define the requirements for quality control and testing of medicines.

2. *Harmonization of standards*: The EDQM plays a crucial role in harmonizing quality standards across Europe. By establishing common requirements and guidelines through the Ph. Eur., the EDQM ensures consistency in the quality control of medicines and healthcare products across different member states. This harmonization facilitates the free movement of these products within Europe's single market.
3. *Expert committees and working groups*: The EDQM convenes expert committees and working groups composed of renowned scientists, regulators, and industry experts. These groups work collaboratively to develop and revise quality standards, ensuring they reflect the latest scientific knowledge and technological advancements. The EDQM engages these experts to evaluate and propose updates to existing monographs and develop new ones as needed.
4. *Scientific research and evaluation*: The EDQM conducts scientific research and evaluation to support the development of quality standards. It actively monitors scientific advancements, emerging technologies, and regulatory developments related to the quality of medicines and healthcare products. This research helps ensure that the Ph. Eur. standards are evidence-based and reflect the latest understanding of quality requirements.
5. *Collaboration with stakeholders*: The EDQM collaborates with various stakeholders, including regulatory authorities, industry representatives, and academic institutions. It engages in consultations, information exchanges, and collaborations to gather diverse perspectives and expertise. This collaboration ensures that the quality standards developed by the EDQM are comprehensive, relevant, and widely accepted across the European healthcare community.
6. *Training and education*: The EDQM provides training programs, workshops, and educational resources to support the understanding and implementation of quality standards. These initiatives help stakeholders, including laboratory personnel, regulatory professionals, and healthcare practitioners, stay updated on the latest standards, testing methodologies, and quality control practices.

4.6.2 Certification, Inspection, and Quality Control Activities by the EDQM for Medicines and Healthcare Products

The EDQM conducts various certification, inspection, and quality control activities to ensure the quality, safety, and efficacy of medicines and healthcare products [37].

Key activities performed by the EDQM in these areas include the following.

1. *Certification of substances*: The EDQM issues Certificates of Suitability (CEPs) for specific substances used in the manufacturing of medicines. A CEP confirms that the substance meets the relevant quality standards outlined in the European Pharmacopoeia. This certification simplifies the

marketing authorization process for manufacturers by providing evidence of compliance with quality requirements.

2. *Inspections*: The EDQM conducts inspections of manufacturers, suppliers, and laboratories involved in the production, distribution, and testing of medicines and healthcare products. These inspections aim to verify compliance with good manufacturing practices, good distribution practices, and good laboratory practices. Inspections help ensure that facilities and processes meet the required quality standards and regulatory requirements.
3. *Pharmacopoeial laboratory activities*: The EDQM operates specialized laboratories that perform quality control testing and analysis of medicines, including biological and biotechnological products. These laboratories contribute to the development and maintenance of the European Pharmacopoeia standards by conducting research, method validation, and analysis of pharmaceutical substances.
4. *Reference standards*: The EDQM provides reference standards for quality control testing. These standards are used by manufacturers, regulatory authorities, and testing laboratories to verify the quality and identity of medicines and healthcare products. Reference standards help ensure consistency and accuracy in the analysis and evaluation of pharmaceutical substances.
5. *Proficiency testing*: The EDQM organizes proficiency testing programs, also known as interlaboratory comparisons, to assess the performance of laboratories involved in quality control testing. These programs enable participating laboratories to evaluate their analytical methods, identify areas for improvement, and ensure the accuracy and reliability of their testing results.
6. *Collaborative quality control activities*: The EDQM collaborates with national and international authorities, organizations, and networks to promote and improve quality control practices. It engages in information sharing, joint research projects, and collaborative initiatives to enhance the understanding and implementation of quality control standards across Europe.

4.6.3 Pharmacovigilance and Post-Marketing Surveillance

Pharmacovigilance systems in the EU are comprehensive frameworks established to monitor and ensure the safety of medicines. These systems involve various stakeholders, including regulatory authorities, marketing authorization holders (MAHs), healthcare professionals, and patients [38,39].

4.6.4 Overview of Pharmacovigilance Systems in the EU

1. *Legal framework*: The EU .pharmacovigilance system operates under a robust legal framework, primarily governed by Regulation (EC) No 726/2004 and Directive 2001/83/EC. These regulations outline the

responsibilities of MAHs, national competent authorities, and the EMA in pharmacovigilance activities.

2. *Pharmacovigilance system master file (PSMF)*: MAHs are required to maintain a PSMF, which provides an overview of their pharmacovigilance system. The PSMF contains detailed information on the organization, personnel, processes, and procedures for monitoring the safety of their medicines.
3. *Reporting of adverse drug reactions (ADRs)*: Healthcare professionals, patients, and other stakeholders are encouraged to report suspected ADRs to national competent authorities or directly to MAHs. These reports are crucial in detecting and evaluating potential safety concerns associated with medicines.
4. *EudraVigilance database*: The EMA operates the EudraVigilance database, which serves as a centralized system for collecting and managing information on suspected ADRs. MAHs submit individual case safety reports to EudraVigilance, and these reports are analyzed to identify potential safety signals.
5. *Signal detection and evaluation*: Regulatory authorities continuously monitor safety data from various sources, including spontaneous reports, clinical trials, literature, and other pharmacovigilance databases, to detect signals or potential safety concerns. Signals trigger further evaluation, including data analysis, signal validation, and assessment of the causal relationship.
6. *Benefit-risk assessment*: Pharmacovigilance systems facilitate the ongoing assessment of the benefit-risk balance of medicines. Regulatory authorities, supported by scientific committees, evaluate safety data and consider the effectiveness and therapeutic benefits of medicines to ensure that their benefits outweigh the potential risks.
7. *Risk management plans (RMPs)*: MAHs are required to develop RMPs for medicines with specific safety concerns. RMPs outline strategies to minimize risks and ensure the safe use of medicines. These plans include risk minimization measures, additional monitoring requirements, and the provision of educational materials to healthcare professionals and patients.
8. *Communication of safety information*: Regulatory authorities and the EMA communicate safety information and updates to healthcare professionals, patients, and the public. This includes issuing safety alerts, updating product labelling with new safety information, and providing educational materials to promote the safe and informed use of medicines.

4.6.5 EU Clinical Trials Regulation (EU-CTR) and Its Impact on Drug Development

The EU-CTR is a regulatory framework that governs the conduct and oversight of clinical trials in the EU. It aims to streamline and harmonize the authorization and supervision of clinical trials, enhance patient safety, and facilitate efficient drug development [40,41].

4.6.6 The EU-CTR Has Several Impacts on Drug Development

1. *Simplified and harmonized procedures*: The EU-CTR introduces a harmonized and streamlined process for the authorization of clinical trials across EU member states. It establishes a single submission portal and a coordinated review process, reducing administrative burden and time delays associated with conducting trials in multiple countries. This simplification fosters efficient drug development and enables quicker access to innovative therapies for patients.
2. *Improved safety monitoring*: The EU-CTR places a strong emphasis on patient safety and pharmacovigilance during clinical trials. It mandates the implementation of robust safety monitoring systems and risk management plans to ensure the timely detection, reporting, and evaluation of adverse events. This focus on safety enhances patient protection and helps generate comprehensive safety data for investigational drugs.
3. *Increased transparency*: The EU-CTR promotes transparency in clinical trial processes and results. It requires the registration and publication of all clinical trial information in the EU Clinical Trials Database (EudraCT). This transparency improves access to trial information for researchers, healthcare professionals, and patients, fostering collaboration, scientific advancement, and informed decision-making.
4. *Simplified and harmonized data requirements*: The EU-CTR introduces simplified and harmonized data requirements for clinical trial submissions. It aligns with international standards, such as the International Council for Harmonisation of Technical Requirements for Pharmaceuticals for Human Use (ICH), promoting data consistency and facilitating the acceptance of trial data in regulatory submissions worldwide. This simplification reduces duplication and supports global drug development efforts.
5. *Strengthened sponsor responsibilities*: The EU-CTR places increased responsibilities on trial sponsors regarding the oversight and conduct of clinical trials. Sponsors are required to ensure appropriate quality and safety standards, adhere to good clinical practice (GCP) guidelines, and maintain accurate and complete trial documentation. This emphasis on sponsor accountability enhances the integrity and reliability of clinical trial data.
6. *Streamlined multinational trials*: The EU-CTR facilitates the conduct of multinational clinical trials within the EU. It enables the coordination and simultaneous submission of trial applications across multiple member states, simplifying the approval process for trials conducted in several countries. This streamlining encourages international collaboration and enables efficient enrolment of patients, leading to faster completion of trials and drug development timelines.

Overall, the EU-CTR has a significant impact on drug development by harmonizing procedures, improving patient safety monitoring, promoting transparency, simplifying data requirements, strengthening sponsor responsibilities, and facilitating multinational trials. These changes contribute to a more efficient and transparent clinical trial environment, ultimately supporting the development of safe and effective medicines for patients in the EU and beyond.

4.6.7 Key Requirements for Conducting Clinical Trials in the EU

Conducting clinical trials in the EU involves meeting several key requirements to ensure patient safety, data integrity, and regulatory compliance. It must obtain ethical approval from an independent ethics committee (IEC) or institutional review board (IRB) before initiation. The IEC/IRB ensures that the trial protocol is scientifically valid, respects the rights of the participants, and adheres to ethical principles [42].

Sponsors or their authorized representatives must submit a clinical trial application to the competent authority of each EU member state where the trial will take place. The application includes comprehensive information about the trial, such as the protocol, investigator credentials, investigational product details, and safety measures. If the trial involves the use of investigational medicinal products, the sponsor must obtain an investigational medicinal product authorization from the competent authority or obtain a waiver if the product is already authorized or exempted. It must adhere to GCP principles, which provide a framework for the design, conduct, monitoring, recording, and reporting of clinical trials. GCP ensures that trials are conducted ethically, with the safety and well-being of participants as the top priority. Informed consent is a fundamental requirement in clinical trials. Participants must provide voluntary, informed, and written consent to participate in the trial after receiving detailed information about the study, its objectives, potential risks, and benefits. The consent process must comply with applicable EU and national laws. Sponsors have a responsibility to monitor and report adverse events occurring during the trial and take appropriate safety measures. They must have a pharmacovigilance system in place to collect, evaluate, and report safety data, ensuring the ongoing assessment of the investigational product's safety profile [43]. Clinical trial data and participant information must be protected and handled in compliance with EU data protection regulations, such as the General Data Protection Regulation. Participants' privacy and confidentiality must be maintained throughout the trial, and data should be anonymized or pseudonymized when appropriate. Clinical trial registration and results reporting are mandatory in the EU. Trials must be registered in the EudraCT, and sponsors are required to publish trial results within specific timelines on publicly accessible databases, promoting transparency and the dissemination of trial information. Competent authorities have the authority to conduct inspections and audits to ensure compliance with regulatory requirements. Sponsors may also perform monitoring visits to trial sites to ensure protocol adherence, data accuracy, and participant safety. After the completion of a clinical trial, participants should have access to any investigational product that has shown positive results and is not yet commercially available, provided it is in their best interest and approved by the relevant regulatory authorities [44].

4.6.8 Pharmaceutical Pricing Policies in the EU

Pharmaceutical pricing policies in the EU can vary among member states, as each country has its own healthcare system and regulatory framework. However, there are some common elements and policy approaches followed in the EU [45].

Many EU countries use reference pricing, where the price of a medication is compared with similar products in the market. A maximum reimbursement amount is set based on the prices of comparable medicines. Patients may have to pay the difference if the price of their prescribed medication exceeds the reference price. Health technology assessment (HTA) is conducted to evaluate the clinical effectiveness, safety, and cost-effectiveness of pharmaceuticals. It helps inform pricing and reimbursement decisions, considering the value and benefits provided by a medication compared with alternative treatments [46]. Some EU countries negotiate directly with pharmaceutical companies to establish pricing agreements. This can involve confidential price negotiations based on factors like the therapeutic value, budget impact, and health benefits of the medicine. External price referencing, where prices are determined by comparing prices in other countries, is also used in some cases. Managed entry agreements (MEAs) are arrangements between payers and pharmaceutical companies to provide access to innovative medicines while managing their cost impact. These agreements can include discounts, rebates, or performance-based agreements, allowing conditional reimbursement or risk-sharing between the payer and manufacturer. Some EU countries implement price controls to regulate the prices of pharmaceuticals. These controls can take the form of price ceilings, profit margins, or price freezes, aiming to ensure affordable access to medicines and control healthcare costs. Transparency measures are implemented to promote openness and accountability in pharmaceutical pricing. This includes the disclosure of prices, discounts, and rebates offered by pharmaceutical companies to payers, as well as the disclosure of clinical trial data and information on research and development costs. Intellectual property rights, including patents, provide pharmaceutical companies with a period of market exclusivity to recoup their investment in research and development. However, there are discussions and policy debates surrounding the balance between intellectual property rights and affordable access to medicines.

4.6.9 Health Technology Assessment (HTA) and Its Role in Pricing and Reimbursement Decisions

HTA is a systematic and multidisciplinary process that evaluates the clinical effectiveness, safety, cost-effectiveness, and broader societal impact of healthcare interventions, including pharmaceuticals, medical devices, and procedures.

HTA plays a crucial role in informing pricing and reimbursement decisions by providing evidence-based information to payers and policymakers [47]. HTA involves the systematic review and synthesis of available evidence on the clinical effectiveness and safety of healthcare interventions. This includes evaluating clinical trial data, real-world evidence, and comparative effectiveness studies to assess the potential benefits and risks associated with a specific intervention. It assesses the cost-effectiveness of healthcare interventions by comparing the costs incurred with the health outcomes achieved. Economic evaluations, such as cost-utility analysis or cost-effectiveness analysis, are conducted to estimate the incremental cost per unit of health benefit gained. This information helps inform pricing and reimbursement decisions by considering the value for money provided by an intervention. It examines the impact of healthcare interventions on patient-relevant health outcomes and quality of life. It considers factors such as disease burden, patient preferences, and the potential for improved health outcomes. This information helps determine the value and impact of an intervention on patient health and well-being. HTA compares the effectiveness of different interventions within a given therapeutic area. It helps identify the relative clinical benefits, risks, and outcomes associated with different treatment options. This information supports decision-making regarding the pricing and reimbursement of specific interventions based on their comparative efficacy [48,49]. It evaluates the potential financial impact of adopting a specific healthcare intervention on healthcare budgets. It considers the costs associated with widespread adoption, patient population size, and potential cost offsets resulting from improved health outcomes. This analysis helps policymakers and payers understand the financial implications of reimbursement decisions. It contributes to the concept of value-based pricing, where the price of a healthcare intervention is determined based on its demonstrated value and benefits. By considering the clinical effectiveness, safety, cost-effectiveness, and broader impact on patients and society, HTA helps establish a fair price for an intervention relative to the benefits it provides. HTA provides evidence-based recommendations and guidance to payers and policymakers regarding the reimbursement and pricing of healthcare interventions [47]. The findings and recommendations from HTA reports inform decision-making, enabling payers to make informed choices on which interventions to include in reimbursement schemes and at what price. It often involves stakeholder engagement, including input from patients, healthcare professionals, industry representatives, and other relevant stakeholders. This ensures that diverse perspectives and values are considered in pricing and reimbursement decisions, enhancing transparency and accountability [49,50].

4.6.10 Patent Protection for Pharmaceuticals in the EU

Patent protection for pharmaceuticals in the EU is governed by various laws and regulations, including the European Patent Convention (EPC) and the EU Supplementary Protection Certificate (SPC) Regulation [51].

4.6.11 Overview of Patent Protection for Pharmaceuticals in the EU

The EPC is an international treaty that establishes a unified patent system for European countries, including most EU member states. Under the EPC, inventors can apply for a European patent, which offers protection in multiple countries simultaneously. In the EU, pharmaceutical inventions can be eligible for patent protection if they meet the criteria of novelty, inventive step, and industrial applicability. This means that the invention must be new, involve an inventive step that is not obvious to a person skilled in the field, and have practical applicability. The standard term of a European patent is 20 years from the filing date of the patent application. However, the effective term of protection for pharmaceuticals can be extended through SPCs. SPCs are a form of intellectual property protection specifically designed for pharmaceutical and plant protection products in the EU [52]. They extend the patent protection beyond the initial 20-year term to compensate for the time required to obtain regulatory approvals for these products. The EU SPC Regulation provides the legal framework for granting and enforcing SPCs in the EU [53]. To be eligible for an SPC, the product must be protected by a basic patent in force, have obtained marketing authorization as a medicinal product, and have not previously been granted an SPC for the same active ingredient. The duration of an SPC is calculated as the period between the date of filing of the patent application and the date of the first marketing authorization in the EU, minus 5 years. The maximum duration of an SPC is 5 years. Patents can be challenged through opposition or invalidity proceedings before the European Patent Office (EPO) or national patent office [54]. Generic or biosimilar manufacturers can also challenge the validity or non-infringement of patents to seek market entry. In exceptional circumstances, EU member states have the right to issue compulsory licenses to allow third parties to use patented inventions without the consent of the patent holder. Compulsory licenses are granted in cases of public health emergencies or when the patent holder has abused their patent rights. Patent protection plays a vital role in incentivizing pharmaceutical innovation by providing exclusive rights to the inventors. It allows pharmaceutical companies to recoup their investment in research and development and fosters a competitive environment for developing new and improved medicines [55].

4.6.12 Supplementary Protection Certificates (SPCs) and Data Exclusivity

SPCs and data exclusivity are two distinct forms of intellectual property protection related to pharmaceutical products [53].

1. *SPCs*: SPCs provide an extension of patent protection for pharmaceutical and plant protection products in the EU. They compensate for the time it takes to obtain regulatory approvals, such as marketing authorization, which can significantly reduce the effective patent protection period. SPCs are granted based on the existence of a valid basic patent and the authorization of the corresponding product as a medicinal or plant protection

product. The duration of an SPC is typically calculated as the time between the filing date of the patent and the date of the first marketing authorization, minus 5 years. The maximum duration is 5 years [56,57].

2. *Data exclusivity*: Data exclusivity refers to a period of protection given to the data submitted by pharmaceutical companies to regulatory authorities to obtain marketing authorization for their products. During the data exclusivity period, other companies cannot rely on the originator's data to obtain their marketing authorization [58]. Data exclusivity is separate from patent protection and provides exclusive rights to the data submitter, preventing generic or biosimilar manufacturers from relying on the originator's data for a specific period. The duration of data exclusivity varies depending on the specific regulations of each country or region but is typically several years [59].

Both SPCs and data exclusivity aim to balance the interests of innovators and generic/biosimilar manufacturers. SPCs extend patent protection, allowing innovators to recover the investment made in research and development, while data exclusivity provides a period of exclusivity for the originator's data, encouraging the generation of new clinical data for regulatory approvals. Together, they contribute to incentivizing innovation and protecting the rights of pharmaceutical companies in the EU.

4.7 CONCLUSION

In conclusion, this chapter on drug regulation in the European Union has provided a comprehensive overview of the regulatory framework governing pharmaceuticals in this region. The European Union has established a robust system aimed at ensuring the safety, efficacy, and quality of medicinal products available to its citizens. Through the EMA and various directives and regulations, the EU has harmonized the drug approval processes, pharmacovigilance, and post-market surveillance across member states. This chapter has highlighted the significance of regulatory cooperation, scientific evaluation, and transparency in maintaining public health and fostering innovation in the pharmaceutical industry. Overall, the EU's drug regulation system serves as a model for other regions aspiring to establish effective frameworks for drug oversight and patient safety.

REFERENCES

[1] European Regulatory System for Medicines. (2023) (cited 30 Nov. 23). Available from www.ema.europa.eu/en/documents/leaflet/european-regulatory-system-medicines_en.pdf.

[2] World Health Organization. (2021). *WHO Expert Committee on Specifications for Pharmaceutical Preparations: Fifty-Fifth Report*. World Health Organization.

[3] World Health Organization. (2003). *Effective Medicines Regulation: Ensuring Safety, Efficacy and Quality (No. WHO/EDM/2003.2)*. World Health Organization.

[4] Lezotre, P. L. (2013). *International Cooperation, Convergence and Harmonization of Pharmaceutical Regulations: A Global Perspective*. Academic Press.

[5] Olson, M. K. (2014). Regulation of safety, efficacy, and quality. In *Encyclopedia of Health Economics* (pp. 240–248). Elsevier. https://doi.org/10.1016/B978-0-12-375678-7.01202-5.

[6] Potts, J., Genov, G., Segec, A., Raine, J., Straus, S., & Arlett, P. (2020). Improving the safety of medicines in the European Union: From signals to action. *Clinical Pharmacology & Therapeutics*, *107*(3), 521–529.

[7] Wilson, J. B. (2011). European union regulations. In *Global Clinical Trials* (pp. 47–62). Academic Press.

[8] European Commission. (2008). *Strengthening Pharmacovigilance to Reduce Adverse Effects of Medicines*. Available from https://ec.europa.eu/commission/presscorner/detail/en/MEMO_08_782.

[9] Santoro, A., Genov, G., Spooner, A., Raine, J., & Arlett, P. (2017). Promoting and protecting public health: How the European Union pharmacovigilance system works. *Drug Safety*, *40*(10), 855–869. https://doi.org/10.1007/s40264-017-0572-8

[10] Vogel, D. (1998). The globalization of pharmaceutical regulation. *Governance*, *11*(1), 1–22.

[11] Lezotre, P. L. (2014). Value and influencing factors of the cooperation, convergence, and harmonization in the pharmaceutical sector. In *International Cooperation, Convergence and Harmonization of Pharmaceutical Regulations* (p. 171). Academic Press.

[12] Rägo, L., & Santoso, B. (2008). Drug regulation: History, present and future. *Drug Benefits and Risks: International Textbook of Clinical Pharmacology*, *2*, 65–77.

[13] European Commission. (2014). *50 Years of EU Pharmaceutical Regulation Milestones* (cited 30 Nov. 23). Available from http://ec.europa.eu/health/50_years_of_eu_milestones/timeline.htm

[14] European Commission. *Legal Framework Governing Medicinal Products for Human Use in the EU* (cited 30 Nov. 23). Available from: https://health.ec.europa.eu/medicinal-products/legal-framework-governing-medicinal-products-human-use-eu_en

[15] Lee, K. S., Ming, L. C., Lean, Q. Y., Yee, S. M., Patel, R., Taha, N. A., & Kassab, Y. W. (2019). Cross-border collaboration to improve access to medicine: Association of Southeast Asian Nations perspective. *Journal of Epidemiology and Global Health*, *9*(2), 93.

[16] Zerhouni, E., & Hamburg, M. (2016). The need for global regulatory harmonization: A public health imperative. *Science Translational Medicine*, *8*(338), 338ed6–338ed6.

[17] Xu, M., Zhang, L., Feng, X., Zhang, Z., & Huang, Y. (2022). Regulatory reliance for convergence and harmonisation in the medical device space in Asia-Pacific. *BMJ Global Health*, *7*(8), e009798.

[18] WHO. *Global and Regional Regulatory Harmonization Initiatives* (cited 30 Nov. 23). Available from www.who.int/teams/regulation-prequalification/regulation-and-safety/regulatory-convergence-networks/harmonization?page=33

[19] European Medicines Agency. (2016). *European Medicines Agency. About Us* (cited 30 Nov. 23). Available from www.ema.europa.eu/docs/en_GB/document_library/Other/2016/08/WC500211862.pdf

[20] European Medicines Agency. (2014). *Mandate and Objectives for the EMA Working Party on Quality Review of Documents (QRD)* (cited 30 Nov. 23). Available from www.ema.europa.eu/en/documents/other/mandate-objectives-european-medicines-agency-working-party-quality-review-documents-qrd_en.pdf

[21] European Medicines Agency. (2023). *European Medicines Agency. About Us* (cited 30 Nov. 23). Available from www.ema.europa.eu/en/documents/other/about-us-european-medicines-agency-ema_en.pdf

[22] European Medicines Agency. (2009). *Procedure for European Union Guidelines and Related Documents Within the Pharmaceutical Legislative Framework* (cited 30 Nov. 23). Available from www.ema.europa.eu/en/documents/scientific-guideline/procedure-european-union-guidelines-related-documents-within-pharmaceutical-legislative-framework_en.pdf

[23] European Medicines Agency. (2022). *Committee for Medicinal Products for Human Use* (cited 30 Nov. 23). Available from www.ema.europa.eu/en/documents/other/chmp-rules-procedure_en.pdf

[24] Enzmann, H., & Schneider, C. (2008). Die rolle des ausschusses für humanarzneimittel (CHMP) bei der europäischen zentralen zulassung [The role of the Committee for Medicinal products for human use (CHMP) in the European centralised procedure]. *Bundesgesundheitsblatt, Gesundheitsforschung, Gesundheitsschutz, 51*(7), 731–739. https://doi.org/10.1007/s00103-008-0579-5

[25] European Medicines Agency. *The Evaluation of Medicines, Step-by-Step* (cited 30 Nov. 23). Available from www.ema.europa.eu/en/human-regulatory/marketing-authorisation/evaluation-medicines-step-step

[26] European Medicines Agency. (2019). *Notice to Applicants Volume 2A Procedures for Marketing Authorisation, Chapter 1 Marketing Authorisation, Revision 11* (cited 1 Dec. 23). Available from https://health.ec.europa.eu/system/files/2019-07/vol2a_chap1_en_0.pdf

[27] European Medicines Agency. (2007). *Notice to Applicants Volume 2A Procedures for Marketing Authorisation, Chapter 2 Mutual Recognization, Revision 5* (cited 1 Dec. 23). Available from https://health.ec.europa.eu/system/files/2016-11/vol2a_chap2_2007-02_en_0.pdf

[28] European Medicines Agency. *Human Regulatory-Pre Authorisation Guidance* (cited 1 Dec. 23). Available from www.ema.europa.eu/en/human-regulatory/marketing-authorisation/pre-authorisation-guidance#1.-types-of-applications-and-applicants-section

[29] European Medicines Agency. *Human Regulatory- Obtaining an EU Marketing Authorisation, Step-by-Step* (cited 1 Dec. 23). Available from www.ema.europa.eu/en/human-regulatory/marketing-authorisation/obtaining-eu-marketing-authorisation-step-step

[30] Kashyap, U. N., Gupta, V., & Raghunandan, H. V. (2013). Comparison of drug approval process in United States & Europe. *Journal of Pharmaceutical Sciences and Research, 5*(6), 131.

[31] Healy, E. M., & Kaitin, K. I. (1999). The European agency for the evaluation of medicinal products' centralized procedure for product approval: Current status. *Drug Information Journal, 33*(4), 969–978.

[32] Walsh, G. (1999). Drug approval in Europe. *Nature Biotechnology, 17*(3), 237–240.

[33] Insuvia.com. *RMS* (cited 1 Dec. 23). Available from https://insuvia.com/glossary/rms/

[34] European Medicines Agency. *Introduction to the SmPC Guideline* (cited 1 Dec. 23). Available from www.ema.europa.eu/en/documents/presentation/presentation-introduction-summary-product-characteristics-guideline_en.pdf

[35] hma.eu. *Human Medicine, Co-Ordination Group for Mutual Recognition and Decentralised Procedures—Human (CMDh)* (cited 1 Dec. 23). Available from www.ema.europa.eu/en/committees/working-parties-domains/coordination-group-mutual-recognition-decentralised-procedures-human-cmdh

[36] European Medicines Agency. *European Directorate for the Quality of Medicines and HealthCare (EDQM) of the Council of Europe* (cited 1 Dec. 23). Available from www.ema.

europa.eu/en/partners-networks/international-activities/multilateral-coalitions-initiatives/european-directorate-quality-medicines-healthcare-edqm-council-europe

[37] edqm.eu. *Council of Europe. Structure* (cited 1 Dec. 23). Available from www.edqm.eu/en/edqm/about/structure#{%22333408%22:[0]}

[38] European Medicines Agency. *Human Regulatory- Pharmacovigilance: Post-Authorisation* (cited 1 Dec. 23). Available from www.ema.europa.eu/en/human-regulatory/post-authorisation/pharmacovigilance-post-authorisation

[39] Gough, S. (2005). Post-marketing surveillance: A UK/European perspective. *Current Medical Research and Opinion*, *21*(4), 565–570.

[40] European Medicines Agency. *Human Regulatory. Clinical Trials Regulation* (cited 1 Dec. 23). Available from www.ema.europa.eu/en/human-regulatory/research-development/clinical-trials/clinical-trials-regulation

[41] Scavone, C., di Mauro, G., Pietropaolo, M., Alfano, R., Berrino, L., Rossi, F., . . . & Capuano, A. (2019). The European clinical trials regulation (No 536/2014): Changes and challenges. *Expert Review of Clinical Pharmacology*, *12*(11), 1027–1032.

[42] Brebou, S. (2023). *Clinical Trials in EU: Definition, Types, Regulatory Framework and Challenges*. International Hellenic University Scholar Works.

[43] Zemła-Pacud, Ż., & Lenarczyk, G. (2023). Clinical trial data transparency in the EU: Is the new clinical trials regulation a game-changer? *IIC-International Review of Intellectual Property and Competition Law*, 1–32.

[44] Flear, M. L. (2016). The EU clinical trials regulation: Key priorities, purposes and aims and the implications for public health. *Journal of Medical Ethics*, *42*(3), 192–198.

[45] Vogler, S., Habimana, K. (2014). *Pharmaceutical pricing policies in European countries*. Gesundheit Österreich Forschungs-und Planungs GmbH, Vienna

[46] Mrazek, M., & Mossialos, E. (2004). Regulating pharmaceutical prices in the European Union. *Regulating Pharmaceuticals in Europe: Striving for Efficiency, Equity and Quality*, *1*, 114–129.

[47] National Library of Medicine. *HTA 101: Introduction to Health Technology Assessment* (cited 1 Dec. 23). Available from www.nlm.nih.gov/nichsr/hta101/ta10103.html.

[48] Oortwijn, W., Mathijssen, J., & Banta, D. (2010). The role of health technology assessment on pharmaceutical reimbursement in selected middle-income countries. *Health Policy*, *95*(2–3), 174–184.

[49] Drummond, M., Jönsson, B., Rutten, F., & Stargardt, T. (2011). Reimbursement of pharmaceuticals: Reference pricing versus health technology assessment. *The European Journal of Health Economics*, *12*, 263–271.

[50] European Medicines Agency. *Partners and Network Health Technology Assessment Bodies* (cited 1 Dec. 23). Available from www.ema.europa.eu/en/partners-networks/health-technology-assessment-bodies

[51] Domeij, B. (2000). *Pharmaceutical Patents in Europe* (Vol. 3). Martinus Nijhoff Publishers.

[52] European Commission. *Supplementary Protection Certificates for Pharmaceutical and Plant Protection Products* (cited 1 Dec. 23). Available from https://single-market-economy.ec.europa.eu/industry/strategy/intellectual-property/patent-protection-eu/supplementary-protection-certificates-pharmaceutical-and-plant-protection-products_en

[53] Bale Jr, H. E. (1996). Patent protection and pharmaceutical innovation. *New York University Journal of International Law & Politics*, *29*, 95.

[54] Mándi, A. (2003). Protection and challenge of pharmaceutical patents. *Journal of Generic Medicines*, *1*(1), 72–82.

[55] Aboy, M., Liddell, K., Jordan, M., Crespo, C., & Liddicoat, J. (2022). European patent protection for medical uses of known products and drug repurposing. *Nature Biotechnology*, *40*(4), 465–471.

[56] Romandini, R. (2022). *Study on the Options for a Unified Supplementary Protection Certificate (SPC) System in Europe*. Romandini, Roberto: European Commission, Directorate-General for Internal Market, Industry, Entrepreneurship and SMEs: Study on the Options for a Unified Supplementary Protection Certificates (SPCs) System in Europe, 23–09.

[57] Roussou, G. A. (2023). *Supplementary Protection Certificates for Medicinal Products*. Edward Elgar Publishing.

[58] European Medicine Agency. *Human Regulatory-Market Authorization. Data Exclusivity/Generics/Biosimilars: Regulatory and Procedural Guidance* (cited 1 Dec. 23). Available from www.ema.europa.eu/en/human-regulatory/marketing-authorisation/guidance-documents/data-exclusivity-generics-biosimilars-regulatory-procedural-guidance

[59] Gaessler, F., & Wagner, S. (2022). Patents, data exclusivity, and the development of new drugs. *Review of Economics and Statistics*, *104*(3), 571–586.

5 Regulations in the United Kingdom

Kumari Neha, Vivekanandan Kalaiselvan, and Faraat Ali

5.1 INTRODUCTION

The Medicines and Healthcare Products Regulatory Agency (MHRA) is in charge of drug monitoring in the United Kingdom. Before medications and medical equipment can be used in the United Kingdom, the MHRA must ensure that they fulfill relevant criteria of security, reliability, and efficacy. The MHRA fulfills its regulation duty by taking into account the benefits and risks of a medicine, which relies on methodical indication from statistical records and clinical studies, data collected through the Yellow Card Scheme (YCS), and new knowledge originating from the medicinal sector. The MHRA or the Marketing Authorisation holder informs healthcare practitioners about negative consequences and the global risk-benefit profile. The General Practice Research Database (GPRD) passed from the Headquarters for National Statistics to the Medicines Control Agency (MCA) in 1999. The MCA and the Medical Devices Agency (MDA) merged to create the MHRA in 2003. It amalgamated with the National Institute for Biological Standards and Control (NIBSC) in April 2013 and remarketed their products with the MHRA moniker being used primarily for the group's administrative organization. More than 1200 individuals work for the business in London, South Mimms, Hertfordshire, and York. Certain medications are under extensive tracking, as indicated by a black triangle in the British National Formulary (BNF), the official prescriptive reference source for healthcare providers in the United Kingdom. The black triangle is often used for newly licensed drugs, medications licensed for a new method or indication, or pharmaceuticals licensed for an innovative combination of active ingredients. Unlike the boxed alarm system, the existence of a black triangle implies increased surveillance but does not suggest the presence of a recognized hazard. The MHRA is split into three primary phases: the first is MHRA Supervisory, which is the authority for the medicinal products and health equipment businesses. The second phase is Clinical Practice Research Datalink, which controls the licensing of anonymized healthcare facts to pharmaceutical corporations, universities, and other regulators for investigation. The third phase is the National Institute for Biological Standards and Control, which is in charge of all aspects of biological medicine standardization and control. The MHRA has numerous impartial advisory groups (Figure 5.1) that provide details and advise to the UK government on the legalization of pharmaceuticals and medical devices. A

DOI: 10.1201/9781003296492-6

Advisory Board on the Registration of Homeopathic Products
Blood Consultative Committee
British Pharmacopoeia
Clinical Practice Research Datalink (CPRD) Research Data Governance (RDG) Process
Commission on Human Medicines
Devices Expert Advisory Committee
Herbal Medicines Advisory Committee
The Review Panel

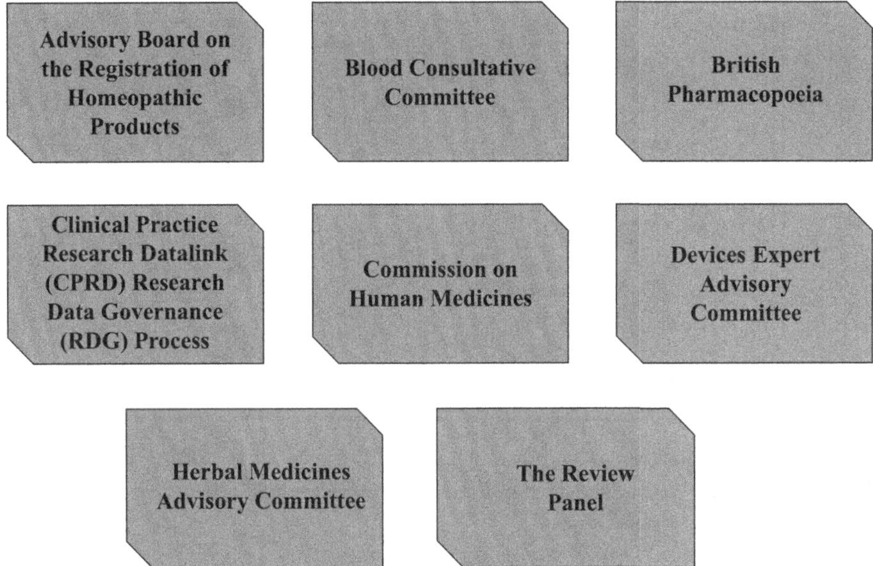

FIGURE 5.1 UK Independent Advisory Bodies.

variety of expert advisory committees are hosted and supported by the MHRA, such as the Commission on Human Medicine (which took over from the Committee on the Safety of Medicines in 2005) and the British Pharmacopoeia Commission. The Early Access to Medicines Scheme (EAMS), established in 2014 to provide access to medications before market authorization in cases where a demonstrable unmet need for medicine exists, is overseen by the MHRA. [1-3]

5.2 UK DRUG REGULATION

The Misuse of Drugs Act 1971, the Medicines Act 1968, and the Psychoactive Substances Act 2016 govern drug legislation in the United Kingdom. The Misuse of Drugs Act 1971 is the key part of regulation leading medicine regulation in the United Kingdom, and it categorizes restricted substances into three categories (A, B, and C). The categorization is based on the chemicals' potential for damage, abuse, and medical use. The Misuse of Drugs Act of 1971 and its rules govern the use of listed drugs, which include both legal and non-medical narcotics. The act also outlines offenses including controlled substance possession, distribution, manufacturing, and smuggling. The Medicines Act 1968 (shown in Figure 5.2) governs the sale, delivery, and advertising of pharmaceutical items. Its primary goal is to confirm the safety, quality, and effectiveness of medications on the market, as well as maintaining public health. The Psychoactive Substances Act 2016 is a piece of UK legislation that intends to tackle the problems of psychoactive chemicals, also known as "legal highs" or "designer drugs." The law was enacted to prohibit the sale, shipping, and manufacture of such substances. [4-5]

1868	Pharmacy Act
1908	Poisons and Pharmacy Act
1916	Defense of the Realm Act 1914
1920	Dangerous Drugs Act
1964	Drugs (Prevention of Misuse Act)
1971	Misuse of Drugs Act
1985	Controlled Drugs (Penalties) Act
1986	Drug Trafficking Offences Act
1991	Criminal Justice Act 1991. Schedule 1A6
1998	Crime and Disorder Act
2000	Criminal Justice and Court Services Act
2003	Criminal Justice Act 2003 & Anti-Social Behaviour Act
2005	Drugs Act
2006	Police and Justice Act
2008	Controlled Drugs (Drug Precursors) (Intra-Community Trade & Community External Trade) Regulations 2008
2016	Psychoactive Substances Act 2016
2017	The Misuse of Drugs Act 1971 (Amendment) (No. 2) Order 634 & 1114
2018	The Misuse of Drugs Act 1971 (Amendment) Order 1356
2019	The Misuse of Drugs Act 1971 (Amendment) Order 323
2021	The Misuse of Drugs Act 1971 (Amendment) Order 868

FIGURE 5.2 UK Drug-related Legislation.

5.3 PHASES OF THE UK REVIEW OF MEDICINES

There were three stages to the review procedure.

- *The methodical review*: The active substances were originally considered, with the goal of reviewing efficacy asserts, dose, the necessity for cautions, limitations, negative possessions, and the necessity for limits on promotion or labeling. Standards for excellence were developed. Provisional suggestions for discussion have been tracked by definite approvals for the active components from license holders and representative organizations. This method proved inefficient because the procedure of discussion, revision, and analysis of distinct licenses took far longer than anticipated. During the first 3 years, only one medication grouping for each time was evaluated. Despite prior consultation, companies routinely refused to take advice for goods and requested to the Board on the Evaluation of Medications and, on certain occasions, the Medications Commission [6].
- *Streamlined systemic review*: In 1979, another stage of systematic evaluation began, allowing the Committee to assess individual goods much earlier and without prior consultation. This process had some issues in maintaining uniformity, but it significantly boosted the rate of review. Because of quality issues, large-volume parenteral fluids were examined independently

at the time. The release of such Panel proposals was later discontinued because this open plan sparked great disagreement and created permissible complications. It was hoped that it would anticipate discussions with distinct license holders and boundary their opportunity to appeal. A quicker appraisal system was established at the time to confirm that risky items were not kept unreviewed over long periods of time.

- *Third phase*: In the last segment, prescription-only medications were allocated with the first, followed by over-the-counter medications. The most recent batch of submissions (Figure 5.1) arrived in 1990. The Medicines Control Agency assigned more professional workers to the work during this stage, and legal guidance was altered to allow for faster progress, particularly in medical assessments. Customer relationship management (CRM, 1986) took a more realistic method to goods with minor restricting indications, engaging with producers to eliminate spurious claims, lessen the number of potent components, and enhance labeling and data. This method contributed significantly to affecting the Assessment in months of the European Communal time frame [7-8].

5.4 YELLOW CARD SCHEME

The YCS is crucial in supporting the MHRA to regulate the safety of all types of medical goods in Britain to ensure their efficacy for both customers and sufferers. It gathers, categorizes, and evaluates complaints of probable ADRs. The strategy allows for the safety of currently available drugs and immunizations to be monitored. ADRs for all pharmaceuticals, such as vaccinations, bloodstream, variables, and immunoglobulins, can be reported, as can botanical goods, homeopathic treatments, any medical device that is accessible through the British market, inadequate medication (those with a low level of quality), bogus or imitation drugs or medical equipment, nicotine-containing cigarette devices, and refill boxes (e-liquids). The YCS history is given in Figure 5.3.

Concerns about medications, medical equipment, and nicotine electronic cigarettes must be informed, because this information assists in the detection of new problems with these goods. The MHRA will assess the invention and, if necessary,

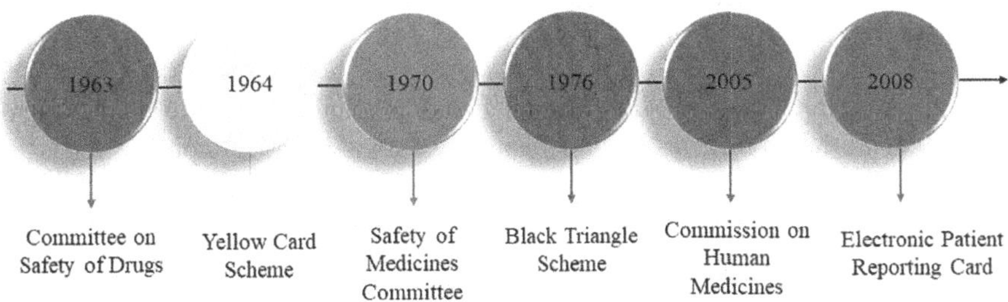

FIGURE 5.3 Timeline of the Yellow Card Scheme.

take steps to decrease risk while maximizing profit to sufferers and the public. The MHRA can also conduct investigations into illegal medications or devices and take action if necessary.

Since its inception in 1964, the MHRA and its predecessor organizations have gathered reports of suspected ADRs via the YCS. It served as the world's initial natural way to report for probable adverse drug reactions, and it continues to serve as the core of post-marketing medicinal product surveillance in the United Kingdom. The effort is entirely volunteer, relying on medical experts and citizens to recognize and disclose adverse drug interactions.

Black triangle scheme: In the package booklet and description of the product's features of new pharmaceuticals and vaccines that are subject to further monitoring, an inverted black triangle symbol (▼) is included, along with a brief text clarifying what the triangle symbolizes—this does not entail the medication is harmful. All suspected ADRs for these goods should be reported. The European Medicines Agency (EMA) oversees updating the checklist of black triangle items for Northern Ireland. The MHRA is in charge of updating the checklist of black triangle items for goods belonging to the United Kingdom [9].

5.5 POST-MARKETING SURVEILLANCE

Post-marketing surveillance (PMS) is the practice that tracks the well-being of pharmaceuticals once they enter the marketplace after the effective conclusion of scientific studies. PMS standards have evolved significantly over the years, with regulatory authorities acknowledging the significance of implementing proper safeguards to curb the rising instances of adverse responses. This has heralded a new period of "proactive methods" as opposed to "reactive tactics," with an emphasis on hazard mitigation and appropriate messaging procedures.

The United Kingdom uses PMS or pharmacovigilance (PV) under the YCS, administered by the MHRA and the Commission on Human Medicines (CHM). One of the initial PV initiatives intended toward minimizing ADRs was the YCS. PV incorporates the following goals:

- Monitoring everyday medication usage with the aim of finding hitherto unknown adverse effects and alterations in harmful impact trends.
- Carrying out risk-benefit evaluations for drugs and suggesting necessary actions.
- Consistently educating consumers and healthcare providers about the appropriate and safe use of drugs.

In addition to the YCS, the MHRA implemented an updated black triangle scheme in 2009, with the goal of raising understanding among healthcare professionals and the general public about medications and vaccinations that required close monitoring. Any potential adverse effects produced by such medications and vaccines were to be reported immediately to the MHRA and the CHM. The emblem, an inverted black triangle, is imprinted alongside the name of the applicable medication product.

The YCS in the United Kingdom satisfies the criterion for impulsive data of ADRs, which is a fundamental process of PV. Documents on Yellow Cards can be delivered, contacted by phone, or submitted online to the MHRA. The primary aim for establishing spontaneously reporting methods is to discover adverse responses to both new and established medications, as experimental trials cannot identify erratic but significant ADRs. A working group comprising the MHRA (which used to be referred to as the Medicines Control Agency), the British Medical Association (BMA), the Committee on the Safety of Medicines, the Royal College of General Physicians, and the Association of the British Pharmaceutical Industry formalized the standards for Safety Assessment Marketed Medicines (SAMM) procedures. This explanation of SAMM strategies includes all reporting supported by the publicizing organization that aims to assess the safety of promoted pharmaceutical goods. These investigations take a neutral approach and can comprise continuous cohort trainings, case-by-case monitoring, and experimental trials [10-11].

5.6 SUBMISSION TO LICENSING BODY

The British system is outlined to track the process of a medicinal corporation's submission to the authorizing body, which is a part of the Division of Social Security & Health (Figure 5.4). They wait in order of receipt until one of the qualified employees is available once their submissions are received. This period of inactivity can last up to 12 months but it is typically 4 to 5 months. Before preparing their report and recommendations, the Secretariat member would normally seek clarification from the sponsoring corporation during their analysis. This summary is included with the application being submitted to the Subcommittee on Noxiousness, Experimental Trials, and Healing Efficacy, which will review the proposal at its subsequent scheduled hearing [12].

The legislation governing medical marketing in the United Kingdom is defined in the Guidelines for Conduct of nationwide business trade organizations. The Association of the British Pharmaceutical Industry (ABPI) constituted the UK Code in 1958. To carry out the standards, the ABPI developed self-supervisory groups that function independent of the various organizations' administrations on every day (Figure 5.5). The Prescription Medicines Code of Practice Authority (PMCPA) was founded by the ABPI in 1993 as a quasi-autonomous institution in charge of implementing the UK Code. It has a two-structured self-regulatory system. Complaints can come from both inside and outside the sector. Employers in the earlier circumstance essential first try to solve issues through inter-organization communication. The Code of Practice (CP) Board in the United Kingdom imposes pecuniary penalties on offending corporations and makes its findings public. Furthermore, the Pharmaceutical Industry's Information Examiner (IGM) can order a firm to publish a remedial declaration. The CP Request Panel and the Information Practices Committee (NBL) handle applications. The CP Board may also submit to the CP Request committee any corporation whose protocol infractions are of significant

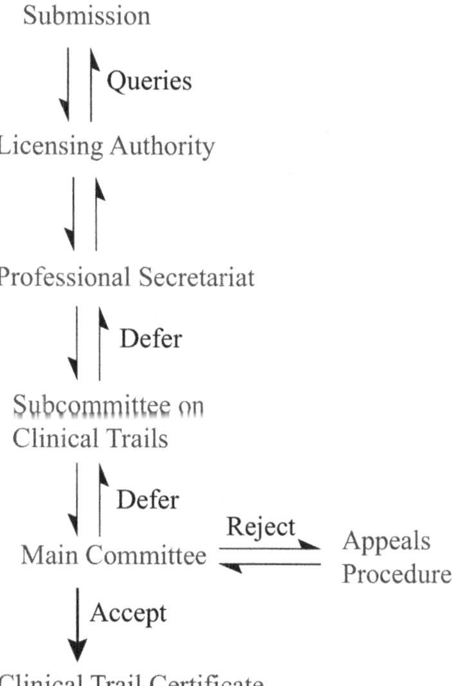

FIGURE 5.4 Submission to Licensing Authority.

warning. The NBL has fewer non-economic disciplinary proceedings than the CP Appeal Board [13].

5.7 DRUG SAFETY WITHDRAWALS

- Withdrawal of rofecoxib.
    - Rofecoxib was pulled off the market in September 2004 because of a seemingly elevated risk of heart disease, and subsequent findings elevated worries that other nonsteroidal anti-inflammatory medicines (NSAIDs) might similarly elevate this hazard. The MHRA distributed precautionary guidance to providers and the general public, as well as postal warnings to consumers, advising that sufferers with developed cardiovascular illness or brain-related disorders ought to transition from a cyclooxygenase-2 selective inhibitor to an alternative pain reliever, though no particular guidance on a suitable substitute was provided. The MHRA reported in January 2010 that high dosages of two frequently used general NSAIDs, diclofenac (150 mg/day) and ibuprofen (1200 mg/day), but studies suggested the menace augmented at 100 mg/day, were associated with an increased cardiovascular risk [14].

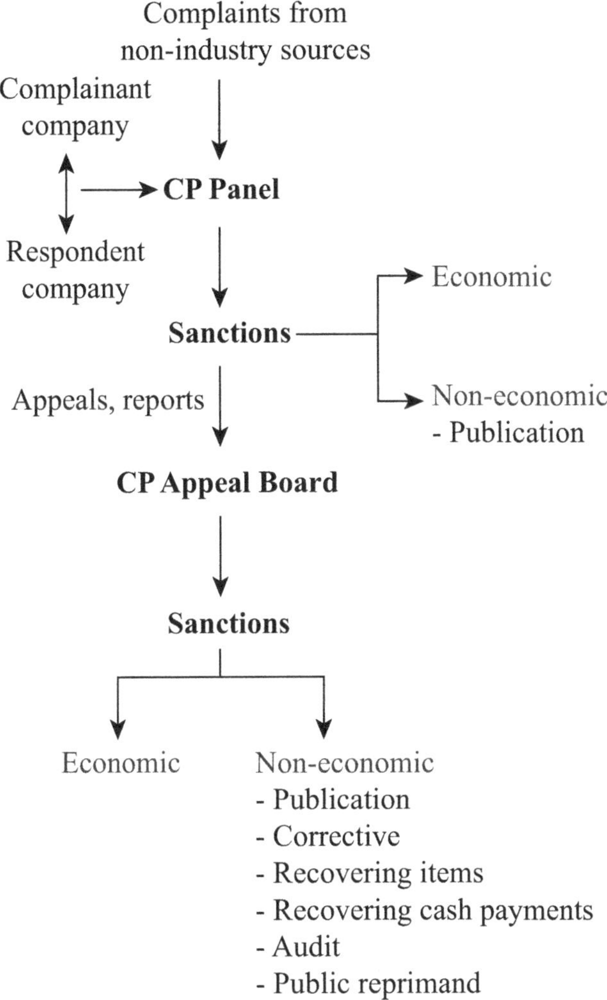

FIGURE 5.5 Systems of Self-regulation in the United Kingdom.

- Contrasting reactions to cautions against the use of second-generation (atypical) antipsychotic medications and thioridazine.
    - The MHRA issued an alert about safety in the month of September 2005 stating that the second-generation antipsychotics risperidone and olanzapine should not be used to address behavioral difficulties in elderly individuals with Alzheimer disease. This trailed an assessment by the Committee the Safety of Medications, which discovered that risperidone raised the risk of infarction in elderly individuals with dementia threefold, and similar worries were expressed for olanzapine. The chief medical officer transmitted the drug safety aware to healthcare providers via the Community

Well-being Agency weblink (later substituted by the National Health Service Central Alerting System), and the MHRA offered guidance to doctors and individuals.

- Stopping the use of co-proxamol and dextropropoxyphene.
  - Co-proxamol is a fixed-dosage formulation of analgesics that combines paracetamol with dextropropoxyphene, the latter of which has long been suspected of having cardiotoxic characteristics. Evidence that co-proxamol overdose is associated with higher mortality as contrasted with acetaminophen alone or other fixed-dose mixture anaesthesia, including co-codamol and co-dydramol, did not emerge in over 20 years of clinical research. The MHRA revoked the marketing permission for co-proxamol, the sole dextropropoxyphene-comprising drug existing in the United Kingdom, in December 2007. Furthermore, this intervention has resulted in a significant decrease in the incidence of co-proxamol overuse, potentially saving 300–400 lives per year in the United Kingdom alone [15-16].

REFERENCES

[1] Winship, K., Hepburn, D. and Lawson, D.H., 1992. The review of medicines in the United Kingdom. *British Journal of Clinical Pharmacology*, *33*, pp. 583–587.

[2] Jefferys, D.B., Leakey, D., Lewis, J.A., Payne, S. and Rawlins, M.D., 1998. New active substances authorized in the United Kingdom between 1972 and 1994. *British Journal of Clinical Pharmacology*, *45*(2), pp. 151–156.

[3] Hans, M. and Gupta, S.K., 2018. Comparative evaluation of pharmacovigilance regulation of the United States, United Kingdom, Canada, India and the need for global harmonized practices. *Perspectives in Clinical Research*, *9*(4), p. 170.

[4] Dunlop, D., 1980. The growth of drug regulation in the United Kingdom. *Journal of the Royal Society of Medicine*, *73*(6), pp. 405–407.

[5] Mossialos, E. and Oliver, A., 2005. An overview of pharmaceutical policy in four countries: France, Germany, the Netherlands and the United Kingdom. *The International Journal of Health Planning and Management*, *20*(4), pp. 291–306.

[6] Rawson, N.S., Kaitin, K.I., Thomas, K.E. and Perry, G., 1998. Drug review in Canada: A comparison with Australia, Sweden, the United Kingdom, and the United States. *Drug Information Journal*, *32*(4), pp. 1133–1141.

[7] Richard, B.W. and Lasagna, L., 1987. *Drug Regulation in the United States and the United Kingdom: The Depo-Provera Story.*

[8] Raj, N., Fernandes, S., Charyulu, N.R., Dubey, A., G. S., R. and Hebbar, S., 2019. Postmarket surveillance: A review on key aspects and measures on the effective functioning in the context of the United Kingdom and Canada. *Therapeutic Advances in Drug Safety*, *10*, pp. 1–13. https://doi.org/10.1177/2042098619865413

[9] Abraham, J. and Davis, C., 2005. A comparative analysis of drug safety withdrawals in the UK and the US (1971–1992): Implications for current regulatory thinking and policy. *Social Science & Medicine*, *61*(5), pp. 881–892.

[10] Alostad, A.H., Steinke, D.T. and Schafheutle, E.I., 2018. International comparison of five herbal medicine registration systems to inform regulation development: United

Kingdom, Germany, United States of America, United Arab Emirates and Kingdom of Bahrain. *Pharmaceutical Medicine*, *32*, pp. 39–49.

[11] Dollery, C.T., 1976. Session V. Regulatory differences and similarities; Drug regulation in the United Kingdom. *Clinical Pharmacology & Therapeutics*, *19*(5part2), pp. 689–693.

[12] Zetterqvist, A.V., Merlo, J. and Mulinari, S., 2015. Complaints, complainants, and rulings regarding drug promotion in the United Kingdom and Sweden 2004–2012: A quantitative and qualitative study of pharmaceutical industry self-regulation. *PLoS Medicine*, *12*(2), p. e1001785. http://doi.org/10.1371/journal.pmed.1001785

[13] Bakke, O.M., Manocchia, M., de Abajo, F., Kaitin, K.I. and Lasagna, L., 1995. Drug safety discontinuations in the United Kingdom, the United States, and Spain from 1974 through 1993: A regulatory perspective. *Clinical Pharmacology & Therapeutics*, *58*(1), pp. 108–117.

[14] Ferner, R.E. and Aronson, J.K., 2023. Medicines legislation and regulation in the United Kingdom 1500–2020. *British Journal of Clinical Pharmacology*, *89*(1), pp. 80–92.

[15] Ceccoli, S., 2002. Divergent paths to drug regulation in the United States and the United Kingdom. *Journal of Policy History*, *14*(2), pp. 135–169.

[16] Waring, W.S. and McGettigan, P., 2011. Clinical toxicology and drug regulation: A United Kingdom perspective. *Clinical Toxicology*, *49*(6), pp. 452–456.

6 Regulations in Canada

Hasan Ali, Sandeep Kumar Singh, Babar Iqbal, Neeraj Kant Sharma, Faraat Ali, and Md. Akbar

6.1 INTRODUCTION

Drug development is a very complex and tedious process, developed from the time of herbals to the time of synthetic chemistry. Developmental transition in this course was essential to milestone scientific development in drugs and pharmaceuticals, because the course of drug discovery and development is subjected to change on the availability and advancement of new information. Hence, drug development is continuously experiencing substantial changes. Over the last ten decades, a number of new chemical entities (NCE) have originated from synthetic chemistry (Ali et al., 2015). Fundamentally, the whole drug discovery needs the intimate collaboration of many scientific fields for a few years. A number of scientific groups are implicated in bringing up a drug discovery through the numerous developmental phases and converting the drug molecule into a potential therapeutic molecule (Somberg, 1996; Stouch, 1996). Drug substance and drug product approval by the law enforcement and regulatory agencies is of prime importance. Among various teams involved from very first step to the translation of NCE in to viable therapeutic molecules, drug regulatory affairs is one of paramount importance (Hägglöf and Holmgren, 2012).

Fundamentally, the regulatory affairs (RA) division of a pharmaceutical organization is accountable for applying, scrutinizing, monitoring, gaining the process of approval for new drug substance and products, and warranting that approval is renewed and continued for as long as the organization desires to keep the product on the market (Hägglöf and Holmgren, 2012). Hence, the RA department serves as the intersection between law enforcement and regulatory agencies and the scientific team involved in the product development; it is the communication channel with the regulatory agencies as the project continues, directing to make sure that plan of the project appropriately forestalls the requirements of regulatory agencies before product approval. Hence, it is the important responsibility of the RA department to keep up to date on knowledge of drug- and health-related legislation, guidelines prescribed by various national and international organizations, filing protocols and time course, and other regulatory understanding (Hägglöf and Holmgren, 2012). Generally, guidelines and rules associated with drug and drug product approval frequently permit some relaxations; moreover, regulatory authorities expect pharmaceutical organizations to take accountability for determining how they should be construed. Additionally, the RA department of the company has an important role in guiding the project team on how best to infer the rules and guidelines. Throughout the drug development process, comprehensive functional relations with the regulatory agencies are essential,

 DOI: 10.1201/9781003296492-7

for instance, to discuss issues such as deviations from guidelines and rules, clinical trials, and product development. The drug RA department, being a participant of the drug development team, also plays an important role in designing the drug development program (Hägglöf and Holmgren, 2012). Furthermore, the RA division evaluates all documents from a regulatory viewpoint, confirming that it is consistent, clear, and complete with explicit conclusions. Also, the RA department writes the fundamental prescribing information, which is the foundation for the product approval, and eventually prepares the ground for marketing. Generally, documentation related to the drug product approval and its sustenance encompass clinical trial applications (CTAs), submission of applications for new drug products and for changes and deviations to already approved products to the regulatory agency (Hägglöf and Holmgren, 2012).

Legislation is required to cater the safe and effective products to the populace, for many countries have set their own drug regulatory agencies and legislation, which are responsible to enforce the regulations and rules and issue the guidelines to control and regulate the drug and drug product development, process, registration, licensing, manufacturing, labeling, marketing, and post-marketing surveillance. Examples are the US Food and Drug Administration (United States), the Medicines and Healthcare Products Regulatory Agency (MHRA; United Kingdom), and the Therapeutic Goods Administration (TGA; Australia) (Van Norman, 2016; Evans and Day, 2005; Ghosh, 2006). For the control and regulation of drug substance and drug products, Canada has its own well-established regulatory agency, Health Canada, accountable for law enforcement, implementation, and regulation of the pharmaceutical industry as a representative of the Government of Canada.

Health Canada imparts its role actively in guaranteeing that the population of Canada have easy access to quality, safe, and effective drug products. Health Canada endeavors to keep an equilibrium between the proposed health benefits and risks exhibited by the drug products. Hence, the Health Canada gives priority to regulate and maintain the balance in the risk-benefit ratio for the sake of public safety. Involving the other related departments of government, manufacturers, healthcare professionals, industrialists, researchers, and patients, Health Canada implicated in the daily activities related to the drug regulation to minimize the health related risk factors to the public, with enhanced safety and efficacy prescribed by the regulatory system for these products. Health Canada also makes efforts to provide its populace with the knowledge they require to make better choices and decisions about their well-being. Health Canada is not a manufacturer or distributor of drugs and health products (Hajizadeh and Keays, 2023).

In this chapter we will highlight the regulatory procedures of drugs and related products, registration, CTA, enforcement, and various laws related to drug and health-related products and their jurisdiction within the ambit of Health Canada.

6.2 DRUG PRODUCTS

Marketing authorization and sale of a drug in the territory of Canada to diagnose, treat, mitigate, or prevent diseases, is controlled by the Food and Drugs Act (FDA). Health Canada analyzes and reviews the quality, efficacy, and safety of the drug products before they are approved for sale in Canada. Fundamentally, drug products encompass prescription and non-prescription medical products and disinfectants (sanitizer). Health Canada requires essential scientific evidence of quality, efficacy, and safety of a drug product(s) from a manufacturer, as mandated by the Food and Drugs Act and Regulations, before the market authorization (Hajizadeh and Keays, 2023).

Hence, before being approved for marketing in Canada, all drug submission and proposals must undertake a strict and demanding scrutiny and completely comply all scientific and technical requirements under the Food and Drug Regulations. Here, the information for the techniques essential for the manufacturers to satisfy with the policies and guidelines prescribed by Food and Drugs Act and Regulations have been established on a number of subjects concerning drugs to deliver further guidance to the stakeholders (Hajizadeh and Keays, 2023).

6.3 COSMETICS

The scope of cosmetics is imperative for dermatologists to comprehend. Patients apply a variety of cosmetics to their face, body, and hair daily. These individuals can consult the health expert for recommendations on particular products, especially the patients having an associated skin condition. However, some of patients may develop dermatological adverse events to the cosmetics they are using, hence, it is imperative to consult with doctors for the diagnosis and treatment for the underlying skin conditions. Overuse or misuse of cosmetics can be implicated into problems associated with hair and skin. It is important that dermatologists and end users understand the particular cosmetic product and its correct use (Holloway, 2003). All cosmetic products sold in Canada must be safe and show no health risks. Product must meet the compliance prescribed by the Food and Drugs Act and Cosmetics Regulations. If necessary, other conditions prescribed by law must also be fulfilled.

6.3.1 Regulation of Cosmetics

According to the underlying legislation that is the Food and Drugs Act, cosmetics include “any substance or mixture of substances manufactured, sold or represented for cleaning, improving or conditioning the skin, skin, hair or teeth, and includes deodorants and perfumes.” These include cosmetics employed in the aesthetic services by professionals, bulk products such as hand sanitizers, disinfectants in school/college washrooms, and handmade cosmetic products sold by businesses in the home (Health Canada, 2023).

All the cosmetic products intended for sale in Canada must comply with the safety and efficacy provisions prescribed by Health Canada. Cosmetic products must fulfil the requirements of the FDA and the Cosmetic Regulations. Cosmetic Regulations and the FDA require that cosmetic products be sold or marketed in the Canada must be manufactured, prepared, preserved, packaged, and stored in clean and sanitary conditions. Moreover, stakeholders must show a list of all the ingredients implicated in the production of the product in question and inform Health Canada that stakeholders are engaged in the product's sale. Other legislation, such as the Consumer

Packaging and Labelling Act, the Canadian Environmental Protection Act 1999, and the Cannabis Act, as well as other relevant laws, must also be followed if applicable (Health Canada, 2023).

6.4 MEDICAL DEVICES

Medical devices encompass a broad range of medical products employed and used in the diagnosis, mitigation, treatment, prevention, and cure of an abnormal physical condition or disease. Examples include stents, artificial heart valves, pacemakers, contraceptive devices, hip implants, artificial skin grafts, and diagnostic kits (Aronson et al., 2020). Because medical devices play an important role to improve and maintain health and well-being, Health Canada, as a representative of the Canadian government, is responsible for enforcing laws and regulations that promote the quality, safety, and efficacy of medical devices used by the Canadian public (Health Canada, 2023).

A fast-track procedure has been established by Health Canada to reinforce the regulation and control of medical devices in Canada to guarantee better health outcomes. Health Canada assesses medical devices for their quality, safety, and efficacy before being approved for sale and marketing in Canada. The Medical Devices Directorate (MDD) assesses and monitors the quality, safety, and efficacy of therapeutic and diagnostic medical devices. Also, Pharmaceutical Drugs Directorate (PDD) (erstwhile the Therapeutic Products Directorate) guarantees the quality, safety, and efficacy of medical devices as much as possible by a systematic way of stringent pre-market appraisal, post-market surveillance, and evaluation of quality systems in the production process. Apart from the MDD, medical devices also need authorization from the Canadian Nuclear Safety Commission (CNSC) before the grant of a license for operational or servicing activities (Health Canada, 2023).

Medical devices in Canada are grouped into four classes depending on the risk assessment. Generally, the medical devices of Class I exhibit the minimum level of possible risks, for instance, a thermometer, whereas medical devices of Class IV showed the maximum level of possible risks, like pacemakers. Stakeholders are required to acquire a medical device licence before the approval of Class II, III, and IV devices for marketing and sale in Canada. No medical device licence is required for Class I devices, and they are generally monitored by establishment licences (Health Canada, 2023).

The Medical Devices Regulations use a risk-based technique to regulate medical devices within its scope by applying the Classification Rules for Medical Devices as per Schedule 1 of the Regulations, which classifies medical devices into the four risk-based categories:

- Class I devices (low risk), for example, wound care and non-surgically invasive devices.
- Class II devices (low to moderate risk), such as contact lenses, needles, and magnetic resonance imaging equipment.
- Class III devices (medium to high risk), such as hip implants, ultrasound diagnostic imaging equipment, and glucose monitors.

- Class IV devices (high risk), such as pacemakers and surgically invasive devices used to diagnose, regulate, or treat a problem with the central cardiovascular system (Health Canada, 2023).

It is the responsibility of the device distributor, importer, or manufacturer to classify the device.

6.4.1 Establishment License

To authorize the manufacturing, distribution, and import the Class I medical devices through a licensed importer or distributor, an Establishment License is required to market the product in Canada. Fundamentally, Establishment Licencing ensures that the nature of establishment that is manufacturing and selling the medical devices is in the knowledge of PPD. Moreover, this license asks the establishments to give the guarantee to the PPD that the post-production activities comply as per the related regulatory requirements. Steps involved in the appraisal procedure for a medical device are discussed in Figure 6.1. The time period of the appraisal process depends upon the class of the medical device. A 15-day period is required for Class II licence applications. Generally, Class III medical device submissions need an appraisal time period of about 75 days, and Class IV medical devices applications require approximately 90 days for review. The licence can be cancelled or suspended, or the producer may be asked to recall the product, if the device is found to be unsafe and ineffective. If the PPD agrees not to issue the license for a medical device, the producer has the chance to re-submit the submission and provide the supplementary information or to appeal the PPD's decision (Health Canada, 2023).

A Special Access Programme (SAP) is developed to provide healthcare workers access to technologies that have not been authorised or licenced in Canada. In general, it is used in medical emergencies or when established treatments have failed, are unavailable, or are inappropriate for treating a patient (Health Canada, 2023).

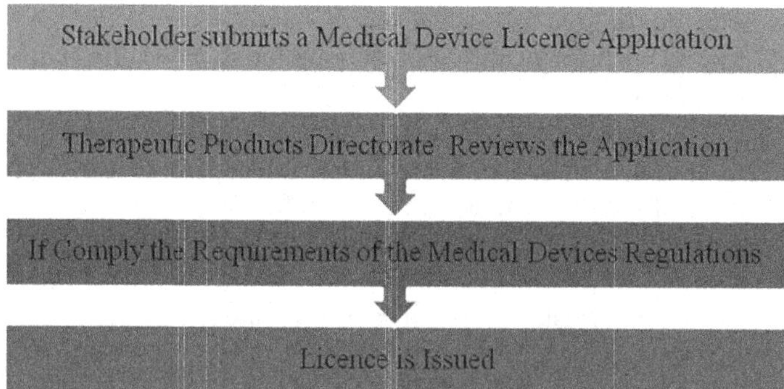

FIGURE 6.1 Flow Chart Depicting the Steps Implicated in the Review Process for a Medical Device.

6.4.2 Nanotechnology-Based Health Products and Food

Implementation of technical knowledge of scientific to control and manipulate the material in the range of nanometers to make use of size, surface, and shape-dependent characteristics and phenomena separate from the properties that are linked with the single atom or molecule as well as with the bulk materials is called nanotechnology (Ali and Singh, 2018). The definition for the nanotechnology products intended for medical use has not been decided, internationally; however, Health Canada has embraced a useful and functional definition for nanotechnology products. Any substance or product generated, as well as any ingredient of a material, device, component, or assembly, is considered a nanomaterial by Health Canada if at least one exterior dimension or internal or surface structure of the material is at or within the nanoscale. Products based on or derived from nanotechnological tools have an extensive range of uses and capacity to influence many areas, encompassing sectors related to health and food. In the healthcare segment, the utility of nanotechnological tools influence drugs, drug delivery systems, novel natural health products, diagnostic and medical devices, and tissue engineering products for better diagnosis and treatment of the disease (Csóka et al., 2021).

Health Canada set up an interdepartmental discussion forum to troubleshoot the disputes related to nanotechnology-based products subjected to sell or market in the Canada, the Health Portfolio Nanotechnology Working Group, which collects the facts and figures (Health Canada, 2023).

Presently, there are no specific regulations for health products involving nanotechnology. For this, Health Canada depends on existing regulatory and legislative frameworks, which need the evaluation of benefits and potential risks of products to health and safety before they can be approved for sale in Canada (Health Canada, 2023).

6.4.3 General Guidance

In Health Canada, it is the stakeholder's duty to identify the product if it is based on the nanotechnology when the application is reporting a nanomaterial or nanoproduct in any form. Revised section 59 permits the stakeholders to report actives and excipients listed under Section 56 or 57 that are nanomaterials. Health Canada motivates stakeholders to inform the concerned regulatory body in the preliminary phase of product development. To categorize and evaluate benefits and potential risks of nanotechnology-based products, Health Canada motivates stakeholders to demand a pre-submission meeting with the concerned regulatory agency to deliberate the type of information that may be needed for their product's safety analysis (Health Canada, 2023). To identify and evaluate the possible benefits and risks of nanomaterials, Health Canada may need the following basic information:

1. Proposed application, purpose and function of the nanomaterial, and evidences related to the final product where it is being employed.
2. Production procedures.
3. Physico-chemical properties and general features of the nanomaterial, such as morphology, identity, composition, and purity.

4. Nanomaterials specific to environmental, metabolic, and toxicological outcomes.
5. Risk evaluation and its approaches to overcome the risks, if significant or applied (Health Canada, 2023).

6.5 BIOLOGICS

Biologics are the drugs that are manufactured and refined from industry-scale cell cultures of animal cells, plants, bacteria, or fungi. Hence, biologics are a class of drugs that encompasses growth factors, immunomodulators, monoclonal antibodies, antisera, vaccines, and human blood–derived products (WHO, 2023; Health Canada, 2023). However, biologics is not a new drug product: erythrocyte stimulating substances, human growth hormone, and insulin have already been developed and have been in use for decades, but with the advent of novel genetic information and new insights of cell signaling, pathogenesis, and disease processes, the targets have increased exponentially. An increasing understanding of cellular processes and genetics has led to the potential new biological (and drug) targets at every step of the protein production process. This leads to the emergence of new treatments, which in turn leads to a new understanding of the disease (Morrow and Felcone, 2004).

Adequate scientific proofs should be collected to exhibit the safety, efficacy, and quality of the biologic before it can be approved for the market authorization. Biologics require more comprehensive manufacturing and chemistry data as compared with the drugs for human use. It is essential to ensure the quality, purity, safety, and efficacy of the product. Biologics encompass, therapeutic products obtained through biotechnology, viral and bacterial vaccines, blood and related products, cells, tissues and organs, gene therapies, xenografts, and radiopharmaceuticals (Health Canada, 2023) (see section 6.6).

As a step of the New Drug Submission (NDS) procedure, stakeholders have to provide Product Specific Facility Information (PSFI) outlining the manufacturing procedure with substantial description, because minor changes can affect the final product. Furthermore, a preliminary audit of the production facility, known as an On-Site Evaluation (OSE), is performed to evaluate the manufacturing technique and location, as these factors, too, have a significant impact on the safety and efficacy of the biologic. If there is sufficient data to support safety, efficacy, or quality claims for an NDS or a Supplement to a New Drug Submission (S/NDS), a Notice of Compliance (NOC) and a Drug Identification Number (DIN) are issued, indicating that the product is authorised for marketing and sale in Canada (Health Canada, 2023).

In general, biologics are monitored for manufacture, testing, inspection, and possible risks. Individual batches of high-risk biologics are quality checked before they are sold. Moderate-risk biologics are occasionally evaluated at Health Canada's discretion, but makers of low-risk biologics are often obliged to contact with Health Canada about batches on the market or to provide assurance of complete and appropriate testing. Health Canada, in collaboration with the Public Health Agency of Canada, monitors adverse effects associated with biologics, inspects complaints, conducts post-approval monitoring, and manages product recalls as appropriate (Health Canada, 2023).

6.6 RADIOPHARMACEUTICALS

As their name suggests, radiopharmaceuticals are both drugs and radioactive substances. Radiolabels are employed in diagnostics as emitters of electromagnetic radiation (X-rays or gamma rays) whose detection allows the quantification of radiopharmaceutical concentrations. Also, radioactive labels can be employed in the clinical applications, where emissions from the decay of radionuclides is implicated in the destruction of cells. The in vivo distribution of radionuclides throughout the body or in particular organs or tissue of the body can be assessed by X-ray or gamma radiation detection employing positron emission tomography or photon emission tomography cameras (Vermeulen et al., 2019).

Radiopharmaceuticals including radionuclide generators, drug products and substances apart from radionuclides employed in the manufacture of radiopharmaceuticals are listed on Schedule C of the FDA of Canada. Health Canada, being a national drug regulatory agency, assesses the quality, safety, and efficacy of drugs listed in Schedule C, for approval to market in Canada. Guidance document related to radiopharmaceuticals is applicable to all the drugs listed in Schedule C of the FDA with few exceptions that include, the ANDS mechanism is not applicable to Schedule C drugs having biological articles, and radiopharmaceuticals emitting positron employed in the fundamental clinical research. Another course of conforming with the data defined in the guidance can be deliberated with suitable technical rationalization. If particular guidelines are not recommended by Health Canada, guidelines of international agencies, like the US Food and Drug Administration or the European Medical Agency, may be used to deliver a justification. This regulatory approach provides wide-ranging inputs about the guideline of radiopharmaceuticals for human use in Canada (Health Canada, 2023).

The Biologics and Genetic Therapies Directorate, a department of Health Canada, controls and regulates the submissions, market approval, and authorization of radiopharmaceuticals intended for human applications based on the adequate assessment of quality, safety, and efficacy of radiopharmaceuticals (Health Canada, 2023).

6.7 INTERFACE PRODUCTS

6.7.1 Drug–Medical Device Interface

Typically, the difference between a drug product and a medical device looks clear. However, there are some situations when the difference between a product being a drug or a device is indistinct (Cutler, 1993; Willis and Lewis, 2008; Donawa, 1996). Fundamentally, healthcare products at the drug-medical device interface do not come under the definitions of “drug” or “device” in Part 2 of the FDA. According to the FDA, these products may be subject to three sets of regulations:

1. Food and Drug Regulations.
2. Natural Health Products Regulations.
3. Medical Devices Regulations.

Classification is the first step in the review of health products by the Health Products and Food Branch (HPFB). If the medical product classification is not clear, in that case, consultation with the Office of Science of PDD is required. The Office of Science of PDD provides guidance on the classification of pharmaceutical products as drugs, medical devices, and drug-medical device interfaces. The classification of nutraceuticals involves rigorous research, analysis, and necessary consultation. This can be complex and resource intensive. In rare cases, the Office of Science may initiate additional consultations with the Therapeutic Products Classification Committee (TPCC). The TPCC includes deputies from all the related fields of Health Canada, both inside and outside of HPFB. This guidance document describes the factors that Health Canada considers when classifying a health product as a device or drug. Product classification should be done carefully to ensure that health products are placed in the appropriate regulatory categories. The level of risk related with the use of the product is not taken into account when determining the regulatory framework into which the product falls. However, a correctly classified product will be integrated into a regulatory tool, which will allow the risks it may represent to be dealt with accordingly. Each set of regulations made under the Food and Drugs Act includes regulatory requirements that provide risk mitigation measures corresponding with the level of risk of health products (Health Canada, 2023).

In addition, pre-market and post-market requirements allow Health Canada to maintain oversight throughout the life cycle of health products, from design/manufacturing quality and pre-market testing to post-market surveillance and operational activities. Health Canada contributes to risk reduction through reviewing and approving CTAs; pre-market implementation and post-market changes of submitted medical products; monitoring the safety and efficacy of medical products placed on the market; communication; and improving industry compliance, such as those related to clinical trials, drug manufacturing, and adverse event reporting. The level of review under the various regulatory regimes under the Food and Drugs Act allows Canadians to avail safe and effective health products at all levels of risk (Health Canada, 2023).

6.7.2 Cosmetic-Drug Interface

These goods may be classified as both "cosmetics" and "drugs" under the Food and Drug Act, making classification problematic. Acne treatment products, antiperspirant products, anti-dandruff products, fluoride products against cavities, skin products, diaper rash products, antibacterial cleansers for skin, skin burn protection products, and skin and teeth whitening products are examples of such products. Based on the composition of the products and the claims made by stockholders, cosmetic drug interface products (CDIPs) in Canada may be regulated under one of three sets of regulations under the Food and Drugs Act: Food and Drug Regulations, Cosmetic Regulations, and Natural Health Products Regulations. Guidelines for Product Classification at the Cosmetic-Drug Interface explain how Health Canada interprets and implements the Food and Drugs Act definitions of cosmetics and pharmaceuticals so that goods are subject to the most suitable regulatory regime for their purpose (Health Canada, 2023).

The rules and criteria outlined in the guidance paper above will be used to establish whether a product comes under the applicable regulatory regime for specified PCDI categories. Each Product Criteria Assessment (PAAC) fundamentally gives a well-described, documented reason for the categorization choice (Health Canada, 2023).

6.8 LEGISLATION

6.8.1 Food and Drugs Act and Its Regulations

Health Canada is in charge of establishing quality, safety, and efficacy standards for all pharmaceuticals, cosmetics, and medical devices sold and marketed in Canada. The Division carries out this mission in accordance with the mandate of the Food and Drugs Act and the Food and Drug Regulations. The Food and Pharmaceuticals legislation is Canadian Parliament legislation that governs the manufacturing, export, import, interprovincial transportation, sale, and marketing of food, pharmaceuticals, medical devices, contraceptives, and cosmetics, including personal cleaning products such as soap and toothpaste (Health Canada, 2023).

The Food and Drugs Act was initially adopted in 1920 and last amended in 1985. Rather than being promoted as food or cosmetics, it strives to guarantee that goods are safe, their components are disclosed, and therapies are effective. It also forbids the general public from promoting pharmaceuticals used to treat Schedule A disorders such as cancer, depression, obesity, asthma, anxiety, sexually transmitted infections, and appendicitis. Part I includes a comprehensive explanation of words and describes each of the conversation subjects covered by the legislation, which are foods, pharmaceuticals, cosmetics, and electrical appliances (Justice Laws Website, 2023).

Part II of the bill focuses on regulation and enforcement, allowing the government to intervene with manufacturers. It includes inspections, seizures and confiscations, analysis, ministerial powers, registration, regulation, interim orders, marketing authorization, offenses and penalties, and enforcement. Parts III (adopted in 1961) and IV (approved in 1969) deal with the execution of the control mechanisms required by the Psychotropic Substances Convention. Part III addresses "controlled" substances having real medicinal use, such as amphetamines, methaqualone, and phenmetrazine. Part IV concentrates on Schedule H "restricted drugs," such as the hallucinogens LSD, DMT, and MDMA, whose only permitted usage is for scientific study. These sections list eight categories of banned drugs, from Schedule A to Schedule H (Justice Laws Website, 2023).

In essence, categorization is the first step in every regulatory action implemented by Health Canada. The FDA and its accompanying rules serve as the framework for classifying foods, pharmaceuticals, cosmetics, and devices, and include Food and Drug rules, Cosmetic Regulations, Natural Health Product Regulations, and Medical Devices Regulations. Figure 6.2 provides a visual overview of the regulations that apply to each product line.

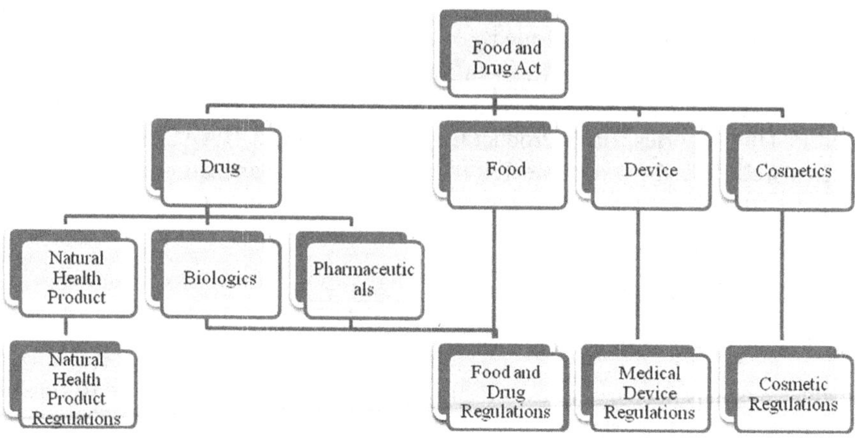

FIGURE 6.2 Visual Representation of the Regulations that Apply to Each Product Line (Health Canada, 2023).

6.8.2 Controlled Drugs and Substances Act (CDSA)

This is an Act to govern and regulate some pharmaceuticals, their chemical precursors, intermediates, and other related substances, as well as to modify existing Acts. The CDSA is Canada's federal drug control statute. Parts III and IV of the Narcotic Control Act and the Food and Drug Act were removed, and eight lists of restricted drugs and two categories of precursors were introduced. "The Governor in Council may, by order, amend any of the sections of Schedules I to VIII, add or delete any section or part of a section therein, if he considers such modification necessary in the public interest," it says. The CDSA was implemented to provide single legislation for the Narcotic Drugs, Psychotropic Substances, and the United Nations Convention against Illicit Traffic in Narcotic Drugs and Psychotropic Substances (Justice Laws Website, 2023).

The law consists of seven parts and nine annexes. Part I covers violations and penalties, Part II covers enforcement, Part III covers penalties, Part IV covers management and compliance, and Part V covers administrative regulations in case of violation of specific regulations. Ministerial orders, crime, punishment, injunctions, evidence, procedure, technical assistance, regulations and exemptions, schedule changes. and other miscellaneous matters are contained in Part VI. Part VII deals with transitional provisions, consequential and conditional amendments, repeals and effects (Justice Laws Website, 2023).

6.9 CLINICAL TRIALS

Fundamentally, clinical trials assist in the estimation of the effectiveness of drugs, drug treatments, surgery, radiation therapy, behavioral interventions, or preventive health strategies. These studies can be conducted with a wide range of participants including healthy subjects, such as in phase I clinical trials, or in patients undergoing a medical or surgical or radiological procedure (Croghan et al., 2015). These studies are conducted to determine the efficacy of evidence-based medical interventions and practices. Evidence-based practice aids enhance the patient safety and therapeutic effects, thereby promoting better population health (Schultz et al., 2019). However, clinical trials are difficult, labor and time intensive, and need meticulous planning in implementation. Each academic unit is supported by four functions: patient care, teaching/training of health professionals, administrative duties, and research (Sackett et al., 1996).

The FDA and its rules provide Health Canada the authority to supervise the sale, import, and export of medications and pharmaceuticals for clinical studies. The conditions for a Clinical Trial Application (CTA) and an Addendum to a Clinical Trial Application (CTA-A) for pharmaceuticals sold and imported into Canada for clinical trials are outlined in Section 5 of Part C of the Act and its Regulations. Section 5 of the Act and Regulations is primarily concerned with the notion and codes of good clinical practice. Furthermore, Health Canada follows International Council for Harmonisation (ICH) efficacy guidelines such as E2A (Definitions and Standards for Expedited Reporting), E6 (Good Clinical Practice), and E8 (General Considerations for Clinical Studies) (Health Canada, 2023).

6.9.1 Clinical Trial Application (CTA)

Stakeholders must submit a CTA before beginning clinical trials for Phase I–III drug research and development, as well as bioavailability and bioequivalence (BA/BE) investigations. This includes applications to conduct clinical trials on commercially available pharmaceuticals when the intended use of the drug product does not satisfy the criteria of an authorised Notice of Compliance (NOC) or Drug Identification Number. (DIN). When conducting a clinical trial in Canada using a product that has received a Notice of Compliance with Conditions (NOC/c), a CTA is also necessary. It is not necessary to submit the CTA to Health Canada to undertake Phase IV of the clinical study. If the application is found incomplete by Health Canada, the stakeholders will be notified within 30 days of its submission. If a CTA is determined to be acceptable, a No Objection Letter (NOL) will be given within the 30 days review period. The CTA includes information and papers that support the purpose and goals of the proposed clinical trial. It also has statistics to back up the quality of the drugs. The clinical and qualitative components of the application will be assessed concurrently, and both must be satisfied before issuing a letter of no objection. Before beginning clinical trials, approval from the institution's local/institutional research and ethics board must be obtained. Changes to an already approved CTA must be submitted to Health Canada as an amendment or notification to the CTA (Health Canada, 2023).

Furthermore, Health Canada examine the clinical trial protocols to analyze the participants' safety and protection; assess the quality of medicines; assure review by the research ethics board; monitor and review adverse drug events; and verify the educational qualifications and experiences of investigators and researchers involved in the clinical trial. Health Canada also considers ethical problems such as standard operating procedures, conflict of interest, informed consent, and financial settlements. Researchers carrying out clinical trials must provide care in accordance with the principles of good clinical practices, observe the adverse drug events, obtain informed consent, and follow approved research protocols (patient screening, dosage, frequency, monitoring, etc.). Adverse drug events should be reported to the stakeholders and the research ethics board (Health Canada, 2023).

6.9.2 Compliance with the Regulatory Framework

Compliance with the regulatory outline is ensured by the evaluation of filed CTA and the monitoring of the trials during the process. The Health Products and Food Inspectorate (HPFI) is accountable for the inspection of clinical trials. About 2% of research is reviewed each year, primarily focused on protecting research subjects. Complaints or concerns sent to Health Canada are also reviewed. CTAs having drugs and their products of synthetic or semi-synthetic source, with the exception of biotechnology/biologics (List D) and radiopharmaceuticals (List C), are submitted to Health Canada. Stakeholders must provide more detailed quality information in later stages of CT, gradually. However, all the requirements of these guidelines are not applied to all the phases of CT. Alternatives to concepts and techniques discussed in the guidance document might be acceptable if backed by substantial and strong scientific evidence. Stakeholders are encouraged to discuss alternative approaches in advance to support their drug submission to avoid denial or withdrawal. Depending on the stage of CT development, a Quality Overall Summary template for pharmaceuticals is applicable to phases I, II, and III. However, for combination protocols (like Phase I/II or II/III), stakeholders must submit quality data in accordance with the next highest CT phase (Health Canada, 2023).

6.9.3 Canadian New Drug Submission (NDS)

Fundamentally, New Drug Submission (NDS) refers to the method and course of action through which new drug products are examined and authorised by Health Canada before their introduction into the Canadian market. In Canada, new medications are typically governed under Division 8 of Part C of the Food and Drug Regulations (FDR) of the FDA. An applicant gains authority to commercialize a novel medicine in Canada by filing an NDS under Food and medicine Regulations section C08.002. The NDS application, together with other information necessary by Canada's FDA and regulations, must be submitted to Health Canada for assessment and approval. Depending on the drug product category, the appropriate division of Health Canada will examine the NDS in line with the applicable regulatory criteria. The FDA issues a Notice of Compliance (NOC) after satisfactory validation of the new drug's quality, safety, and effectiveness, allowing the stakeholders to advance to the next step of market access. A Supplemental New Drug Submission (SNDS) is essentially an extra request made to Health Canada to report changes that may have a detrimental effect on the identity, strength, quality, purity, or effectiveness of a pharmaceutical product (Health Canada, 2023).

6.9.4 Abbreviated New Drug Submission (ANDS)

ANDS is a request in written form to Health Canada requesting authorization to market a generic drug. Before the sale and marketing of generics in the Canada under Canadian food and drug regulations, ANDS must be approved by Health Canada, the federal agency responsible for national healthcare. Fundamentally, ANDS provides the information to the Health Canada, needed to assess the safety and effectiveness of generic drugs compared with their brand name equivalents. For a generic drug to be approved, it must be as safe and effective as the innovator product. Simplified administration of new drugs for generic drug approval. This contrasts with a New Drug Submission (NDS), which is required to get the approval for a new drug. Moreover, ANDS contains the relevant drug name, chemical name, manufacturer name, drug form and strength (Health Canada, 2023). This indicates whether the drug has been approved for marketing in the United States, EU, Australia, Singapore, and/or Switzerland. It also deals with issues related to drug impurities and drug stability.

- ANDS requires approval to sell generic drugs in Canada.
- Submissions offer important relevant data, such as information from comparative studies of generic drugs to the innovator's product and bioavailability data.
- Many ANDS applications approved can serve as data points for biotech stakeholders to assess the profitability potential of pharmaceutical companies (Health Canada, 2023).

Essentially, generic medicines are bioequivalent to the innovators products. Generic products are comparable with innovators product in terms of use, strength, dosage form, quality, route of administration, and overall performance characteristics of the product. Because ANDS are labeled as "abbreviated," clinical data is generally not necessary to prove safety and effectiveness of the final product. Moreover, ANDS provides data obtained from the studies from generic products for the comparison with the innovator's products, also known as "reference drug." Moreover, for delivery devices, the ANDS indicates whether there are studies comparing the physical and operational characteristics of a branded device to those of a proposed generic device. ANDS also delivers the data on studies comparing the bioavailability of brand name drugs and offered generic drugs and on the results of bacterial endotoxin testing of sterile drugs. Applicants must pay the required fee with their ANDS (Health Canada, 2023).

6.10 FUNDING AND FEES

Health Canada has been taking fees under the FDA for some services and activities like regulation of drugs, biologicals, medical devices, and veterinary drugs since 1990. These fees apply to activities like pre-market regulatory assessment, compliance and enforcement through Health Canada's inspection programs, and ongoing post-market product monitoring. There is a separate fee provision for different type of products like human drugs, medical devices, and veterinary drugs. Health Canada has also provided a list of regulation documents that have been revised to provide updates on information of fees, rules, and mitigations steps. For the sustenance and support of small business ventures, Health Canada has taken significant steps to reduce the influence of fees on small business ventures. Eligible companies may obtain a 50% discount on pre-market assessment fees and a 25% discount on right to sale fees, as well as a 25% discount on establishment licenses. Fees will be waived for companies submitting their first pre-market product in Canada (Health Canada, 2023).

6.11 DRUG REVIEW PROCESS

Once a drug has passed the drug review process, it is approved for marketing and sale in Canada. Drug applications are reviewed by scientists from Health Canada's Health Products and Food Branch (HPFB), and sometimes external experts, to evaluate the safety, efficacy, and quality of the drug. The HPFB is a national agency accountable for regulation, evaluation, and monitoring of the quality, safety, and efficacy of therapeutic and diagnostic products accessible to the population of Canada. These include drug products, medical devices, sanitizers, and disinfectants. Before beginning the review of drugs, it is essential to review and understand the scope of the term *drug* in the context of the regulatory mechanism. Thus, "drugs" encompass both over-the-counter and prescription drugs; products of biological origin, like blood products, vaccines, tissues, organs, disinfectants, radiopharmaceuticals, and biotechnologically produced products. According to the FDA,

> A drug contains any substance or mixture of substances produced, marketed, or represented for use in the:
>
> - prevention, mitigation, treatment, and diagnosis of a disease, abnormal body condition, disorder or symptoms of human and/or animals,
> - correction, restoration, or changing of organs function of human or animal, and/or
> - disinfection of premises in which food is produced or stored.

Natural health products, such as vitamin and mineral supplements and herbal products, are also included as drugs under the FDA, if they claim some therapeutic value; otherwise, they are regulated under the Natural Health Products Regulations, but not a drug under the Food and Drug Regulations (Health Canada, 2023).

6.11.1 Drug Development Process: An Outline

Research into new drugs starts when research scientists develop a new chemical substance. As the newly synthesized substance is isolated and purified, it is used in tissue cultures or various experimental animal species to observe if there are any substantial medicinal effect. If encouraging outcomes are attained from these preliminary studies, perform various animal laboratory tests to investigate the other effects of the drug substance and determines the dose to be given to achieve a particular pharmacological effects. If these preclinical experiments show that the new chemical substance yields the expected results and is safe enough, the stakeholder may apply to the HPFB for authorization to conduct a clinical trial in Canada. The purpose of a clinical trial is to study and gather information about the dosage, efficacy, and safety of a drug in humans. Prior consent from the volunteers involved in the clinical trial is essential to comply good clinical practices. It provides a controlled environment in which medication administration procedures and outcome assessments are closely monitored (Health Canada, 2023).

Before the start of clinical trials in Canada, HPFB will review the data submitted in the CTA. This CTA appeals to permit the trial drug to distribute to the accountable clinical investigator indicated in the CTA. Some of the data included in a CTA are preclinical trial results, type dosage forms, manufacturing procedure and information about the researchers who will conduct the trials. If trial study indicate that a drug has promising therapeutic effects that outweighs the risks related to its use (e.g., adverse effects, toxicity), the stakeholders may choose to file a NDS with HPFB (Health Canada, 2023).

6.11.2 Steps in the Review Process for a Drug in Health Canada

A flow chart depicting the various steps involved in the appraisal process for a drug in Health Canada for the market authorization in Canada is shown in Figure 6.3. The HPFB will not grant marketing authorization to a drug if there is insufficient data to support claims regarding quality, safety, and efficacy. All drugs approved for the marketing in Canada are reviewed to guarantee to comply the requirements of the FDA. Approval is at the discretion of HPFB: if HPFB decides not to grant

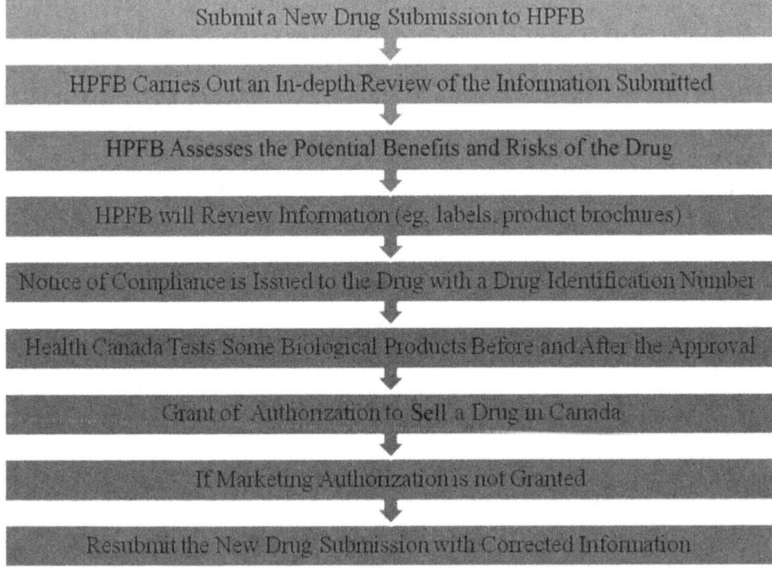

FIGURE 6.3 Flow Chart Depicting the Steps Implicated in the Review Process for a Drug in Health Canada for the Market Authorization in Canada.

registration, the stakeholders can choose to provide additional information, resubmit their additional data at a later date, or ask HPFB to reverse their decision or reconsider. The HPFB has established internationally competitive performance targets for inspections. Moreover, review time depends on the product submitted and the size and quality of the submission and is influenced by HPFB's workload and human resources (Health Canada, 2023).

The HPFB has a priority review programme that expedites the assessment and licensing of promising medicines for the treatment of life-threatening or severely debilitating diseases such as cancer, AIDS, or Parkinson disease, for which few viable treatments are available. Because Health Canada already erased the information, if the applicant wishes to market a product that precisely matches the monograph, the approval procedure will be accelerated. The Product Licensing System of the Natural and Nonprescription Health Products Directorate (NNHPD) allows applicants to cite monographs on certain nonprescription drugs to support the safety and efficacy of these products, allowing DIN registration/authorization applications to be reviewed in a timely manner. The HPFB Special Access Program enables doctors to get drugs that are not currently accessible in Canada. If the Special Access Program authorizes the drug, a doctor may administer it to certain patients if conventional therapy is deemed to have failed or is ineffective. The drug will be released only when the HPFB has determined that there is a real need and a qualified physician has been engaged. Furthermore, drug manufacturers must promise to deliver the medicine to competent, experienced practitioners (Health Canada, 2023).

6.11.3 Monitoring Drugs after Approval

Once a medicine is on the market, regulatory oversight continues. Any new information concerning adverse drug occurrences, side effects, or the medicine not working as planned should be reported by drug distributors. Distributors should also notify the HPFB of any new safety studies and request clearance for any substantial modifications to the drug's production method, dosage regimen, or suggested usage. The HPFB monitors adverse reaction reports, examines complaints and issue reports, and handles recalls as warranted. Furthermore, as a requirement of the license, the HPFB gives licences to most pharmaceutical production units and conducts frequent inspections (Health Canada, 2023).

6.11.4 Drug and Medical Product Submissions under Review

Submissions under Review (SUR) mostly comprise new drug submissions including novel active compounds (i.e., drugs and biological products containing active substances not approved in Canada). The list also contains NDS and S/NDS submissions that have been expressly accepted for evaluation. The list of Generic Submissions under Review (GSUR) contains a fresh list of accepted generic medicine submissions ANDS. The NDS under review, supplementary NDS under review, NDS previously reviewed, and supplementary NDS previously reviewed elements constitute the SUR (disclaimer) list. The four item lists are updated on a monthly basis. When a substance is completed (withdrawn or finalized), it is transferred from the list of submissions currently under review to the list of previously reviewed submissions (Health Canada, 2023).

6.11.5 Decision

When a submission is cancelled or a final decision is made, it is removed from the list of submissions currently under review and added to the list of previously reviewed submissions; if the submission is approved, it is no longer reviewed and can be viewed in the Notice of Compliance database. The Regulatory Decision Summary (RDS) contains information on decisions (both positive and unfavorable) and cancellations. More information is available in the Summary Basis of Decision (SBD) documents, if required (Health Canada, 2023).

6.12 NOTICE OF COMPLIANCE

The Notice of Compliance (NOC) is issued under paragraph C.08.004(1)(a) demonstrating that a manufacturer has fulfilled the requirements mentioned in the paragraph C.08.002 or C.08.003 and C.08.005.1 of FDR. After satisfactory review of the submission, an NOC will be issued to the manufacturer. There are two ways to find NOC information. The NOC's online data reporting is updated weekly on Friday. Compliance and enforcement activities are key elements in the protection of pharmaceuticals and health products offered to the population of the Canada. Essentially, Health Canada is accountable for monitoring compliance and enforcement actions related to drug products to substantiate that requirements related to the drug regulations are being implemented properly. It is Regulatory Operations and Enforcement Branch (ROEB) that develops and execute enforcement plans in these areas. The Health Products Compliance and Enforcement Policy (POL-0001) is related to Health Canada's compliance and enforcement activities for health products covered by the FDA. These products encompass blood for transfusion or employed in drug manufacturing, cells, tissues and organs, drugs (human and veterinary), medical devices, and natural health products (Health Canada, 2023).

6.12.1 Post-Authorization Link

For current market conditions, a supplemental Drug Products Database (DPD) is available on the Health Canada website. The DPD is a list of medications marketed in Canada that guides stakeholders in their choice to commercialize the drug. The website Notices, Advisories, Warnings, and Alerts, produced by the Marketed Health Products Directorate (MHPD), PPD, but not the Biologics and Genetic Therapies Directorate (BGTD), provides safety alerts, press releases, and other industry notifications for stakeholders. The Veterinary Pharmaceuticals Directorate (VDD) issues Notices, advisories, cautions, and Alerts about the safety and efficacy of veterinary pharmaceuticals authorized for use in animals, as well as the safety of people who handle these products or eat food from animals treated with these treatments (Health Canada, 2023).

6.12.2 Enforcement

The Health Products and Food Branch Inspectorate is in charge of Food and Drug Administration Act compliance and enforcement. The quality, health, and safety standards, sale conditions, and fraud prevention of human and veterinary medications, medical equipment, natural health products, biological, and biotechnology-related items are governed by this Act and its supporting rules. Most laboratory activities are inspected, investigated, and licensed as instances of enforcement and compliance measures. The degree of danger to Canadians' health, as well as the risk management decision-making principles contained in Health Canada's decision-making framework, control the Inspectorate's decision-making process. Compliance and enforcement actions should be aimed at the point of distribution as soon as possible for maximum impact and efficiency. Prioritization will be based on risk, whether compliance issues are detected through corporate or customer complaints, or through other ways. If an inspector reports a violation to a regulated party, the regulated party must take timely and appropriate action to comply with legal and regulatory duties. The Inspectorate reviews noncompliance cases to determine the appropriate course of action (Health Canada, 2023).

6.12.3 Summary Basis of Decision (SBD)

The Summary Basis of Decision (SBD) document outlines why Health Canada has granted permission for the sale of certain pharmaceuticals and medical devices in Canada. Regulations, safety, efficacy, and quality are all documented (chemistry and manufacturing). SBDs for pharmaceuticals, biologics, and medical devices are now exclusively accessible through the Drug and Health Product Registry (DHPR) on at the website www.Canada.ca (Health Canada, 2023).

6.12.4 Advertising: Regulatory Requirements

Only Health Canada–approved health items for sale in Canada may be marketed. Advertising for prescription drugs must meet specific criteria. The national regulator of healthcare product advertising is Health Canada. It creates standards for the interpretation of rules, offers strategies for effective regulation of health goods in the marketplace, and monitors regulated advertising. Health Canada is dedicated to ensuring that the information presented in health product marketing is not untrue, misleading, or deceptive. It has the authority to act if the advertisement creates a substantial safety concern, if a resolution cannot be achieved through an independent complaint procedure, if prescription pharmaceuticals are illegally advertised to the public, or if unapproved health items are marketed. An impartial agency reviews and pre-approves advertisements for health items. The list of Canadian preclearance agencies contains contact information and functions for Canadian preclearance agencies (Health Canada, 2023).

- Over-the-counter medicine and natural health product consumer advertising materials are assessed and pre-approved by an independent agency that has publicly proven conformity with Health Canada's recommended certification requirements.
- Advertisement materials for all health-related goods (excluding exempt natural health products) designed for healthcare professionals are examined and pre-approved by Health Canada's recognized independent organization, the Pharmaceutical Advertising Advisory Board (PAAB).
- The Advisory on Prescription Drug Consumer Information and Health/Disease Educational Materials: PAAB, like Advertising Standards Canada (ASC), provides advice on providing prescription drug information to consumers and educational materials dealing with medical conditions/diseases to ensure regulatory compliance (Health Canada, 2023).
- To promote awareness of illegal drug and medical device marketing, Health Canada has established an online portal called Stop Illegal Marketing of Medicines and Devices that explains product advertising regulations in Canada and a fast and easy mechanism for reporting suspected deceptive marketing activities to Health Canada (Health Canada, 2023).

6.12.5 Product Recall

Regarding medical products other than medical devices, the corporation shall not sell, use, or fix disseminated items that represent a health risk to consumers or breach relevant medical product and food sector rules and regulations. Compliance and enforcement actions should be focused as soon as possible at the point of distribution for maximum impact and efficiency. Prioritization will be based on the degree of risk, whether compliance issues are detected through corporate or customer complaints, or through other sources. If an inspector notifies a regulated party of a violation, that party must take quick and appropriate action to comply with legal and regulatory responsibilities. The Inspectorate assesses noncompliance problems to determine the appropriate course of action (Health Canada, 2023).

6.13 CONCLUSION

Health Canada is the government department accountable for drug and drug-related laws in Canada. It aids in the enforcement of national laws in a number of activities related to drug development. Health Canada is also involved in the substantial coordination with a variety of other bodies within the jurisdiction of Health Canada to guarantee the safety of food and drugs, as well as the regulation and supervision of drug-related research, manufacturing, and testing. Health Canada provides regulatory roadmap for the registration, approval, market authorization, and product recall for drugs and drug-related substances. It also offers a mechanism of filing of CTAs, guidelines-related clinical trials, and numerous laws pertaining to drugs and drug-related products under the jurisdiction of Health Canada's authority. Health Canada also offers a special access programme through which healthcare practitioners can request pharmaceuticals that are not currently commercially accessible in the country. Conclusively, Health Canada is accountable for assisting the Canadian populace to maintain and improve their health by guaranteeing the high quality health services works to reduce health risks.

REFERENCES

Ali, H., & Singh, S.K. (2018). Preparation and characterization of solid lipid nanoparticles of furosemide using quality by design. *Particulate Science and Technology*, *36*(6), 695–709. https://doi.org/10.1080/02726351.2017.1295293

Ali, H., Singh, S.K., & Verma, P.R.P. (2015). Preformulation and physicochemical interaction study of furosemide with different solid lipids. *Journal of Pharmaceutical Investigation*, *45*(4), 385–398. https://doi.org/10.1007/s40005-015-0191-2

Aronson, J.K., Heneghan, C., & Ferner, R.E. (2020). Medical devices: Definition, classification, and regulatory implications. *Drug Safety*, *43*(2), 83–93. https://doi.org/10.1007/s40264-019-00878-3

Croghan, I.T., Viker, S.D., Limper, A.H., Evans, T.K., Cornell, A.R., Ebbert, J.O., & Gertz, M.A. (2015). Developing a clinical trial unit to advance research in an academic institution. *Contemporary Clinical Trials*, *45*(B), 270–276. https://doi.org/10.1016/j.cct.2015.10.001

Csóka, I., Ismail, R., Jójárt-Laczkovich, O., & Pallagi, E. (2021). Regulatory considerations, challenges and risk-based approach in nanomedicine development. *Current Medicinal Chemistry*, *28*(36), 7461–7476. https://doi.org/10.2174/0929867328666210406115529

Cutler, I.R. (1993). The drug-device interface. *Medical Device Technology*, *4*(5), 48–51.

Donawa, M.E. (1996). The European regulation of drug-delivery devices. *Medical Device Technology*, *7*(8), 12–16.

Evans, S.J.W., & Day, S.J. (2005). Medicines and healthcare products regulatory agency (MHRA) (Formerly MCA). In *Encyclopedia of Biostatistics*. Academic Press. Peter Armitage & Theodore Colton, 110-124

Ghosh, D., Skinner, M., & Ferguson, L.R. (2006). The role of the Therapeutic goods administration and the medicine and medical devices safety authority in evaluating complementary and alternative medicines in Australia and New Zealand. *Toxicology*, *221*(1), 88–94. https://doi.org/10.1016/j.tox.2005.12.023

Hägglöf, I., & Holmgren, Å. (2012). Regulatory affairs in drug discovery and development. In R.G. Hill & H.P. Rang (Eds.), *Churchill Livingstone* (2nd ed., pp. 285–301). Elsevier Ltd.

Hajizadeh, M., & Keays, D. (2023, March). Ten years after the 2015 Canada Health Transfer reform: A persistent equity concern of insufficient risk-equalization. *Health Policy*, *129*, 104711. https://doi.org/10.1016/j.healthpol.2023.104711

Health Canada. (2023). *Government of Canada*. www.canada.ca/en/health-canada.html

Holloway, V.L. (2003). Ethnic cosmetic products. *Dermatologic Clinics*, *21*(4), 743–749. https://doi.org/10.1016/s0733-8635(03)00089-5

Justice Laws Website, Government of Canada. (2023). https://laws-lois.justice.gc.ca/eng/acts/c-38.8

Morrow, T., & Felcone, L.H. (2004). Defining the difference: What makes biologics unique. *Biotechnology Healthcare*, *1*(4), 24–29.

Sackett, D.L., Rosenberg, W.M., Gray, J.A., Haynes, R.B., & Richardson, W.S. (1996). Evidence based medicine: What it is and what it isn't. *BMJ*, *312*(7023), 71–72. https://doi.org/10.1136/bmj.312.7023.71

Schultz, A., Saville, B.R., Marsh, J.A., & Snelling, T.L. (2019). An introduction to clinical trial design. *Paediatric Respiratory Reviews, 32*, 30–35. https://doi.org/10.1016/j.prrv.2019.06.002

Somberg, J.C. (1996). The evolving drug discovery and development process. In P.G. Welling, L. Lasagna & U.V. Banakar (Eds.), *The Drug Development Process Increasing Efficiency and Cost Effectiveness* (vol. 76, pp. 13–38). Marcel Dekker.

Stouch, T.R. (1996). Computer aided drug design. In P.G. Welling, L. Lasagna & V. Banakar (Eds.), *The Drug Development Process Increasing Efficiency and Cost Effectiveness* (vol. 76, pp. 204–217). Marcel Dekker.

Van Norman, G.A. (2016). Drugs, devices, and the FDA: Part 1: An overview of approval processes for drugs. *JACC. Basic to Translational Science, 1*(3), 170–179. https://doi.org/10.1016/j.jacbts.2016.03.002

Vermeulen, K., Vandamme, M., Bormans, G., & Cleeren, F. (2019). Design and challenges of radiopharmaceuticals. *Seminars in Nuclear Medicine, 49*(5), 339–356. https://doi.org/10.1053/j.semnuclmed.2019.07.001

Willis, S.L., & Lewis, A.L. (2008). The interface of medical devices and pharmaceuticals: Part II. *Medical Device & Technology, 19*(3), 38–43.

World Health Organization (WHO) (2023). Geneva, Switzerland. www.who.int/health-topics/biologicals#tab=tab_1

7 Regulations in Australia and New Zealand

Kumari Neha, Faraat Ali, Gaurav Pratap Singh Jadaun, and Yayra Timothy Tuani

7.1 INTRODUCTION

Globalization affects legal systems tasked with governing the marketing of medicinal items in a variety of ways. Globalization has a role and has worsened the issues faced by regulatory bodies in many complex or contentious parts of drug regulation, such as clinical trials, the regulation of complementary and alternative treatments, and direct-to-consumer pharmaceutical advertising. As the sector becomes more globalized, there is an increasing push to standardize regulatory standards and processes. Harmonization, and more broadly, regulatory convergence, can take several forms, ranging from informal collaboration to full integration of similar regulatory procedures. This research will look at a variety of harmonization aims and models in the field of healthcare product regulation, with an emphasis on a unique proposal in Australia and New Zealand to form a combined therapeutic goods authority. The Australia New Zealand Therapeutic Goods sovereignty project will be examined to characterize the framework of integration that it reflects and to describe the competing priorities that have hampered the project's completion, despite the fact that it is likely the best model to meet the relevant objectives [1].

Both nations have comparable legislative framework for the practice of medicines and therapeutic devices, and they are aiming to develop unified procedures. Although the operations used in both countries to evaluate pharmaceuticals, devices, and services, which would include processes, in New Zealand, the responsibility for pharmaceutical estimation has been merged with that of organizing (which would include purchasing) medical products within a covered budget and has been conferred on a solo government organization (PHARMAC), which also will soon be liable for equivalent handling of healthcare devices.

Although Australians and New Zealanders may see their medicine subsidy regimes as separate, substantial connections emerge when viewed from the other side of the Pacific, both regimes offer a consistent public subsidy to make commonly used pharmaceuticals more accessible and affordable to the public. Other OECD (Organization for Economic Co-operation and Development) nations, such as Canada and the United States, have yet to achieve this level of cooperation [2]. In fact, Australia and New Zealand have distinct spending management systems, resulting in

DOI: 10.1201/9781003296492-8

significant expenditure disparities. Yet, the health results are expected to be comparable. Contracting with pharmaceutical manufacturers is becoming more common, and the use of several legislative measures by the two nations appears to be converging.

Australia and New Zealand are widely recognized across the world for enacting national drugs rules that aim to provide fair entrée to profitable and safe medications. The nations, though, took different paths. In 2011, Australia paid twofold extra than what New Zealand did per capita on medications. The Pharmaceutical Management Agency of New Zealand (PHARMAC) works on a tight budget, which contributes to the disparities. As a result, it pits new drugs contrary to one other and counter to universal entrée to all treatments. The Pharmaceutical Benefits Advisory Committee (PBAC) in Australia likewise analyses the profitable new pharmaceuticals in comparison to the present standard of treatment, but there is no set budget.

The majority of medications financed in Australia but not in New Zealand were extensions to established healing classes rather than novel treatments with significant therapeutic advantages. There is now a proposal to unify medical regulation in Australia and New Zealand through the establishment of an Australia New Zealand Therapeutic Goods Agency, however there are no present tactics to harmonize finance structures.

In Australia, the PBAC makes all of its rulings public, although the judgments imbedded or implicit in these conclusions are rarely disputed. Although there is broad gratification in Australia with admittance to pharmaceuticals, there are worries regarding delayed financing for innovative therapies. Industry-backed organizations such as the Oncology Industry Taskforce and the Cancer Medicines Alliance say that the number of new cancer medications included on the Pharmaceutical Benefits Scheme (PBS) is alarmingly low and advocate for changes to the present financing mechanisms. Yet, Australia recompenses extra over other nations for pharmaceuticals such as statins, which might have been purchased more economically and freed up funding for innovative medicines.

Concerns have been raised in New Zealand concerning availability to expensive pharmaceuticals, red tape in obtaining unpublicized therapies for particular patients, and equal entrée for Māori and Pacific Islanders [3]. Several comments to PHARMAC's community discussion cited poor experiences with medicine shortages and that the economic effect of choices trumped attention of other measures [4]. PHARMAC has declared that it will produce a change proposal in response to this consultation.

The Office of Medicines Safety Monitoring (OMSM) (usually associated with Adverse Drug Reaction Advisory Committee), a division of the Therapeutic Goods Administration (TGA), monitors drug safety in Australia. Medsafe is the supervisory specialist in New Zealand in control of drug care/pharmacovigilance operations. The objective of both regulatory organizations is fulfilled by implementing a system that assures advantages in the use of medicinal items while minimizing possible hazards [5,6]. Both governing bodies possess their own pharmacovigilance regulations and has composed work with other nationwide monitoring premises and the WHO's Global Drug Monitoring Program repository. Since 2012, the European Medicines Agency and the European Commission have had secrecy agreements in place with the TGA of the Australian Administration Branch of Well-being and geriatic to permit the parties to swap data as part of their regulatory and scientific programmes [7].

7.2 AUSTRALIA

Since 2001, the Australian prescription medicine business has seen some variations because of the introduction of several generic medications succeeding the termination of patent protection. A slew of studies published in the years thereafter have found that Australian generic medicines are more expensive than those in other similar nations, with costs approaching those of the corresponding original products. For example, nine Pharmaceutical Benefits Scheme (PBS) drugs were discovered to be more extortionate in Australia than integrated New Zealand and the United Kingdom [8]. Furthermore, research associating the fees (balanced by means of procuring power parity ratios) of 34 medicines in Australia with those in New Zealand, including 12 medications with generic forms accessible, found that Australians paid more for 11 generic medicines than New Zealanders, resulting in an overall cost variance of extra than A$460 million.

Moderately competing on medication price discounts to the government, generic medicine producers competed on giving cheap drug costs to pharmacies. Consequently, the management compensated the chemists at a greater rate than they were rewarded [9,10]. To close the gaps, the Australian administration implemented extensive improvements in PBS administration in August 2007, including changes to compensation agreements amid drugstores and pharmaceutical wholesalers, as well as estimating PBS-registered drugs. This pricing policy change mandated the formation of two different formularies for PBS drugs, F1 and F2, as well as the implementation of price transparency and mandatory price reductions. The Australian government issued a second round of amendments in December 2010, with significant price discounts for medications itemized on the F2 formulary and for first-period enumerated generic drugs [11].

The Expanded and Expedited Price Disclosure strategy required amount revelation for all medicines on the F2 formulary and decreased the amount revelation period from 24 to 18 months. Between April 2012 and August 2014, 160 pharmaceuticals had price reductions as a result of this initiative, with an average price drop of 42% [5]. With the adoption of the Simplified Price Disclosure rule in October 2014, the cycle was further decreased to 12 months, allowing PBS prices to be changed to market pricing extra swiftly.

Even though the change has focused on the generic drug market, concerns have been made about the high pricing negotiated by the pharmaceutical sector for numerous new medicines. As a result, controlled entry contracts have been put in place to provide entrée to select new medications with particular profitable medical manifestations, but with restricted usage outside these scientific suggestions. Some contracts are valuing arrangements in which a cost or capacity deduction is in home, whilst others are performance- or outcome-founded contracts in which attaining specified therapeutic outcomes is required for continuous payment.

TGA is an agency of the Australian Administration's Bureau of Health. The TGA's branches are separated into three key divisions: Market Authorisation, Surveillance and Conformance, and Legal Support. The TGA National Director serves on the US Department of Healthcare Executive Committee and is assisted by a Senior Clinical Consultant and a Primary Administrative Consultant. Australian Public Assessment Reports (AusPARs) include valuation summaries of the medicine's excellence, safety, and effectiveness based on reports made as portion of the TGA's review and managerial process [12]. The TGA follows the Therapeutic Goods Act 1989 and Therapeutic Goods Regulations, which is accountable for the quality, well-being, efficacy, and suitable approachability of medications and medical devices in Australia. The TGA's goal is to guarantee that society as a whole has timely access to medical advancements. No healthcare item is fully hazard-free, and medicines with prescriptions pose the most danger. Prescription drug assessment is the communal image of the TGA, some of the function of TGA. The TGA too controls over the counter drugs, therapeutic devices, vitamin, dietary and herbal goods. There are around 48,000 goods comprised on the Australian Register of Therapeutic Goods (ARTG). This total contains almost 21,000 devices and 27,000 drugs, of which only 3500 are enumerated prescription-only products [13].

The TGA may first become aware of a medicine when a request for commercialization is received or whenever an Australian clinical trial is arranged. In the case of clinical studies, the sponsoring business may submit initial information to the TGA for examination (CTX scheme) or inform the TGA (CTN scheme) if the study has been authorized by an organization's ethic council. Figure 7.1 depicts the drug assessment procedure for novel molecular entities. The chemistry, toxicity, and clinical use of the medicine are examined using data provided by the sponsoring firm. The TGA conducts the majority of the reviews, but external evaluations are permitted. The Australian Drug Evaluation Committee (ADEC) considers the application once all of the data has been assessed. The Minister appoints this committee of doctors to advise on the suitability of medications for marketing in Australia. When reaching a final decision, the TGA considers the recommendations provided by the ADEC.

Prior to the Baume report, the ADEC evaluated practically all medicinal product applicants. Because these kinds of uses typically entail difficult clinical concerns, the ADEC is now only considering novel pharmaceutical entities, new methods of treatment, new fixed arrangements, new treatment signs, and modifications in patient populations. Unless the TGA has advised the denial of the proposal or there are medical difficulties that necessitate the ADEC's guidance, generic medicines, fresh formulations, new abilities, and reformulations involving current drugs are no longer forwarded to the ADEC. TGA functions in pre-marketing evaluation process and also after the marketing of drug. It also helps in conservation of the Australian Register of Therapeutic Goods for the registration and listing of products. It also regulates drug and device exports from Australia. It monitors post-marketing investigation and adverse drug response. It reports complaining about medical device, drug, and device advertising controls.

The TGA has approved the subsequent European Union/International Conference on Harmonisation (EU/ICH) criteria for contaminants in novel chemical entities created by the synthesis of chemicals and their resulting medicinal products:

1. Standards for novel drug substances and innovative drug products approval criteria falls under (CPMP/ICH/367/96 Corr) ICHQ6A.
2. Contaminants testing: contaminants in novel substances for drugs under (CPMP/ICH/2737/99) ICHQ3A(R).
3. Contaminants in new medications (CPMP/ICH/2738/99) ICHQ3B(R2).
4. Genotoxic impurity limitations (CPMP/SWP/5199/02).

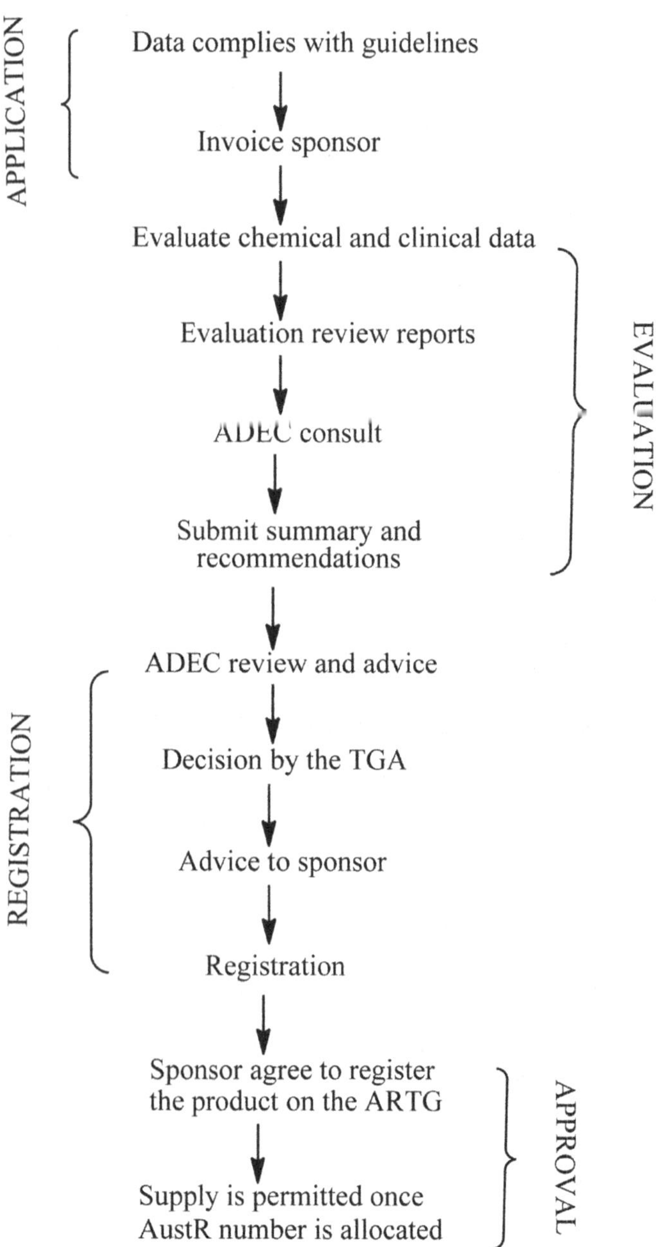

FIGURE 7.1 Drug Evaluation and Registration Process.

The Authorized Prescriber System (APS) and the Special Access Scheme (SAS) are two programs in Australia that allow doctors to use unapproved drugs, biologicals, and medical devices. A doctor is permitted by the APS to administer a certain unapproved substance (or a class of drugs) to specific patients suffering from a specific ailment. A bioethics committee or an expert in a discipline related to the proposed treatment must approve an application for the use of an illegal drug [14]. Unauthorized medications may be used in extreme clinical conditions in single patients in the SAS on a case-by-case basis. All permitted therapy options should have been exhausted before the use of an unauthorized medicine. Also, the doctor must seek the patient's informed consent. SAS is divided into three groups. SAS category A is a notification pathway meant for the action of individuals suffering from potentially fatal conditions. SAS category B is an submission process that doctors can use if their patients do not match the conditions of category A and the medicine is not authorized for supply under category C. TGA must accept Category B applications. An application must include, among other things, a complete scientific explanation, details as to why an approved drug cannot be used in a certain patient, and appropriate evidence on the safety in addition effectiveness of the illegal drug. SAS category C is a notification mechanism that allows clinicians to use medications with a known usage history.

7.3 NEW ZEALAND

Drug price increases were a big issue in New Zealand throughout the 1980s, with some years seeing a 20% increase. Drug price increases have squeezed out other components of healthcare spending. In June 1993, PHARMAC was originated to regulate the administration's expenses on medications in the limits of available funds. PHARMAC's establishment amplified the value struggle between pharmaceutical makers, lessening medicine amounts. The reference pricing system, in which administration reimbursement is secure for all medications within a healing federation, was an important policy employed in achieving price discounts. This strategy requires the producer to either match the reference price for a cluster of medications or risk victim and prescribers selecting a dissimilar treatment because victims pay the difference if the real amount of a drug is greater than the federal reimbursement. Moreover, PHARMAC has been presenting sole source agreements for generic tablets for a quick time in the meantime 1997 to excite the growth of less costly generic forms of off-patent drugs. In reality, tenders are used to acquire half of the entire amount of reimbursed pharmaceuticals [15,16].

One of PHARMAC's rebate techniques is expenditure caps, which operate as risk-division contracts to guarantee that if a listed pharmaceutical's sales volume surpasses an agreed-upon amount, the pharmaceutical maker is answerable for absorbing all or portion of the increased expenses. In the case of cross-product (hustling) treaties, PHARMAC would exchange a price reduction on single or more presently registered medications offered by the pharmaceutical producer who appeals for the entry of a novel medicinal that is clinically useful but not profitable. After the implementation of the National Hospital Pharmaceutical Strategy in 2002, PHARMAC began to undertake the responsibility of functioning the economic plan for inpatient medical products within district health boards (DHBs), enabling each DHB to create its own inpatient medicinal rule judgements and to oversee its own inexpensive budget for inpatient medications. This shift, however, highlighted apprehensions about entrée disparities founded on a patient's location (mentioned as postcode lottery). In July 2013, PHARMAC changed all DHB pharmaceutical rules with the Hospital Medications List, a statewide inpatient pharmaceutical formulary. PHARMAC's reformatory hard work has led to noteworthy investments for numerous medicines over the years, with the amount of statins, for instance, dropping to a fraction of what they were in Australia. According to a Canadian government study, the amount of generic medications in New Zealand is fewer than a fifth of what it is in Canada. Also, patented medications were around 10% less expensive in New Zealand than in Canada [17].

In count to assessing medicine eminence, protection, and effectiveness, the TGA must also examine drug affordability. The ADEC is governed decision over new chemical entities and applications that necessitate professional assessment. Although the ADEC can offer suggestions, the TGA is ultimately responsible for registering a medicine for use in Australia [18-19].

7.4 REGULATION OF HERBAL MEDICINES AND OTHER NATURAL HEALTH PRODUCTS IN AUSTRALIA

The Australian National Medicines Dogma [20] expressly covers herbal medicines (HMs), and the nationwide rule's standards spread equally to the value, harmlessness, and effectiveness of HMs, as well as the excellence practice of other complementary medicines (CMs) in the Australian healthiness scheme. The large percentage of HMs are accessible in Australia as over-the-counter (OTC) medications and are regulated by the TGA. Australia has an associated legislative structure in place, with CMs classified as an overall lesser menace or increased menace. Less hazardous drugs are classified as "Listed" goods, whereas more hazardous medications are classified as "Registered" products. Entire medications in these two classes bear the AUST L or AUST R mark and are appropriate for listing on the Australian Registry of Therapeutic Goods (ARTG) [21]. A handful of HMs are classed as "Exempt" items and are not covered by the ARTG. Australia has about 12,000 CM preparations classified on the ARTG as Itemized items and about 200 CMs as Registered goods [22,23]. Figure 7.2 describes the important characteristics that control whether an HM artefact is classed as Enumerated, Registered, or Relieved. The TGA conducts post-market regulatory operations on both Listed and Registered HMs, such reporting of undesirable events, inspection of producers, and test center examination of goods, in direction to ensure high standards of eminence, safety, and effectiveness of medications. CM marketing is governed by governing rules outlined in the Therapeutic Products Publicity Code 2005 [24]. A plethora of

Application

Inspect to determine if the information adheres to Australian standards [19]
Invoice the sponsor for 75% of the evaluation price.

Assessment

- Examine pharmacological and chemical information;
  Examine animal pharmacology and toxicity information; and
  Examine clinical information
  The assessment unit evaluates reports (and, if necessary, arranges external evaluations), writes a summary, and offers an preliminary suggestion.
  Discussion with the patron prior to ADEC meetings
  Preparation of authorized product information (PI) and consideration of consumer product information (CPI)
  Deliver closing summary and recommendation set to ADEC (6 meetings each year)

Sanction

- ADEC analysis and recommendation to the TGA
- TGA final choice
- Finalize registration requirements
- Assistance to sponsor, invoice final 25% of assessment fee
- For novel chemical entities, guide medication management centers, forensic laboratories, etc.

Registration

- Sponsor submits an application to register the product on the ARTG
- Supply is authorized after an AustR number is assigned

FIGURE 7.2 The Procedure for Evaluating and Registering Drugs (ADEC Stream).

commerce organizations (Australian Self Medication Industry and Complementary Medicines Australia) similarly regulate promotion over the enforcement of intended rules of training (own-supervisory cryptographs). The Act supports the requirement for balanced and accurate promotion of therapeutic items, endorses excellence practice of medications, and urges Australian people not to self-medicate for healthiness concerns that require proficient assistance. Publicity items with instructions for usage for an alarming healthiness illness (such as stomach or duodenal ulcer, HIV contagion, and tumor) is forbidden, particularly where a finding needs communication with a highly competent health expert [25].

CM labeling is likewise strictly controlled. Labeling of HM goods in Australia must adhere to a set of norms and laws, which include a number of particular restrictions [26]. In Australia [27], info on the label of HM goods essentially be presented in English and should include the title of the artefact, its sign for use, suggested dose, and medicinal instructions for practice, altogether potent therapeutic components or elements, and in the instance of natural health products (NHPs), the herbal fragment used and the dosages or parched mass correspondent dose, as well as the individuality and stages of any predefined ingredients. Labels should also carry cautionary or warning words that are required for proper product usage, which might comprise inadequate or constrained usage in particular demographic segments of the people, such as prenatal or nursing females.

7.5 NZ'S CURRENT CONTROLLING OUTLINE FOR HMS AND OTHER NHPS

Herbal remedies are currently classified as a special subcategory of treatments in New Zealand, as definite in section 2 of the Medicines Act 1981 [27]: herbal medicine means a medicine (not being or consisting a prescribed medication, constrained medicine, or pharmacy-only medicine) comprised of (a) any ingredient generated by exposing a herbal to drying, pulverizing, or any other comparable procedure; or (b) a mixture containing 2 or more such compounds only; or (c) a combination of one or more of these compounds with water, ethanol, or another inert material.

Ministry agreement is not mandated for the dispersion of a herbal therapy that is traded or delivered deprived of any suggestion as to its usage and where the labeling cooperates with the necessities of section 28 of the Medicines Act; nevertheless, governmental permission is needed for the transmission of a herbal therapy that is sold with an advice for usage for a medical applications (however, this is overlooked by few dealers and is not continuously obligatory by the supervisory form). Consequently, herbal medications are excluded from the necessity to get premarket legislative permission based on adequate proof of superiority, safety, and effectiveness, and are not now obliged to comply to good manufacturing practice norms (GMP) [28].

An additional exclusion, known as the herbalists exception, under section 28 of the Medicines Act, allows anyone to make and sell or contribute medicinal herbs for government if the therapy is to be traded or distributed underneath a certification that clarifies only the shrub from which it is created and the method to which the herb has been exposed throughout the manufacturing of the cure, and does not implement any other term to the medicine; and deprived of any documented suggestion (whether through a branded vessel or suite or a pamphlet or in any other technique) as to the usage of the therapy [27]. A supplementary exclusion underneath section 32 situations that any normal health professional or other individual may produce and sell, wrap, listing, by department stores, or deliver in conditions correlating to commercial sale, any drug that is an over-the-counter medication, a constricted drug, or a pharmacy-only drug, for administering to a specific individual after being invited by or on behalf of that individual to practice their particular opinion as to the conduct needed. These exclusions are meant to let natural healthcare and extra clinicians to manufacture herbal mixtures and other personalized ordinary health therapies for individuals, not to allow large-scale HM production.

The majority of additional NHPs are now controlled as "dietary supplements" (few of which might comprise plant-based components) under the Dietary Supplement Rules 1985 and the Food Act 1981 [29,30]. The Dietary Supplement Rules 1985 impose limited limits on dietary supplement components, and no beneficial privileges are permitted; similarly, to "herbal remedies," the production of dietary extras does not need GMP compliance or premarket consent.

In March 2010, modifications to the Dietary Addition Ordinance 1985 limited the description of nutritional additives to therapeutic-type goods only, and culpability for these goods was passed from the New Zealand Food Safety officialdom to Medsafe, New Zealand's regulatory specialist for medications and medical tools [31]. This came after ideas for a combined Australia New Zealand Therapeutic Products Authority (ANZTPA) failed to get legislative approval in New Zealand [32]. The combined authority would have been in charge of regulating pharmaceuticals in Australia and New Zealand, counting CMs/NHPs, medical machines, and blood products. Because Australia already has CM laws, ANZTPA would have imposed CM regulations in New Zealand.

The ANZTPA plan was resurrected in 2011, but NHPs were initially excluded [33]; NZ then announced its intention to implement national laws for this type of goods [34]. The Australian and New Zealand governments reached an agreement in November 2014 to end attempts to establish a combined medicinal goods regulator (Figure 7.3) [35].

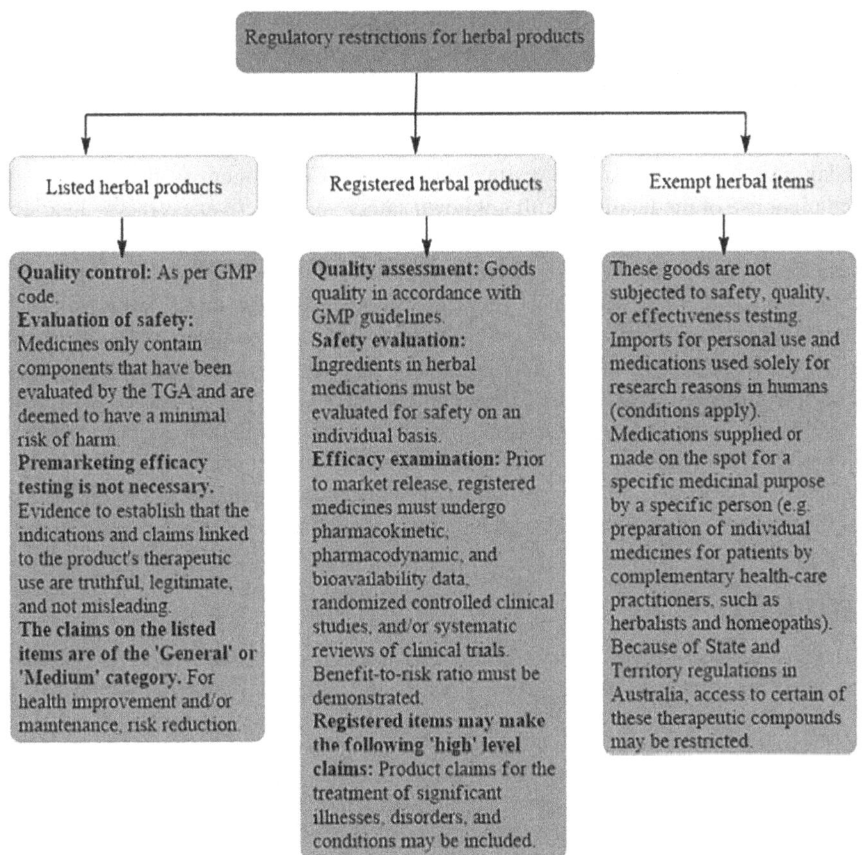

FIGURE 7.3 Australian Supervisory Boundaries for Herbal Remedies, Containing the Associated Circumstances.

7.6 CONCLUSION

In conclusion, this study has revealed crucial insights into drug users' attitudes toward legal drug source models and controlled drug marketplaces, counting sustenance for such replicas, as well as worry and skepticism about the régime's role in drug parameter and their lives. These results compel us to explore how drug supply management may systematically regulate drug users, therefore repeating and strengthening oppression against this group. To guarantee that their different viewpoints are taken into account, one method to minimize the maintenance of these organizational harms may be to expressively incorporate individuals who use medicines in the debate, design, and provision of a safer drug stream. A significant minority of defendants in this model of Australian festivalgoers indicated fright consumption and core concealment of unlawful drugs (in reply to drug patrolling). These answers add to the indication that castigatory drug enforcement somewhat lowers the likelihood of drug-linked damage. These discoveries support the shift away from disciplinary medication strategies at jubilees and toward policies centered on public health. Crucially, the statistics indicate that drug exoneration containers must not be considered as an satisfactory approach to prevention harms or as a replacement for other outcomes-based measures (e.g., drug examination).

Australia has implemented regulatory laws that allow clinicians to employ unapproved pharmaceuticals (most commonly investigational drugs undergoing clinical trials); and treatment using investigational medical equipment is permitted. Yet, medicinal use of medications with unknown safety and effectiveness raises a variety of moral concerns. Physicians considering compassionate usage should be aware of these issues; the Declaration of Helsinki and several nationwide codes of remedial ethics offer rules that may assist them in establishing high moral values of such therapy. NZ must review its worldwide keenness in the countless workings of the drug expansion worth chain and create reliable plans to provision the country's drug development industry's continued development.

NZ should strengthen its partnership with Australia to benefit on both nations' strengths. They ought to work together to establish strong partnerships with other nations in Asia-Pacific that have excellent drug discovery capabilities, as well as market the region's competence to the global pharmaceutical sector in a coordinated way.

REFERENCES

[1] Babar, Zaheer-Ud-Din, Vitry, Agnes. Differences in Australian and New Zealand medicines funding policies. *Aust Prescr.* 2014;37:150–151. http://doi.org/10.18773/austprescr.2014.059

[2] Organisation for Economic Co-operation and Development. *Health at a Glance 2013. OECD Indicators*. Paris: OECD Publishing; 2013 [cited 2014 Jun 20]. Available from: www.oecd.org/els/health-systems/Health-at-a-Glance.2013.pdf

[3] Babar, Z., Francis, S. Identifying priority medicines policy issues for New Zealand: A general inductive study. *BMJ Open* 2014;4:e004415

[4] Pharmaceutical Management Agency. *PHARMAC's Decision Criteria: Summary of Submissions*. Wellington: PHARMAC; 2013 [cited 2014 Jun 20]. Available from: www.pharmac.health.nz/assets/decision-criteria-summary-of-submissions-2013-12.pdf

[5] Dr. Arlene Amor, Pharmacovigilance in Australia and New Zealand. Available from: www.pharmoutsourcing.com/Featured-Articles/37484-Pharmacovigilance-in-Australia-and-New-Zealand/#:~:text=Drug%20safety%20in%20Australia%20is%20regulated%20via%20the,agency%20responsible%20for%20overseeing%20drug%20safety%2F%20pharmacovigilance%20activities
[6] Tga [Regulatory Requirements for Clinical Trials. A Comparison of Australia and the US. 2020]. Available from: https://novotech-cro.com/sites/default/files/2020-02/Australia%20Reg%20and%20Tox%20requirements_March%202020.pdf
[7] www.ema.europa.eu/en/partners-networks/international-activities/bilateral-interactions-non-eu-regulators/australia
[8] Hasan, S.S., Kow, C.S., Dawoud, D., Mohamed, O., Baines, D. Pharmaceutical policy reforms to regulate drug prices in the Asia Pacific region: The case of Australia, China, India, Malaysia, New Zealand, and South Korea. *Value Health Reg Issues* 2019;18:18–23.
[9] Lofgren, H. Generic medicines in Australia: Business dynamics and € recent policy reform. *South Med Rev* 2009;2(2):24–28.
[10] Bulfone, L. High prices for generics in Australia: More competition might help. *Aust Health Rev* 2009;33(2):200–214.
[11] Australian Government, Department of Health and Ageing. *The Impact of PBS Reform: Report to Parliament on the National Health Amendment (Pharmaceutical Benefits Scheme) Act 2007.* Barton, Australia: Commonwealth of Australia; 2010.
[12] Papathanasiou, P., Brassart, L., Blake, P., Hart, A., Whitbread, L., Pembrey, R., Kieffer, J. Transparency in drug regulation: Public assessment reports in Europe and Australia. *Drug Discov Today* 2016;21(11):1806–1813.
[13] Vaughan, G. The Australian drug regulatory system. *Aust Prescr* 1995;18:69–71.
[14] Borysowski, J., Górski, A. Compassionate use of unauthorized drugs: Legal regulations and ethical challenges. *Eur J Intern Med* 2019;65:12–16.
[15] Pharmaceutical Management Agency. *Operating Policies and Procedures of PHARMAC (the Pharmaceutical Management Agency)* [cited 2017 Jun 1]. Available from: https://www.pharmac.govt.nz/about/operating-policies-and-procedures
[16] Pharmaceutical Management Agency. *Our History* [cited 2018 Jan 13]. Available from: www.pharmac.govt.nz/about/our-history/
[17] Pharmaceutical Management Agency. *Prescription for Pharmacoeconomic Analysis: Methods for Cost-Utility Analysis* [cited 2017 Aug 1]. Available from: www.pharmac.govt.nz/assets/pfpa-2-2.pdf
[18] Vaughan, G. The Australian drug regulatory system. *Aust Prescr* 1995;18(3). http://doi.org/10.18773/austprescr.1995.068
[19] Therapeutic Goods Administration. *Australian Guidelines for the Registration of Drugs. Volume 1: Prescription and Other Specified Drug Products.* Canberra; 1994. Available from: www.nps.org.au/australian-prescriber/articles/the-australian-drug-regulatory-system#
[20] Australian Government, Department of Health. *National Medicines Policy* [cited, 2016 Feb 18]. Available from: www.health.gov.au/nationalmedicinespolicy
[21] Australian Government, Department of Health. *An Overview of the Regulation of Complementary Medicines in Australia, Therapeutic Goods Administration* [cited 2016 Feb 18]. Available from: https://www.tga.gov.au/overview-regulation-complementary-medicinesaustralia
[22] Expert Committee on Complementary Medicines in the Health System. *Complementary Medicines in the Health System, Report to the Parliamentary Secretary to the Minister for Health and Ageing*, Commonwealth of Australia; 2003 [cited 2016 Feb 10]. Available from: www.tga.gov.au/sites/default/files/com mittees-eccmhs-report-031031.pdf
[23] Sansom, L.D.W., Horvath, J. *Expert Review of Medicines and Medical Devices Regulation—Stage Two, Report on the Regulatory Frameworks for Complementary Medicines and*

Advertising of Therapeutic Goods [cited 2016 Feb 18]. Available from: www.health.gov.au/internet/main/publishing.nsf/Content/Expert-Review-ofMedicines-and-Medical-Devices-Regulation

[24] Australian Government, Department of Health, Therapeutic Goods Administration. *Therapeutic Goods Advertising Code* [updated 2015 Nov; cited 2016 Feb 10]. Available from: www.tga.gov.au/publication/therapeutic-goods-advertising-code

[25] AustralianGovernment,DepartmentofHealth.TherapeuticGoodsAdministration.*Advertising of Complementary Medicines, Australian Regulatory Guidelines for Complementary Medicines (ARGCM)*, Version 5.3 July 2015 [cited 2016 Feb 18]. Available from: www.tga.gov.au/book/complementary-medicinesexemptexcluded-certain-regulatory-requirements

[26] Australian Government, Department of Health, Therapeutic Goods Administration. *Exempt Medicines, Australian Regulatory Guidelines for Complementary Medicines (ARGCM)*, Version 5.3 [cited 2016 Feb 10]. Available from: www.tga.gov.au/book/complemen tary-medicines-exemptexcluded-certain-regulatory-requirements

[27] Medicines Act 1981 as at 1 July 2014 [cited 2016 Feb 10]. Available from: www.legislation.govt.nz/act/public/1981/0118/latest/whole.html

[28] Barnes, J., McLachlan, A.J., Sherwin, C.M.T., Enioutina, E.Y. Herbal medicines: Challenges in the modern world. Part 1. Australia and New Zealand. *Expert Rev Clin Pharmacol* 2016. http://doi.org/10.1586/17512433.2016.1171712

[29] Dietary supplement regulations 1985 (SR 1985/208). Reprint 2010 Mar 31 [cited 2016 Feb 10]. Available from: www.legislation.govt.nz/regulation/public/1985/0208/latest/DLM102109.html

[30] Food Act 1981. Reprint 2014 Jun 24 [cited 2016 Feb 10]. Available from: www.legislation.govt.nz/act/public/1981/0045/latest/DLM48687.html

[31] Dietary supplements amendment regulations 2010 [cited 2016 Feb 10]. Available from: www.legislation.govt.nz/regulation/public/2010/0005/latest/whole.html

[32] Australia New Zealand Therapeutic Products Authority (ANZTPA) postponed. 2007 [updated 2015 Nov 6; cited 2016 Feb 10]. Available from: www.tga.gov.au/media-release/australianew-zealand-therapeutic-products-authority-anztpa-postponed

[33] Australia New Zealand Therapeutic Products Agency (ANZTPA). *Trans Tasman Ministerial Council Agrees Foundations for Joint Therapeutic Products Regulator* [cited 2016 Feb 10]. Available from: www.medsafe.govt.nz/hot/anztpa.asp

[34] Ministry of Health, The Development of a Natural Health Products Bill. *Agency Disclosure Statement. Regulatory Impact Statement* [cited 2016 Feb 18]. Available from: www.health.govt.nz/system/files/documents/pages/natural-health-products-bill-ris_0.pdf

[35] Joint statement by Hon Peter Dutton MP, Minister for Health for Australia, and Hon Dr Jonathan Coleman, Minister of Health for New Zealand, regarding ANZTPA. 2014 Nov 20 [updated 2015 Aug 11; cited 2016 Feb 10]. Available from: www.tga.gov.au/media-release/joint-statement-hon-peter-dutton-mp-minister-health-australia-and-hon-dr-jonathan-coleman-minister-health-new-zealand-regarding-anztpa

8 Regulations in China

Varisha Anjum, Khushboo Sharma, Pritya Jha, Irina Potoroko, and Rishi Kumar

8.1 INTRODUCTION

China's regulatory climate has always been quite difficult. On the other hand, the China Health Authority started revamping the regulatory environment to bring China's medical products up to international standards in 2015 to increase the public's demand for drugs and to develop the process of access to novel drugs and therapies worldwide in terms of efficiency, safety, and quality. However, adjustments are made to ensure that procedures for developing new pharmaceuticals go smoothly, including adopting general standards and technology criteria, enhancing review and approval openness, and speeding up the review and approval of new drugs.

China's well-being authority has likewise delivered rules to direct medication improvement in terms of correspondence for drug advancement and specialized assessment, electronic normal specialized record execution, and post-endorsement security observation. China's well-being authority has likewise delivered guidelines including need survey and endorsement, and information security system, imported drug enrollment, and new synthetic medication characterization to support innovative medication advancement [1]. After the United States, China has the second-largest global pharmaceutical market, which is constantly expanding. With a typical growth rate of 5%, it is predicted that it will reach $161.8 billion in 2023 and capture 30% of the global market. A variety of opportunities are presented to the drug industry by the quickening pace of new medicine access, altering administrative landscapes of different classes, rapidly developing Chinese society, and consequently increasing clinical needs. The criteria and regulations for enlisting pharmaceuticals have seen some adjustments after 13 years, according to the Chinese administration. The progress made is to decrease the intricacy and coordinate with the other worldwide controllers [2].

The China Food and Drug Administration (CFDA), which is greatly impacted by the Drug Administrative Organization section for service of well-being, is the national drug administrative power in China. The CFDA was founded by the Chinese Ministry of Health in March 1998. Previously known as the State Food and Drug Organization of China (SFDA), the CFDA primarily oversees medication production, trade, and enrollment. The establishment of a single drug administrative authority was a crucial step in organizing unrestricted access; the CFDA also has affiliated divisions that play a crucial role in the Drug Administrative Organization. The CFDA is continuously improving despite its awareness of its limitations and is trying to uphold its standards in accordance with EU, US, and Japanese regulations. CFDA is placing importance on developing

DOI: 10.1201/9781003296492-9

innovative drugs in addition to traditional medications (which are bioequivalent to those in trendsetter drugs) to advance drug guidelines and ensure security and practical use. The Chinese administrative authority is continuing to uphold its insurance of protected innovations and further putting forth more efforts on administrative lucidity [3].

The purpose of this chapter is to give a detailed account on the major administrative changes starting around 2015 that occurred in China to accelerate the new medication advancement and enrollment in accordance with worldwide principles and to carry Chinese clinical items to the worldwide level [1].

8.1.1 Affiliated Organizations and Their Functions

China's regulatory body is the China Food and Drug Administration (CFDA), formerly the State Food and Drug Administration (SFDA). In March 2013, the administrative body was renamed and rebuilt as the CFDA to upgrade it to a clerical level agency. By substituting a huge number of covering controllers with an organization like the Food and Drug Administration of the United States, the CFDA simplified the procedures for creating guidelines for the security of food and drugs. The People's Republic of China's State Council is directly responsible for extensive oversight over the executives of food, well-being food, and beauty care products, and the China Food and Drug Administration is the competent power of medication guidance in the country's central region.

The FDA, which is under the regulated control of the service of well-being, inspired the creation and modernization of the Chinese Drug Administrative Power, which was designed to replace the state Drug Organization. The CFDA oversees all drug enrollments and endorsements. To make the activities more convenient, the CFDA has five associated units, as shown in Table 8.1 [4].

8.1.2 Key Ministries

NHFPC: The Ministry of Health and the National Family Planning Commission merged to form this agency in 2013, and it oversees regulating medical treatment. The executives of the Essential Drug List (EDL), include medicine choice and offering, organization of the New Cooperative Medical Schemes (NCMS), general direction for medical service change, advancement of public clinic and critical consideration change.

NDRC: The National Development and Reform Commission's (NDRC's) primary responsibility is to monitor, foresee, and control the cost of pharmaceuticals, medical equipment, and clinical benefits. It houses the High-Innovation Industry Office, which organizes important steps toward the advancement of new companies. Additionally, it used to impose price ceilings for medications up until June 2015, but those were eliminated.

Ministry of Human Resources and Social Security: This service deals with the Urban Employee Basic Medical Insurance (URBMI) and Urban Employee Basic Medical Insurance (UEBMI) plots and is additionally answerable for the National Reimbursement Drug List (NRDL).

8.1.2.1 Supporting Ministries

Ministry of Finance: The NHFPC, the Ministry of Human Resources and Social Security, and the Ministry of Civil Affairs all have expenditure plans that are drafted

TABLE 8.1
Affiliated Units of CFDA and Their Functions

S. No	Affiliated Units of CFDA	Functions
1	NICPBP	The National Institute for the Control of Pharmaceutical and Biological Products (NICPBP) primarily examines drug samples and confirms the standards for drug goods.
2	CDE	In conducting scientific reviews including pharmacology data reviews, toxicological data reviews, clinical related data reviews, and pharmacy related reviews, the Centre for Drug Evaluation (CDE) department is crucial.
3	CCD	The Chinese Drug Regulatory Authority established the Certification Committee for Drugs (CCD Committee) to develop standards for good laboratory practices (GLP), good clinical practices (GCP), good agricultural practices (GAP), good supplying practices (GSP), and good manufacturing practices (GMP). It also conducts inspections on the specifications for conducting studies.
4	CDR	The Centre for Drugs Re-evaluation (CDR) Committee was primarily established to offer technical assistance to the CFDA. It is charged with re-evaluating drugs, reviewing their safety on the market, eliminating unsafe drugs, and keeping track of adverse drug reactions.
5	CPC	The Chinese Pharmacopoeia Commission (CPC) primarily creates the Chinese Pharmacopoeia, an official compendium of drugs that provides details on each drug based on purity, potency, storage, and dosage form criteria.

by the Ministry of Finance. Additionally, they collect information on various health insurance schemes and deal with how the central government sponsors local governments to support healthcare.

Ministry of Civil Affairs: The Ministry is responsible for maintaining a social safety net for the most vulnerable people in urban and rural areas, a responsibility that extends to granting access to medical care.

Ministry of Industry and Information Technology: This Ministry also directs the use of rankings of drug organizations for carrying out the drug portion of the 12th Five Year Plan. The Ministry provides the plan for making antibodies, supports the board responsible for supplying essential medications, and oversees the main reform of the pharmaceutical industry.

Ministry of Commerce: The Antimonopoly Bureau and the Market Order Office, both of which are responsible for testing restraint infrastructures, managing local protectionism, and collaborating with other divisions to combat licensed innovation freedoms, encroachment, forging, and other types of misrepresentation, perform the bulk of the Ministry of Commerce's duties in the field of healthcare. Additionally, the Ministry controls commodities and imports, which affects imported pharmaceuticals.

Chinese Insurance Regulatory Commission: The Commission oversees commercial health insurance regulation.

8.1.2.2 Other Key Government Agencies

The CFDA is crucial because it is the main regulatory body for pharmaceuticals. It is in charge of registering and examining medicines, medical equipment, food, and cosmetics in China. It is where the Centre for Drug Evaluation (CDE), the CFDA's technical evaluation branch, is situated. It offers policies on GMP and GLP in addition to rules for GSP and GCP. To ensure compliance, it performs inspections. It establishes the norms of practice for clinical chemists, oversees their registration, and controls the regulation of Traditional Chinese medicine (TCM).

State Intellectual Property Office: The Office oversees China's patent and intellectual property laws and carries out court orders in cases involving these matters.

State Administration for Industry and Commerce (SAIC): The Ministry of Commerce is better able to combat monopolies, unfair business practices, and illegal activities including bribery and smuggling.

State Administration of Traditional Chinese Medicine: This is the agency responsible for coordinating and promoting the research and development (R&D) of TCM and in formulating TCM-related policies.

Non-State Council actors: The involvement of two actors who are not State Council members must be mentioned. The Anti-Corruption Office, a part of the Supreme People's Procuratorate, the highest court in China, deals with bribery and graft, misappropriation of public funds, as well as other acts of corruption and criminal behavior. The People's Liberation Army, the country's armed forces, operates a few military hospitals. For instance, there are provincial food and drug administrations, health and family planning commissions, development and reform commissioners, and human resources and social services departments.

8.2 DRUG REGULATION AND LAWS

Prior to 1989, the Chinese Ministry of Health (MOH) had already set up ten pilot monitoring centers around China; the data were mostly acquired through written studies, case reports from healthcare facilities, and patient interviews. The MOH designated the Adverse Drug Reaction (ADR) Monitoring Centre with oversight of both classes of medications in 1989. In 1998, the Center signed up for the World Health Organization International Drug Monitoring Program. In 1999, China's organizational, associational, and regulatory frameworks were enhanced by the National ADR Monitoring Centre. For locating, logging, and managing occurrences involving drug safety, the ADR monitoring system is essential.

The performance of the Centre has improved thanks to several rules issued by MOH and CFDA between 1999 and 2011. The Adverse Drug Reaction Reporting and Monitoring Provision (MOH and CFDA, 2011) underwent a significant amendment in 2011. Additionally, it improved the technical standards for ADR assessments to promote ADR research, reinforced the roles of drug manufacturers, and most significantly, it introduced the concepts of focus monitoring and ADR information management. For example, the Good Manufacturing Practice for Drugs (2010 Revision) (MOH and CFDA, 2010) chapter 10 section "Complaints and Adverse Reaction Reports" was created specifically to strengthen the accountability of pharmaceutical manufacturers with demands for a dedicated ADR monitoring team to collect, inspect, and manage ADR reports, take charge of pharmaceutical risk management, and report ADRs to the Pharmaceutical Supervisory and Administrative Department.

8.2.1 Reinforcing Regulation during and after Drug Administration

The Chinese government has pushed for broad reforms "to streamline administration, delegate powers, and improve regulation and services" to encourage innovation in regulatory concepts, systems, and procedures and to establish and further develop a new administrative framework linking the entire administrative cycle when medications are promoted. The recently passed Drug Administration Law stipulates that "departments for drug administration will generate records of the reliability of drug safety, boost the amount of supervision and inspections for entities with a record of unreliability, and possibly implement joint punishment in accordance with State regulations." The law specifies an information sharing system and a medication traceability system. To achieve drug traceability, promote drug safety regulation, and increase regulatory competency, reliability and information regulation are used.

8.2.2 Developing and Improving Extensive Laws and Regulations on Drug Administration

In comparison to the previous version, the new Drug Administration Law's (DAL) goals, chapters, organization, logic, and guiding principles have all undergone significant revision. In comparison to the 2015 revision's 10 chapters and 104 articles, the new DAL has 12 chapters and 155 articles. Chapters on organizations allowed to sell drugs, drug stocks and supply, drug post-marketing management, and other subjects are now included in the new law.

8.2.3 Embodying the Rule of Law and Flexibly Controlling and Regulating Drug Administration

The pharmaceutical industry is at the forefront of innovation and study. Problems spanning law, science, and technology continue to emerge as a result of the fast growth of information technology and artificial intelligence. In addition to restating the legal definition of drugs, the new DAL also adopts a "general" legislative definition of drugs for the first time, as opposed to a "specific" definition.

The DAL has undergone numerous changes, ranging from conceptual changes to substantive changes, as part of a scientific approach to lawmaking, or "from tweaks to extensive revision." This enhanced the logical coherence of the legal framework, the thoroughness of the amendments, and the viability of the legal provisions. Therefore, new legal safeguards for domestic drug control have been enacted, and China's pharmaceutical affairs legislation has been revised and improved [5].

8.3 ORGANIZATION

Thirty-four province level monitoring branches were also formed by the CFDA National Adverse Drug Reaction Monitoring Centre, which is associated with the

Chinese Ministry of Health. The number of people using electronic submissions has been rising rapidly in recent years. In 2010, there were roughly 40,826 registered users (pharmaceutical firms and healthcare organizations), of which 21,785 (53.40%) were healthcare organizations, 15,919 (39.0%) were firms, and 3122 (7.50%) were other users and people. The general public can also telephone or fax case reports to local or provincial monitoring centers; the personnel will fill out a report form (CFDA, 2011) [6].

8.3.1 New Drug Application and Approval Procedures

The registration and licensing of new pharmaceuticals for sale in the People's Republic of China region are referred to as New Drug Applications. Applications for altered medication formulations, altered administration and release routes, altered illness severity indicators, and altered drug indications are just as well considered as those for novel drugs. According to the Drug Administration Law of the People's Republic of China, a new drug cannot be made available on the market until it has obtained all required CFDA approvals, which include those for the clinical trial approval (phases I, II, and III), the Certificate for New Drug, the New Drug Registration Certificate, and the Drug GMP (good manufacturing practices) Certificate. Each stage is meticulously examined and assessed by an expert team that has been given permission by the CFDA. The Chinese central government encourages innovation and has established a speedy evaluation and approval process for groundbreaking new drugs and other crucial drugs that are meant to treat serious emerging and reemerging diseases that pose a serious threat to public health, such as AIDS, cancer, and other diseases.

For the examination and approval of novel pharmaceuticals, China has two phases. The application and approval of a new drug's clinical trial research constitute the first stage. The second step covers the registration permission to produce a unique drug for market launch. The sponsor of a novel pharmaceutical development project must complete preclinical investigations before applying for clinical trial research. The following factors play a role in the process of creating a new drug, the extraction method, the physicochemical properties, purity, formulation assessment, prescription screening, manufacturing process, testing procedures, quality control reference standards, stability, pharmacology, toxicity, and animal pharmacokinetics are all covered in preclinical studies. Researchers should strictly abide by the regulations that the CFDA imposed on preclinical studies and gene therapy products. SiBiono GeneTech and the National Institute for the Control of Pharmaceutical and Biological Products [NICPBP], 2004) recommend considering human gene therapy and product quality control. To seek the beginning of a clinical study for a novel drug, the applicant must complete the necessary papers, provide the necessary data, and submit a product sample to the nearby FDA office. The applicant should conclude the examination within 30 days and submit an assessment of the new drug's intellectual property status in the application form. The provincial FDA office is required to organize and conduct a site visit within five working days of receiving the application, and to complete the inspection within 30 days, to assess the circumstances surrounding the creation of the new medicine. Three successive sets of product samples must be inspected and tested against a reference standard as per the NICPBP requirements. In addition to informing the applicant, the NICPBP must give the CFDA the assessment results, inspection report, and application materials within 60 days. The CDE of the CFDA convenes an expert panel to assess the new drug application after receiving all application materials. In a period of 120 days (or 100 days for a fast-track review), the CDE is obligated to submit the findings of the evaluation to the CFDA.

It takes 195 days (155 days for fast-track assessment) to examine and approve a clinical trial study for a new medicine. The CFDA strictly regulates the requirements for clinical trial investigator groups. Clinical trial studies can only be carried out by recognized medical facilities or those that take part in the National Base for Clinical Trials of New Drugs. The Good Clinical Practice (GCP) Quality Control Guidelines for Drug Clinical Studies should be followed when conducting clinical studies. The facility where the medication for the clinical trial is made must meet the Quality Control Guideline for Drug Manufacturing standards. Patients shall make up at least as many recruits as specified by the Code of Regulation for Drug Registration. The sponsor of the new medicine may apply for registration, production, and approval of the new drug when the phase III clinical trial study is over. The applicant is required to submit the clinical trial results, together with any other materials—such as directions for the production and quality control of the drug—to the local CFDA office for review once the phase III clinical trial study is over. Three manufacturing cycles must result in three times as many testing samples as are needed for product release testing. Before being transported to the NICPBP for analysis, the samples are sealed. The timely delivery of assessment findings, inspection reports, and application documents to the CFDA is overseen by the provincial FDA office. After receipt of all assessment reports, the CFDA has 30 days (20 days for fast-track evaluation) to notify the sponsor of unqualified and rejected applications. For successful applications, the CFDA provides the sponsor with a Drug Registration Certificate and a New Drug Certificate. A sponsor may also be awarded an approval number at the event provided they are qualified to produce the newly authorized medication and have previously secured a Drug GMP Certificate. After receiving an approval number from the CFDA, a sponsor is permitted, in accordance with the People's Republic of China Regulation for the Implementation of the Drug Administration Law, to ask for a Drug GMP Certificate. The CFDA gives the producer this certificate after concluding that the field inspection of the manufacturing facility was successful. After getting the Drug GMP Certificate, the applicant is required to submit its revised drug-pricing strategy for approval to the State Pricing Bureau. To conduct the phase IV clinical study after the product is introduced to the market, the business must register with the CFDA [7].

8.3.2 Classification of Drug Registration Application

1. New drug application;
2. Application for the drug standardized by the state (which used to be called generic drugs). These are roughly equivalent to Abbreviated New Drug Applications in the United States or Submissions in Canada;
3. Import drug application;
4. Supplementary application.

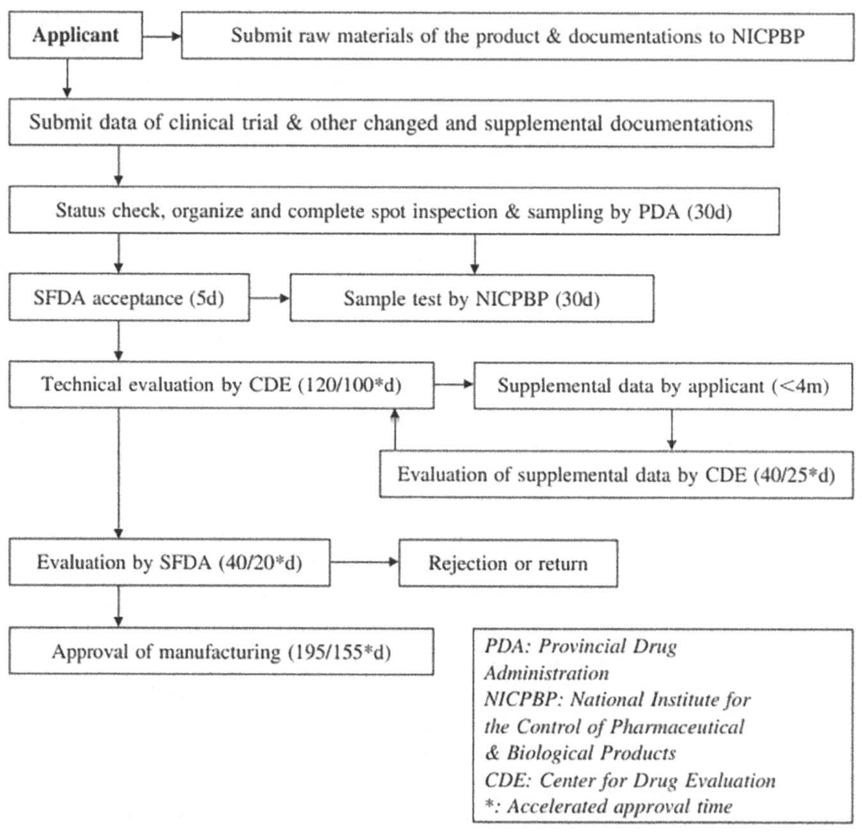

FIGURE 8.1 Diagrammatic Representation of New Drug Evaluation and Approval in China.

8.3.3 Protection of the Undisclosed Trial Data in Drug Application

The state safeguards the information obtained by the manufacturer or distributor of drugs that include novel chemical substances and for which a manufacturing or distribution license has been granted and approved, including unpublished trial findings and other data. It is forbidden to exploit the secret trial and other confidential information for nefarious commercial endeavors. Within a period of 6 years of the drug manufacturer or distributor receiving acceptance for the production or dispersal license of the drug that included the new chemical entity, the drug regulatory authorities will not permit the use of the proprietary data to apply for the manufacture and distribution of the new chemical entity without the licensee's consent. This is the guarantee needed to be granted a privilege in connection with China's World Trade Organization participation [8].

8.3.4 Role of Regulation and Stages Involved in Development of Drugs

Even though the industry is still in its infancy, China is one of the largest pharmaceutical marketplaces in the world. This fact may be attributed to the magnitude of the country's population. Within the next 10 years, the country may become a more sophisticated market because of the dynamics of economic and demographic development, government stimulus, increased public health awareness, market consolidation, and improved R&D capabilities [9].

8.4 DRUG APPROVAL PATHWAY IN CHINA

The Drug Registration Regulation, which debuted in 2007 and underwent revision in 2013, lays out the rules governing the existing procedures for medicine endorsement in China [10]. The CFDA's route determines the timeline for new medications to be approved [11]. Clinical preliminary applications are necessary; this is similar to the investigational new drug framework in the United States. After preliminaries are finished, organizations are then ready to present a New Drug Application (NDA) for survey. NDAs are explored by the CDE, the CFDA's specialized arm. The CFDA has its own principles for GCP, GLP, and GMP. Although these principles have been improving since their foundation in 1999, they do not yet arrive at global guidelines [11]. In China, there are many routes for NDAs, which are often divided into synthetic, organic, and TCM. Pharmaceuticals produced locally (exclusive or nonexclusive) first seek approval through a common food and medication organization unit and then require CFDA approval, but pharmaceuticals produced by international organizations go directly through the CFDA [12]. The CFDA recently released guidelines for evaluating biosimilars, a market with enormous potential in China [13]. There are six distinct application paths [1,11,14] for compound drugs.

8.4.1 Category Description

I. A novel medicine that has not yet received approval in any other countries.
II. Drugs seeking clearance for a novel method of administration that has not received approval elsewhere.
III. Drugs that are authorized in other nations but not in China.
IV. Drug created by altering the metallic components or acidic or alkaline radicals in the salt of a medication licensed in China without altering the medication's original pharmacological effects.
V. A medicine licensed in China that was given a different dose form without altering the way it was administered.
VI. A generic medication in China that satisfies national norms.

The most often looked for routes are multiregional clinical preliminary I, III, VI, and a combination of I and III. Note with the worldwide application situation, organizations foster another medicine totally outside of China, get a declaration of drug item, and afterward can look for endorsement inside China by means of a class III application [15].

Class I applications are the most resource intensive and require completing China's whole drug development procedure. Class III applications cost less money but must be begun after receiving the global drug item testimony. Multiregional clinical preliminary applications fall about evenly into classes I and III and are becoming more and more well known, but recently the public authority has mandated the submission of an additional clinical preliminary application after the approval of a medication item and before the NDA, posing serious obstacles [10]. Ultimately, class VI applications require a type of restricted bioequivalence testing (and, surprisingly, this was not needed before 2007). Organizations face critical deferrals in trusting that the CFDA will support both new and nonexclusive drugs on account of the enormous number of uses consistently, a huge existing excess, and deficient staff to manage the responsibility. The CFDA put up another draft regulation necessitating the creation of new enrollment classes for synthetic drugs in November 2015 [6]. There will be five classes for new medicine enlistments under the suggested framework. Classes I and II, which will be used independently, will be for novel drugs that have not been promoted elsewhere and for "moved along" pharmaceuticals that have not been promoted anywhere (such as modifications in structure, measurement structure, course of organization, etc. that have a clear therapeutic advantage). Classes III through V would be for nonexclusive medications, or characterized drugs that are as of now sold somewhere else. Curiously, this intends that on-patent medications promoted abroad yet not in China would enter as a class III nonexclusive rather than a class I or II creative medication [16-17]. Under China's present framework, getting market approval is dependent upon having an assembling office prepared to do really delivering the medication. This has restricted the capacity of R&D associations (e.g., colleges) from commercializing the medications they create and has prompted an unreasonable measure of assembling limits.

8.4.2 Drug Registration Process

The main regulatory body in charge of managing drug registration, establishing drug registration terms, and setting up drug registration review and approval is the National Medical Products Administration (NMPA). Drug clinical trial uses, drug marketing authorization applications, supplementary applications, and drug re-registration applications for pharmaceuticals produced overseas are all reviewed by the CDE. The Marketing Authorization Holder (MAH) may submit applications for drug clinical trials, drug marketing authorization, re-registration, and supplemental applications.

8.4.3 Medicinal Product Registration Categories in China

The necessities to develop and register a medicinal product in China depend on further classification:

1. Chemical medicine
2. Biological products
3. TCM.

Each type is then grouped into three enlistment classifications, which decide the materials that the candidate should give as a component of its enrollment application model clinical preliminary application, advertising approval application, and so forth.

Registration Categories for Chemical Medicines

1. Innovative drugs
2. Improved new drugs
3. Generics.

Registration Categories for Biologics

1. Innovative biological products
2. Improved new biological products
3. Marketed biological products (including biosimilars).

The relevant application material criteria are based on the product attributes, level of innovation, and review management requirements of the registered medications. Depending on the drug class an applicant chooses to register under, the evaluation and approval procedure for clinical trial applications is established. The clinical trial application is governed by NMPA. A period of 5 years is required for the marketing authorization holder's pharmaceutical enrollment endorsement to be valid. The MAH should be responsible for the welfare, viability, and quality controllability of the recorded medications during the validity period and should apply for drug re-enrollment 6 months before the validity period expires.

8.4.4 Registration Fees for Review and Approval

A charge must be paid by the applicant in accordance with any applicable laws. The NMPA collects drug registration fees to examine and approve clinical studies as part of the medication registration process. The prices vary depending on the following kinds of medications.

- New medications produced in China and those produced elsewhere.
- Generic medications produced both inside and outside of China.

8.4.5 Highlights of China's New Provisions and Opportunities for Drug Registration

The highlights of new provisions made by the Chinese regulators are as follows (Figure 8.2):

- The 60-day window for Clinical Trial Application (CTA) endorsement in accordance with international standards.
- Streamline procedures between medication registration and manufacturing authorization to ensure GMP.
- Clearly defined deadlines for reviewing and approving various types of drug registration applications.
- Enhancing communication between applicant and CDE for a successful CTA procedure.

- The adoption of comparable risk-based site inspections and lab test registration transfers.
- In China, a breakthrough, conditional approval during the clinical trial stage, and priority review during marketing approval expedite the registration of drugs and address unmet medical needs [18].

8.5 STAGES INVOLVED IN DEVELOPMENT OF GENERIC DRUGS

The term "generic drug" refers to a "drug product that is similar to the quantitative and qualitative composition of brand/reference listed drug." A generic product needs to meet certain requirements before it can be approved for marketing in China by the CFDA.

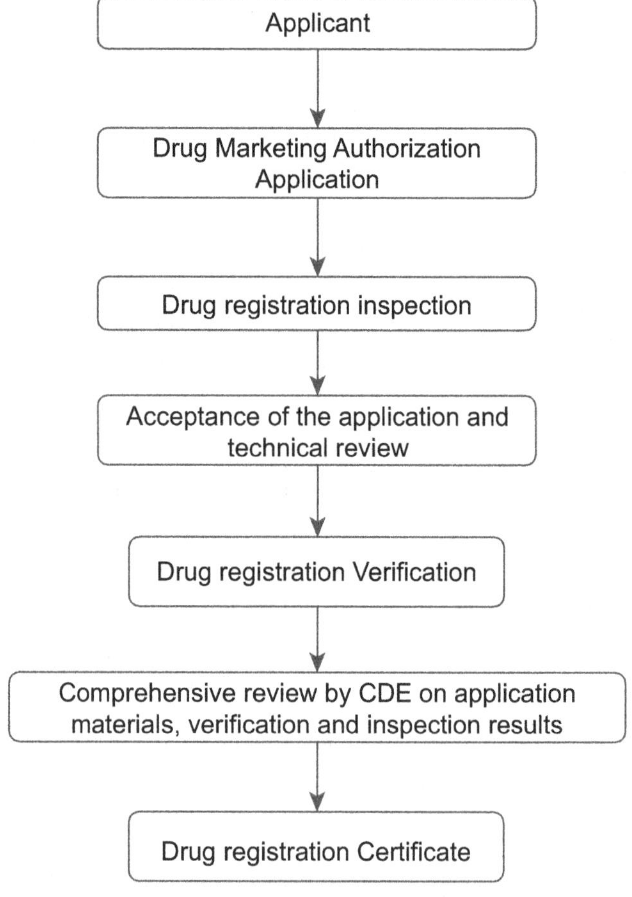

FIGURE 8.2 Drug Registration Process in China.

8.5.1 Steps Involved in Registration of Imported Drugs in China

In China, a representative may approve the registration of a generic product. Pharmaceutical product makers from abroad not having legal representation in China must use agent services to register their products. The CDE conducts the assessment process after receiving an application from the CFDA (Figure 8.3) [19–21].

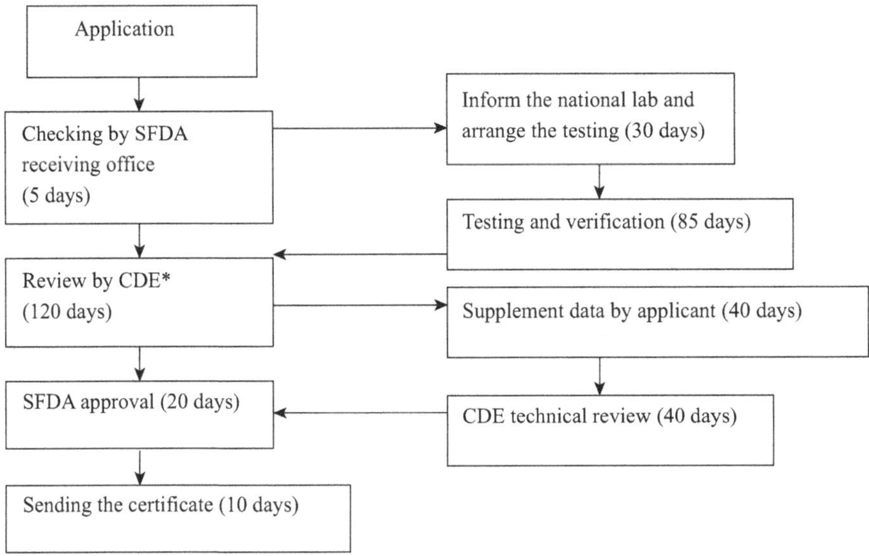

FIGURE 8.3 Imported Drug Registration Process (Before Clinical Study).

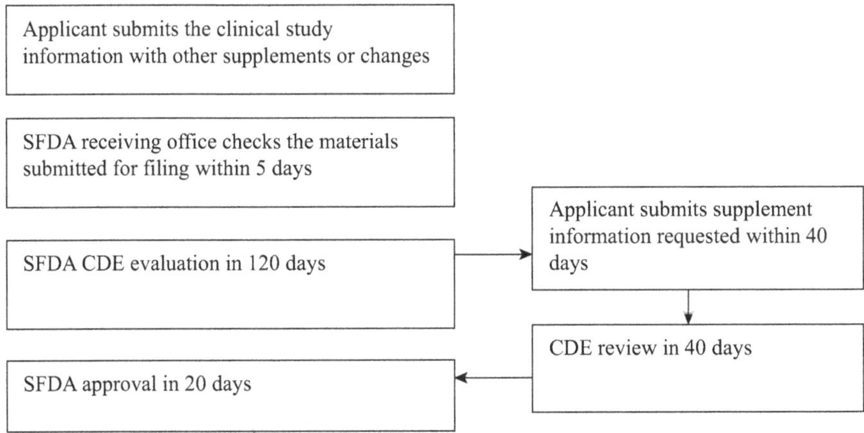

FIGURE 8.4 Imported Drug Registration Process (After Clinical Study).

8.5.2 Requirements for Drug Registration

In China, the registration file or dossier is submitted to the CFDA in accordance with the International Council for Harmonisation–Common Technical Document format specifications [22,23] This format specifies that the registration file or dossier must include five modules, which are shown in Table 8.2.

8.5.3 Regulation of Advertising

China forbids direct-to-consumer (DTCA) advertising for prescription pharmaceuticals, which is one of the key contrasts between China and the United States in terms of how drug advertising is regulated. Pharmaceutical businesses are allowed to market to customers under the US Constitution's protection of commercial free speech [24]. Considering this industry resistance, the destiny of the proposition stays muddled. Commercials of physician-recommended drugs are restricted to state-endorsed clinical and drug proficient distributions. Two offices under the State Council, the managerial office for well-being (up to this point, the Ministry of Health), and the medication administrative division (presently, the CFDA) mutually assign the rundown of endorsed distributions. China additionally rigorously directs notice content and requires endorsement preceding send-off. According to Section 60 of the DAL, any advertisements for prescription or over-the-counter (OTC) drugs must first have

TABLE 8.2
Modules of Registration File or Dossier

S. No.	CTD Modules Content	Description
1.	Administrative (legal) information and prescribing information	Contains legal information and records of application forms or labels that are being considered for usage in the region.
2.	Summaries of CTDs	A major portion of a CTD is the general introduction to pharmaceutical and pharmacological classes, which includes information on business names, medication products, dosage strengths, drug administration methods, safety, effectiveness, and quality.
3.	Quality information reports	For the production, chemistry, and controls of drug products, the required quality papers are built with pharmaceutical, chemical, and biological information on quality provided in a structural format.
4.	Reports of nonclinical study	According to M4S's recommendations, the safety should be available in a specified structured manner that includes a typical analysis of non-clinical data.
5.	Reports of clinical study information	The M4E standard requires that effectiveness data be given in a structured fashion that includes summaries of clinical information on pharmacodynamics, clinical pharmacology, clinical safety and efficacy, pharmaceuticals, and pharmacokinetic studies.

Provincial Food and Drug Administration (PFDA) approval in the territory, independent local, or area where the candidate is found. For medicine advertisements, it is essential that the claims made be true, accurate, and supported by information available in the recommended package insert [25]. Prohibited explanations incorporate security or viability correlations with different medications or depictions of paces of viability (e.g., fixed rates) [26]. Likewise, notices should incorporate the medication's nonexclusive name, the commercial endorsement number, the medication fabricating endorsement number, and other explicit explanations.

If the product is a prescription drug, the advertisement must state that "this advertisement is only for medical or pharmaceutical professionals." If the drug is an OTC medication, the advertisement must include "please purchase and use in accordance with the drug instructions or under the supervision of a pharmacist" and contain the OTC symbol. Even though advertising is strictly regulated, enforcement is hampered by ambiguous legal language, relatively weak fines, and a lack of government resources. In the Administration Law (AL) and Drug Administration Law (DLA), the definition of "advertisement" is not entirely clear. The AL defines the word as "commercial advertisements that, directly or indirectly, and through particular media or forms, publicize some kind of commodities or services at the expense of the suppliers of the commodities or services" [27]. The concept does not clearly distinguish between advertising and non-commercial promotion in addition to being self-referential. Self-printed fliers that advertise drugs are subject to regulations [28].

According to Chinese regulations, the administrative penalties for running drug advertisements without prior approval from the relevant PFDA are limited to (1) the issuance of an administrative order to cease advertising; (2) the confiscation of funds or fees for the advertisement; (3) the issuance of a fine equal to one to five times the advertisement fee; (4) the temporary suspension of drug sales regionally or nationally; and (5) the issuance of a public notice about the violation [29]. The punishment is only necessary—and is only imposed—when unapproved medication marketing encourages off-label usage, substantially inflates efficacy, or seriously misleads consumers [30], even though the temporary suspension of sales can be a significant deterrent. When the makers or distributors make the required remedial announcements on local television or in newspapers, the sales suspension is often removed. As an illustration, Jiangsu's PFDA lifted its sales ban 2 months after the firm published clarifications in two newspapers [31]. The SAIC or the local Administration for Industry and Commerce (AICs) may administer penalties (1) through (3), but only the CFDA or the PFDAs may impose penalties (4) and (5).

Due to their superior industry expertise and experience, the CFDA and PFDAs often undertake drug advertisement violation inspections. If the local AIC has the power to impose the desired punishment, the CFDA or PFDA will transfer the matter to that AIC for administration. Manufacturers may face criminal sanctions for "false advertisement" if they generate a sizable illicit profit, injure consumers significantly, or engage in other severe behavior [32] Criminal fines and/or up to 2 years in jail are the possible penalties under Article 222 of the Criminal Law. There are not many reported convictions for deceptive drug promotion, and even fewer reported criminal charges. For instance, three people were charged in 2012 in what was reportedly China's first criminal case using a televised misleading drug advertisement [33].

Commercial pre-approval and, to a certain extent, enforcement are handled provincially as opposed to nationally, and this results in varying degrees of regulations and enforcement because of disparities in provincial resources and government ability. Nonetheless, regulators are working harder. For running unlawful marketing, the PFDAs have shut down the sales of an increasing number of medications over the previous 5 years [34].

8.5.4 Regulation of Non-Advertising Promotion

Because professional magazine advertising is severely prohibited in China and the DCTA is also prohibited, practically all promotion of prescription medicines is done without the use of advertising. Contrary to the United States, there are no legislative restrictions on the non-advertising promotion of medications. Consumer protection laws in China only provide a general prohibition on deceptive and false advertising of any kind of goods [35]. Although this requirement superficially resembles the criteria in the United States, they are not the same in practice. The fundamental distinction is that promotional content is not required by law or regulation to convey relevant facts or to provide accurate information. According to a legal interpretation from the Supreme People's Court of China, the following advancements may be deemed false and deceptive: (1) a biased promotional introduction of a product; (2) the presentation of speculative scientific theories or phenomena as defensible; and (3) the use of any other deceptive techniques in a promotion. The Chinese Supreme People's Court has provided important advice on what is considered "false and misleading," but the SAIC has not. Advertising that is blatantly exaggerated to prevent confusing the general public is not regarded as deceptive advertising, according to the legal perspective.

8.6 CONCLUSION

China is currently one of the top producers of medicines in the world thanks to the creation of a regulatory structure based on the FDA, which has resulted in the construction of a centralized system and increased openness in healthcare regulatory propaganda. Over the last 30 years, China has effectively built up a very efficient drug regulatory system from almost nothing thanks to its national agenda of reform and opening-up. The CFDA and its affiliated units are crucial to this system because they evaluate drug registration applications and make decisions regarding approvals. The CFDA is constantly improving and correcting its shortcomings while maintaining its standards in accordance with those of the top regulatory principles of the EU, United States, and Japan. It was determined that these associated departments or units are very important in the assessment of drug registration requests.

In this chapter we learned the requirements and rules for enrolling in conventional medicine in China from the review. To be authorized for promotion in China, a generic product must meet the standards defined by the China Food and Drug Administration (CFDA). As a result, we divided the registration criteria for nonexclusive medications in China in our agenda, which we established at the conclusion of the emphasis. The future will see further expansion of non-exclusive medicine advertising due to China's most rising commercial sector. So, when focusing on this market, one should constantly consider the nature of Active Pharmaceutical Ingredient (API) and continually ask the API provider/manufacturer from China for the Drug Master File (DMF) or specialized record for API.

Every drug development paradigm has advantages and disadvantages depending on the regulatory climate in China today. Companies should evaluate and choose the model that best fits their pipeline items for development in China early in the drug advancement development process. This assessment should be done while considering the company's portfolio, primary concern, competitors, specifics of the product or programme, and assets from both a global and Chinese perspective. Important success factors for making an informed decision and designing and implementing a China development program include having the "trust factor" with regulatory agencies, the capacity to add regulatory insight, develop sound regulatory strategies, and navigate the Chinese regulatory system, as well as strong local medical and drug development proficiency.

REFERENCES

[1] Yi Yang, Novartis. China NMPA Reform and New Regulations/Guidelines/Requirements. PharmaSUG, 2019; SS-14.
[2] https://credevo.com/articles/2021/02/25/china-drug-registration-process/
[3] Department of State Food and Drug Administration (SFDA) Guidelines on Data Required for Approval for Marketing a New Drug [Internet]. 2014 [cited 2014 Jan]. Available from: www.sfdaChina.com/info/80-1.html
[4] Nadipineni AK, Dileep KG, Ravindra CK, Suthakaran R. An overview of Chinese drug regulatory system: A review. *International Journal of Drug Regulatory Affairs*. 2018;2:14–18.
[5] www.ncbi.nlm.nih.gov/pmc/articles/PMC6929591
[6] www.sciencedirect.com/science/article/pii/S0378874112001122
[7] hum.2006.17.970.pdf.
[8] Zhen LH. The drug registration application. *Journal of Pharmaceutical Sciences*. 2003;6(2):211–214. Available from: www.ualberta.ca/~csps
[9] CHINA—Growing and Distinctive Pharmaceutical Market [Internet] CFDA [updated 2015 Feb; cited 2014 Dec 15]. Available from: http://eng.sfda.gov.cn/WS03/CL0756/
[10] McTiernan R. Regulatory infarction: CFDA clogs new drug pipeline. *CPB Review*. 2014c;87:18–23.
[11] https://studylib.net/doc/18893289/optimizing-drug-registration-in-china—category-i-route
[12] https://cms-lawnow.com/en/ealerts/2016/03/new-chemical-drug-registration-classification-applied-in-china
[13] McTiernan R. E-retailing: Alibaba or the forty thieves. *CPB Review*. 2014b;82:24–28.
[14] China CFDA (SFDA) Regulations [Internet]. 2014 [cited 2014 May]. Available from: www.sfdaChina.com/
[15] Su L. Drug development models in China and the impact on multinational pharmaceutical corporations. *Food and Drug Law Institute Update*. 2013:19–23.
[16] https://cms-lawnow.com/en/ealerts/2016/03/new-chemical-drug-registration-classification-applied-in-china
[17] https://cms-lawnow.com/en/ealerts/2018/11/extension-of-pilot-period-of-mah-holder-system

[18] Yan J. *An Overview: New Drug Registration System and Approval Process in China.* Beijing: Covance Pharmaceutical; 2013.

[19] Registration Categories of Drugs and Applications [Internet] CFDA; 2013 Dec 6 [cited 2014 Dec 18]. Available from: http://eng.sfda.gov.cn/WS03/CL0769/98158.html

[20] Steps Involved in Registration of Imported Drugs in China [Internet] CFDA; 2013 Dec 6 [cited 2014 Dec 17]. Available from: http://eng.sfda.gov.cn/WS03/CL0769/98162.html

[21] General Requirements for Application Dossiers [Internet] CFDA; 2013 Dec 6 [cited 2014 Dec 12]. Available from: http://eng.sfda.gov.cn/WS03/CL0766/61638.html#01

[22] Hulianwang yaopin xinxi fuwu guanli banfa [Measures Regarding Internet Information Services for Drugs] (promulgated by CFDA, May 28, 2004, effective July 8, 2004), Art. 10 (P.R.C.). Available from: www.sfda.gov.cn/WS01/CL0053/24486.html

[23] Ma FJ, Lou N. Regulation of Drug Promotion in China. *Update.* 2013:6–9.

[24] Yaopin guanli fa [Drug Administration Law] (promulgated by StandingComm. Nat'l People's Congr., Feb. 28, 2001, effective Dec. 1, 2001), Art. 61 (P.R.C.). Available from: http://former. sfda.gov.cn/cmsweb/webportal/W45649037/A48335975.html

[25] Guanggao fa [Advertisement Law] (promulgated by Standing Comm. Nat'l People's Congr., Oct. 27, 1994, effective Feb. 1, 1995, Art. 14, Law Info China (last visited March 3,2013) (P.R.C.).

[26] Yaopin Guanggao Shencha Fabu Biaochun [Standards of Review of Applications for Drug Advertisements], Art. 8.

[27] Bulletin Publicizing Violations of Rules on Advertisements for Health Food, Drug and Medical Device. Available from: www.sfda.gov.cn/WS01/CL0085/

[28] Weifa guanggao gongshi zhidu [Establishment of the Publicity System for Illegal Advertisements] (promulgated jointly by CFDA, SAIC, the Ministry of Health and a Number of Other Government Agencies, Nov. 21, 2006). Available from: www.law-lib. com/law/law_view.asp?id=181703

[29] Yaopin guanggao shencha banfa [Measures for Review of Applications for Drug Advertisements] (promulgated by CFDA, May 1, 2007), Art. 21. Available from: http:// eng.sfda.gov.cn/WS03/CL0768/61649.html

[30] See Jiechu zanting xiaoshou yi qi congming wan de gonggao [Notice of Removal of Sales Suspension of "Yiqi Conming" Pills] (promulgated by Jiangsu PFDA, Jan. 31, 2012). Available from: www.jsfda.gov.cn/art/2012/2/1/art_325_95908.html

[31] See Criminal Law, Art. 222; see also Zuigao renmin jianchayuan, gonganbu guanyu gongan jiguan guanxia dexingshi anjian lian zhuisu biaozhun diguiding [Supreme People's Procuratorate and the Ministry of Public Security's Prosecution Standards for Criminal Cases under the Jurisdiction of the Public Security Organs], Art. 75. Available from: www.mps.gov.cn/n16/n1282/n3493/n3778/n4303/2417768.html

[32] http://zqb.cyol.com/html/2012-06/28/nw.D110000zgqnb_20120628_1-08.htm

[33] See Jiangsu zanting xiaoshou "nujin dan wan" deng qi zhong weifaguanggao yaopin [Jiangsu Suspends Sales of Seven Drugs that Violate Drug Advertisement Laws]. ChIna Med. Rep. Available from: www.chinamsr.com/2012/0703/52820.shtml

[34] Xiaofei zhe quanyi baohu fa [Law on the Protection of Rights and Interests of Consumers] (promulgated by the Standing Comm. Nat'l People's Cong., Oct. 31, 1993, effective Jan. 1, 1994), Arts. 19, 50, Law Info ChIna (last visited March 3, 2013); *see also* Fan bu zhengdang jingzheng fa [Anti-unfair Competition Law] (promulgated by the Standing Comm. Nat'l People's Cong., Sept. 2, 1993), Art. 9, Law Info ChIna (last visited March 3, 2013).

[35] Guanyu shenli bu zhengdang jingzheng minshi anjian yingyong falu ruogan wenti de jieshi [Judicial Interpretation on Application of Anti-Unfair Competition Law at Trials] (issued by Sup. People's Ct., Jan. 12, 2007), Art. 8. Available from: www.court.gov.cn/ qwfb/sfjs/201006/t20100609_5953.htm

9 Regulations in India

Arvind Kumar Sharma, Tarani Prakash Shrivastava, Meghna Amrita Singh, Jitin Ahuja, and Ramesh K. Goyal

9.1 HISTORY AND EVOLUTION OF DRUGS REGULATION IN INDIA

India has an interesting past of traditional medicines and herbal remedies dating back thousands of years [1]. As the country progressed and modernized, the need for robust drugs regulation became increasingly evident. Over the years, India has implemented various measures to ensure the safety, efficacy, and quality of drugs available to its vast population [2]. India's ancient medical systems, such as Ayurveda, Siddha, and Unani, laid the foundation for healthcare practices in the country. These systems emphasized the use of natural remedies and plant-based medicines. During this period, regulation primarily occurred through personal expertise and informal community-based practices, with knowledgeable individuals serving as healers and practitioners [2,3].

9.1.1 Colonial Era and the Birth of Drug Regulation

With the arrival of the British in the 17th century, western medicine and pharmaceutical practices gained prominence in India. The establishment of the Bengal Chemical and Pharmaceutical Works in 1901 marked the first step toward organized drug manufacturing [4]. The British government introduced the Indian Medical Council Act in 1933, which aimed to regulate medical education and standardize medical qualifications. After gaining independence in 1947, India recognized the need for a more comprehensive drug regulatory system. The Drug Control Authority (DCA) was established in 1940 under the Drug Control Act of 1950, which served as the primary legislation governing drug regulation. The DCA's role included licensing, inspection, and quality control of pharmaceutical products. However, the system faced challenges because of limited resources and evolving pharmaceutical practices [5].

9.1.2 Establishment of Drug Jurisdictions

The British India government formed the Drug Enquiry Committee under the Chairmanship of Col. R.N. Chopra on August 11, 1930, to study the issues related to the profession of pharmacy and its various aspects in India. This committee was later known as the Chopra Committee [6]. The committee studied the extent to which

DOI: 10.1201/9781003296492-10

drugs and chemicals of impure quality or defective strength, particularly those recognized by the British Pharmacopoeia, are imported, manufactured, or sold in British India and to make necessary recommendations for controlling such activities in the interest of the public. Further, the committee also examined the need for qualified professionals to practice the profession of pharmacy and generate legislation for these concerns. In 1931, the committee submitted its report that there is no organized and self-contained profession of pharmacy in India, compounders were merely trained in the pharmaceutical sciences and were only able to read English written on the prescriptions [7]. The Drug Enquiry Committee also recommended the compilation of Indian Pharmacopoeia containing monographs on drugs, pharmaceuticals, and indigenous preparations. However, these recommendations could not be implemented for various reasons. Later in 1932, Prof. Mahadeva Lal Schroff initiated pharmacy education in Banaras Hindu University, several other universities followed suit and started degree courses in pharmacy [7,8].

Based on the recommendations of the Chopra Committee Report, the Government of India brought out the Import of Drugs Bill in 1937. However, this Bill was severely criticized as the major recommendations were not adopted, and it was withdrawn because of this criticism [6].

In 1940, the British Government of India presented the Drugs Bill with the objective of regulating the import, manufacture, sale and distribution of drugs in the country. After taking public opinion and screening through a selection committee, this Bill was finally adopted as the Drugs Act, 1940. Drugs rules to this Act were further published in 1945. In its first amendment, in 1962, the Drugs Act became the Drugs and Cosmetics Act (D&C Act) by incorporating cosmetics within its purview. The D&C Act has been amended several times since then [9].

In 1961, the Indian government enacted the D&C Act, which marked a significant turning point in drugs regulation. Under this Act, the Central Drugs Standard Control Organization (CDSCO) was established as the primary regulatory body. The CDSCO took charge of drugs approval, clinical trials, licensing, and ensuring adherence to quality standards of drugs. During the 1970s and 1980s, India witnessed a surge in pharmaceutical research and development. The country became known for its generic drug manufacturing capabilities, making essential medicines more affordable and accessible. However, the need for stricter regulations became apparent as the pharmaceutical industry grew rapidly, leading to concerns about quality and safety [9,10].

India's Patents Act of 1970 played a key role in shaping drugs regulation [11]. This act allowed the country to produce generic versions of patented drugs, which helped maintain affordability and access to essential medicines. However, the Trade-Related Aspects of Intellectual Property Rights (TRIPS) agreement signed in 1995 obligated India to strengthen its patent laws, leading to subsequent amendments in the Patents Act. In 1997, the National Pharmaceutical Pricing Authority (NPPA) was established as an independent regulatory body under the Department of Pharmaceuticals, Ministry of Chemicals and Fertilizers. It is responsible for fixing and regulating the prices of essential drugs in India [12,13].

Recently, in 2019, New Drugs and Clinical Trials Rules have helped to streamline the approval process for new drugs and clinical trials that paved the way for seamless business opportunities in pharmaceutical sector seeding innovations, patient safety, and ethical practices in the process of drug development [14].

9.2 PHARMACEUTICAL REGULATION FRAMEWORKS

Drugs regulation in India is a composite process managed by law, mainly the Drugs and Cosmetics Act of 1940, and by multiple ministries, including the Ministry of Health and Family Welfare. The law creates a web of regulatory authorities to govern the process at both the central and the state level. Further, to this act there are various other specified acts and regulations that form the mesh of the legal ecosystem for drugs and other medical products in India [15].

9.2.1 Acts and Rules Governing Drug Regulation

The D&C Act, 1940, deliberates the central government with the authority to regulate the importation, production, and sale of drugs and cosmetics in India [9,10,16]. This includes defining standards for quality and establishing regulations for the identification of misbranded, adulterated, and spurious drugs products. Moreover, the central government possesses the power to impose restrictions or regulations on the import, production, sale, and distribution of drugs products in the interest of the public, and to issue directives to state governments as necessary. State governments, on the other hand, are responsible for implementing the D&C Act, 1940, and rules 1945 thereunder. The D&C Rules 1945 provide further elaboration on various matters such as the appointment, powers, and responsibilities of government analysts and drug inspectors, as well as regulations pertaining to licensing, storage, sale, display, inspections, and confiscations.

9.2.1.1 Objectives of the Drugs and Cosmetics Act, 1940

The D&C Act aims to hold medical technology and pharmaceutical companies accountable for negligence and sub-standard services provided by them. A major objective of enacting this legislation was to prevent adulteration in medicines. Some other objectives are also discussed below:

1. To regulate the sale, import, and distribution of drugs and cosmetics by means of licensing.
2. To ensure that only qualified individuals are involved in the import, distribution, and sale of drugs and cosmetics.
3. To prevent substandard quality of drugs to maintain high medical treatment standards.
4. To regulate the production and sale of Ayurvedic, Siddha, and Unani drugs.
5. To form a Drugs Technical Advisory Board (DTAB) and Drugs Consultative Committees (DCC) for allopathic and allied drugs, as well as cosmetics.

9.2.1.2 Wings under the Drugs and Cosmetics Act, 1940

The Drugs and Cosmetics Act established three wings with proper authorities to ensure accurate regulation and administration of the Indian pharmaceutical industry. These wings are:

1. Advisory wing, which consists of two bodies:
   a. Drugs Technical Advisory Board (DTAB)
   b. Drugs Consultative Committee (DCC).
2. Analytical wing, which consists of the following bodies and individuals:
   a. Central Drug Laboratory
   b. Government analysts
   c. Drug testing laboratories for the states.
3. Administrative wing, which consists of individuals who are responsible for the administration of drugs and cosmetics regulations:
   a. Drugs Controller General of India (DCGI)
   b. Drugs Control and Licensing Authorities of States
   c. Drug Inspectors of central and state governments.

9.2.1.3 Drugs Technical Advisory Board (DTAB)

DTAB is a statutory board established by the central government under the provisions of the D&C Act to advise the central government and state governments on all technical matters pertaining to the Act, as well as to establish guidelines for types of formulations as and when requested by the central government. It is a technical advisory body composed of members who are ex officio, nominated, and elected. The DTAB has a total of 18 members who represent various aspects of the pharmacy and medical professions in the country. The Chairman of the DTAB is the Director General of Medical and Health Services, Government of India, and the Member Secretary is the Drugs Controller General of India. The DTAB's headquarters is located at the Ministry of Health and Family Welfare, Government of India, Nirman Bhavan, New Delhi. The term of office for elected and nominated members is 3 years. Ex officio members hold office so long as they are in that specific position. Even if they are not members of the DTAB, they can form sub-committees and co-opt member experts for specific assignments. The DTAB makes policy decisions on technical aspects of the Drugs and Cosmetics Act and Rules and forwards its recommendations to the Ministry of Health and Family Welfare for approval. DTAB meets twice a year but can be summoned with one week's notice for certain urgent matters. The Ministry of Health and Family Welfare may decide on very urgent matters on a priority basis at times. However, such government decisions must be ratified by DTAB within 6 months.

9.2.1.4 Drugs Consultative Committee (DCC)

The DCC is the Advisory Body appointed by the central government under Section 7 to advise the central and state governments, as well as the DTAB, on matters pertaining to the uniform implementation of D&C Act and Rules provisions. The

DCC is made up of two representatives nominated by the central government and one representative each from the state government and the union territory. The state government or union territory usually appoints the Director of Drug Control Administration or Drug Controller of State to this Council.

9.2.1.5 Central Drug Laboratory (CDL)

According to Section 6 of the Act, a Central Drug Laboratory (CDL) was to be, and its director would be chosen by the central government. The Statutory Analytical Laboratory for Drugs and Cosmetics under the D&C Act is the organization whose analysis-related decisions are considered final by courts. CDL is responsible for various functions such as analysis of drugs and cosmetics samples sent by customs collectors and courts; performance of analytical tests on samples sent by central, state, and union territory governments; support of research and development (R&D) activities of developing innovative techniques for analytical testing of drugs and cosmetics; and so on.

9.2.1.6 Drugs and Cosmetics Rules, 1945

The Drugs and Cosmetics Rules, 1945, were enacted to respond to the Drugs and Cosmetics Act 1940. The rules classify medicine as per the timetable and guide the storage, sale, display and prescription guidance for each timetable.

The Rules include clauses that classify the drugs into the schedule and provide guidelines for storing, selling, displaying, and prescribing each schedule. The guidelines for the storing, selling, displaying, and schedules are prescribed under Rule 67 of the Drug and Cosmetics Rules, 1945. Rule 97 provides rules for labeling restrictions.

9.2.2 Central Drugs Standard Control Organization (CDSCO)

Regarding regulations, the main governing body is the Central Drugs Standard Control Organization (CDSCO), which is led by the Drug Controller General of India (DCGI) [16]. The CDSCO's primary role is to coordinate the activities of the State Drug Regulatory Authorities (SDRAs), develop policies, and ensure consistent implementation of the D&C Act across India. The DCGI holds responsibility for various tasks including product approval, setting approval standards, overseeing clinical trials, facilitating the introduction of new drugs, and granting import licenses for new drugs. Manufacturing licenses for drugs can only be obtained in a state after receiving approval from the CDSCO. Its main functions and responsibilities include the following:

1. *Drug regulatory authority*: CDSCO is the primary regulatory authority for approving and regulating pharmaceutical products in India. It evaluates and approves the safety, efficacy, and quality of drugs before they can be marketed in the country.
2. *New drug approvals*: CDSCO plays a main role in the approval process of new drugs and clinical trials in the country. It evaluates applications from

pharmaceutical companies for the conduct of clinical trials and grants permissions based on ethical and scientific considerations.

3. *Drug safety monitoring*: CDSCO monitors the safety profile of approved drugs in the market. It collects, analyzes, and assesses adverse drug reactions (ADRs) reported by healthcare professionals and the general public. CDSCO takes appropriate measures, such as labeling changes or product recalls, to ensure patient safety.
4. *Quality control and inspections*: CDSCO regulates the quality of drugs and ensures compliance with good manufacturing practices (GMP). It conducts inspections of drug manufacturing facilities, both domestically and internationally, to ensure adherence to quality standards.
5. *Medical device regulation*: CDSCO is responsible for regulating medical devices and ensuring their safety, quality, and efficacy. It classifies medical devices, issues guidelines for their import, manufacture, and sale, and monitors their post-market surveillance.
6. *Cosmetics and diagnostics regulation*: CDSCO also regulates cosmetics and diagnostics products in India. It sets standards for their safety, quality, and labeling requirements to protect consumer health and safety.

9.2.3 State Drug Regulatory Authorities (SDRAs)

SDRAs established under the D&C Act are responsible for licensing of manufacturing establishments and sale premises, undertaking inspections of such premises to ensure compliance with license conditions, drawing samples for testing and monitoring of quality of drugs, taking actions like suspension/cancellation of licenses, surveillance over sale of spurious and adulterated drugs, instituting legal prosecution when required, and monitoring of objectionable advertisements for drugs [16,17]. The State Drug Controller (SDC) heads the SDRA and reports to a joint secretary in the health department of the state government. A typical SDRA has Drug Inspectors reporting to the Deputy Drugs Controller who also acts as the Licensing Authority for the state. Administrative matters such as departmental budgeting, appointments, training of officers, and allotment of funds and resources for inspections fall under the jurisdiction of the state governments. This report found that a number of SDRAs were conjoined with the food regulatory departments (FDAs) of the state, making it difficult to clearly demarcate the available funds and resources between the two.

9.2.4 Pharmacy Act and Other Legislation

The Bhore Committee, chaired by Sir Joseph Bhore, published its report in 1946 addressing the need for an act to safeguard the interests of qualified pharmacists and protect the health of public. The committee discovered that unqualified individuals were handling drugs, causing harm to society. To address this issue, the committee recommended that the pharmacy profession should be exclusively reserved for trained pharmacists, limiting their scope of work to professional activities. Additionally, the committee advised against allowing pharmacists to engage in functions such as prescribing medications and administering anesthesia. Furthermore, the committee highlighted the unsatisfactory standard of pharmacy education in the country and recommended a revision to improve the training provided to aspiring pharmacists [18].

Based on the recommendations of the Chopra Committee and the interim findings of the Bhore Committee, the British Government of India brought out the Pharmacy Bill in 1945, further it took the shape of the Pharmacy Act 1948 [6]. The first Pharmacy Council of India was constituted in 1949 under the provisions of the Pharmacy Act. Under the Pharmacy Act, the Pharmacy Council of India (PCI) is authorized to establish the standards known as Education Regulations (ER) and present them to the central government for approval. These ER enable the PCI to set the minimum requirements for admission to pharmacy courses such as D. Pharm, B. Pharm, M. Pharm, and so on. They also determine the duration of the courses, the type and duration of practical training, the subjects to be included in the curriculum, the necessary equipment and facilities to be provided by educational institutions, and the conditions to be met by academic institutions, examination authorities, and entities offering practical training to students. According to the Pharmacy Act of 1948, each state is mandated to establish a Pharmacy Council. Additionally, the act allows for the creation of Joint State Pharmacy Councils for a specified or unspecified duration. The State Pharmacy Council comprises three categories of members, similar to the PCI: elected members, nominated members, and ex officio members [6,19].

9.3 PROCESS OF APPROVAL OF PHARMACEUTICAL PRODUCTS

The D&C Act assigns CDSCO with various responsibilities. These include the approval of new drugs, regulation of clinical trials, establishment of drug standards, quality control of imported drugs, oversight of SDRAs, and providing advisory services to ensure consistent enforcement of the D&C Act [9,10].

CDSCO evaluates and grants approval for new drugs (Figure 9.1) by considering non-clinical data, clinical trial results (emphasizing safety and efficacy) obtained from both domestic and international sources, and the regulatory status of the drug in other countries. The specific regulations governing new drugs approvals are outlined in different sections of Schedule Y of the D&C Rules, such as Rules 122 A, 122 B, 122D, 122 DA, 122 DAA, 122 DAB, 122 DAC, 122 DB, 122 DD, and 122 E [9,16].

In certain circumstances, the D&C Act allows for exemptions from conducting local clinical trials if the Licensing Authority deems it in the public interest to grant permission for the importation or manufacturing of the new drug based on data available from other countries.

In cases involving life-threatening or serious diseases, or diseases of particular significance in the Indian health context, the law allows the Licensing Authority to expedite, postpone, or even waive the requirement for certain clinical data. This flexibility is provided to ensure timely access to necessary treatments.

Applications for the approval of new drugs are assessed by the Subject Expert Committee (SEC), previously known as the New Drug Advisory Committee (NDAC). These committees consist of experts selected from government medical colleges and

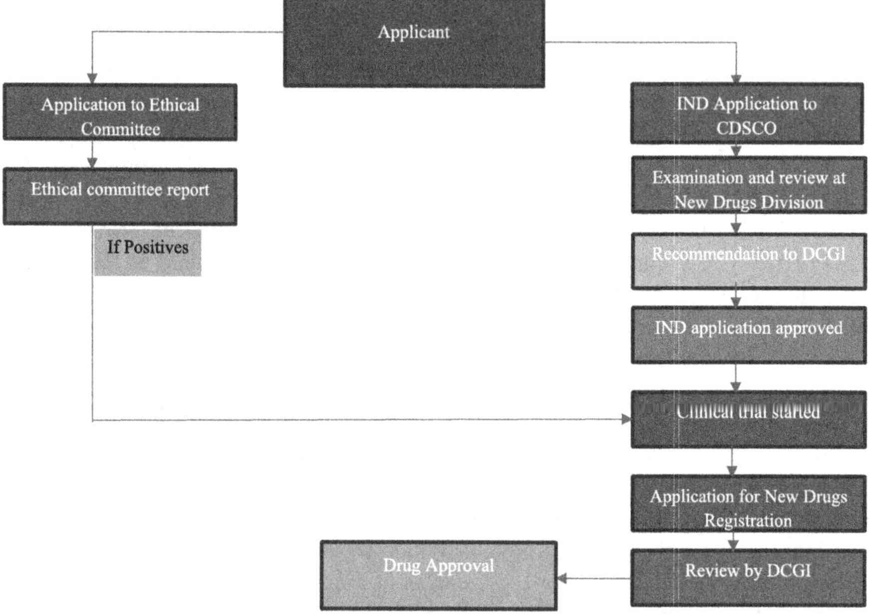

FIGURE 9.1 Process of Drug Approval by DCGI. (IND, Investigational New Drug; NDA, New Drug Application; ANDA, Abbreviated New Drug Application.)

institutes across India. The approval or rejection of the applications is based on the recommendations provided by these expert committees. Their proficiency and evaluation play a fundamental role in the decision-making process [14,16].

9.3.1 Process of Regulation and Licensing of Drugs/Biologicals

CDSCO holds the rights to govern the overall process of regulation and licensing of drugs/biologicals as per the D&C Act [10,14,16]. Table 9.1 represents necessary forms and formats required for submission of licensing and other application. There are several steps of this process as explained herein.

9.3.1.1 New Drug Discovery and Development

- companies undertake R&D to discover and develop new drugs.
- Preclinical studies: Companies conduct extensive laboratory and animal studies to assess the safety and efficacy of the new drug candidate.
- Clinicaltrials: If the preclinical studies show promising results, the drug undergoes clinical trials in humans. These trials are conducted in three phases: Phase I, Phase II, and Phase III.
- New Drug Application (NDA): After successful completion of clinical trials, the pharmaceutical company submits an NDA to the CDSCO for regulatory approval.

TABLE 9.1

Application Forms and Formats for Manufacture, Licensing and Sales of Pharmaceutical Products Prescribed under the Drugs and Cosmetics Act, 1940, and Rules, 1945

Application Type	Description
Form 14A	Application from a purchaser for test or analysis of a drug under Section 26 of the Drugs and Cosmetics Act, 1940
Form 19	Application for grant or renewal of a licence to sell, stock, exhibit or offer for sale, or distribute drugs other than those specified in Schedule X
Form 19A	Application for grant or renewal of a restricted licence to sell, stock or exhibit or offer for sale, or distribute drugs by retail by dealers who do not engage the service of a qualified person
Form 19B	Application for licence to sell, stock or exhibit or offer for sale, or distribute homoeopathic medicines
Form 19C	Application for grant or renewal of a [licence to sell, stock, exhibit or offer for sale, or distribute] drugs specified in Schedule X
Form 24	Application for the grant of or renewal of a licence to manufacture for sale or for distribution of drugs other than those specified in [Schedule C, C (1) and X]
Form 24A	Application for grant or renewal of a loan licence to manufacture for sale or for distribution of drugs other than those specified in Schedule C, C (1) and X
Form 24B	Application for grant or renewal of a licence to repack for sale or distribution of drugs, being drugs other than those specified in Schedule C and C (1), excluding those specified in Schedule X
Form 24C	Application for the grant or renewal of a licence to manufacture for sale [or for distribution] of homoeopathic medicines or a licence to manufacture potentised preparations from back potencies by licensees holding licence in Form 20-C
Form 24F	Application for grant or renewal of a licence to manufacture for sale or for distribution of drugs specified in Schedule X and not specified in Schedule C and C(1)
Form 27	Application for grant or renewal of a licence to manufacture for sale or for distribution of drugs specified in Schedule C and C (1) excluding those specified in part XB and Schedule X
Form 27A	Application for grant or renewal of a loan licence to manufacture for sale or for distribution of drugs specified in Schedule C and C (1) excluding those specified in part XB and Schedule X
Form 27B	Application for grant or renewal of a licence to manufacture for sale or for distribution of drugs specified in Schedules C, C (1) and X
Form 27C	Application for grant/renewal of licence for the operation of a blood bank for processing of whole blood and/or preparation of blood components
Form 27D	Application for grant or renewal of a licence to manufacture for sale or for distribution of large volume parenterals/sera and vaccines excluding those specified in Schedule X
Form 27DA	Application for grant or renewal of a loan licence to manufacture for sale or for distribution of large volume parenterals/sera and vaccine/recombinant DNA (R-DNA) derived drugs excluding those specified under Schedule X

(Continued)

TABLE 9.1 *(Continued)*

Application Forms and Formats for Manufacture, Licensing and Sales of Pharmaceutical Products Prescribed under the Drugs and Cosmetics Act, 1940, and Rules, 1945

Application Type	Description
Form 27E	Application for grant/renewal of licence to manufacture blood products for sale or distribution
Form 27F	Application for grant or renewal of licence
Form 30	Application for licence to manufacture drugs for purpose of examination, test or analysis
Form 31	Application for grant or renewal of a licence to manufacture cosmetics for sale or for distribution
Form 31A	Application for grant or renewal of a loan licence to manufacture cosmetics for sale [or for distribution]
Form 36	Application for grant or renewal of approval for carrying out tests drugs/ cosmetics or raw materials used in the manufacture thereof on behalf of licensees for manufacture for sale of drugs/cosmetics
Form 44	Application for grant of permission to import or manufacture a new drug or to undertake clinical trial
Form 3F	Application for grant of recognition to medical institution

9.3.1.2 Review and Evaluation

- *NDA review*: The CDSCO reviews the NDA to assess the safety, efficacy, and quality of the new drug.
- *Expert Committee*: An Expert Committee is constituted to evaluate the data provided in the NDA. The committee comprises subject experts from various fields, such as medicine, toxicology, pharmacology, and chemistry.
- *Site inspection*: The CDSCO may conduct inspections of the manufacturing facilities and clinical trial sites to ensure compliance with good manufacturing practices (GMP) and good clinical practices (GCP).
- *Evaluation report*: The Expert Committee prepares an evaluation report based on the data provided in the NDA, clinical trial results, and inspection findings.

9.3.1.3 Regulatory Decision

- *Subject Expert Committee* (SEC): The evaluation report is reviewed by the SEC, which recommends whether the drug should be granted approval or not.
- *Drug Controller General of India* (DCGI): The DCGI, who heads the CDSCO, reviews the SEC recommendations and makes the final decision regarding the approval of the new drug.

- *Approval or rejection*: The DCGI may grant approval for marketing the new drug, request additional information, or reject the application. In case of approval, the drug is assigned a unique brand name.

9.3.1.4 Post-Approval

- *Post-approval studies*: The CDSCO may require post-approval studies to gather more data on the drug's safety and efficacy in real-world settings.
- *Manufacturing and quality control*: The drug manufacturing facilities must comply with GMP regulations. The CDSCO conducts regular inspections to ensure adherence to quality standards.
- *Post-marketing surveillance*: Once a drug is approved and available in the market, the CDSCO monitors its safety and effectiveness through post-marketing surveillance. Adverse events, product quality issues, and drug interactions are reported by healthcare professionals, manufacturers, and patients. Pharmaceutical companies and healthcare professionals are required to report any adverse events or side effects associated with the drug to the CDSCO. The CDSCO takes necessary actions, such as product recalls or label revisions, to ensure patient safety.
- The Pharmacovigilance Programme of India (PvPI) is a nationwide initiative aimed at ensuring safety of drugs and promoting patient welfare. It was launched by the Indian Pharmacopoeia Commission (IPC) in 2010 and is actively involved in monitoring and reporting of adverse drug reactions (ADRs) in India. PvPI encourages healthcare professionals, pharmaceutical companies, and consumers to report any suspected ADRs associated with the use of drugs through regional ADR monitoring centers across India or through its online reporting system. Through continuous monitoring, analysis, and dissemination of drug safety information, PvPI contributes significantly to safeguarding public health and promoting the rational use of medicines in India. The CDSCO takes necessary actions whenever necessary, such as product recalls or label revisions, to ensure patient safety [20].

9.3.1.5 Licensing of Generic Drugs

In India, generic drugs play a significant role in providing affordable healthcare. The process for generic drug approval is as follows:

- *Bioequivalence studies*: Companies seeking to market generic drugs must conduct bioequivalence studies to demonstrate that their product is therapeutically equivalent to the reference drug.
- *Abbreviated New Drug Application* (ANDA): The company submits an ANDA to the CDSCO, containing data on bioequivalence studies, manufacturing processes, and labeling.
- *Review and approval*: The CDSCO reviews the ANDA and grants approval for marketing and sale if the generic drug is deemed bioequivalent and meets quality standards.

9.3.1.6 Import and Export

The import and export of drugs in India are regulated by the CDSCO. Imported drugs must comply with Indian drugs regulatory standards, and companies must obtain necessary licenses and permissions.

- *Standards of quality*: The term standard quality for import is in concerning medicine and cosmetics means that medicine and cosmetics should comply with the specification of imports. The standards set by the D&C Act are set out under the Second timetable. Section 12 and Section 13 of the Act grant the central government the power to make rules regarding testing and examination methods that can get used to assess the standard quality of the medication. Section 10 of the D&C Act gives the power to the central government to ban the import of medicines that are not of standard quality or misbranded, adulterated or spurious. To import any product, license is required. No drugs or cosmetics can be imported without a license in the country.
- *Rule-making about import of drugs and cosmetics*: The central government can draw the laws related to the importation of medicinal products and cosmetics after the board's consultation or recommendation. It includes regulations that define the drugs or class of drug or cosmetics for which a license gets issued for importation. The forms and conditions of the issuance, suspension or revocation of licenses and the fees payable are demanded and prescribed.
- *Penalties for importing prohibited drugs or cosmetics*: The D&C Act, 1940 Section 13, which talks about the importation of adulterated drugs or cosmetics, is punishable by imprisonment for 3 years and fines up to 3 years. The fine could be up to 5000 rupees. In the case of medicine or cosmetics that include dangerous ingredients, the penalty is similar as prescribed [16,21].

9.3.2 Process of Regulation and Licensing of Cosmetics

The regulatory framework under D&C Act 1940 ensures the safety, quality, and efficacy of cosmetic products in the Indian market [16,22]. The process of regulation and licensing of cosmetics products in India is as follows:

- *Definition of cosmetics*: The D&C Act defines cosmetics as any substance used for external application on the body, including skin, hair, nails, lips, etc., for the purpose of cleansing, beautifying, promoting attractiveness, or altering appearance.
- *Importer/manufacturer registration*: The first step for selling cosmetics in India is to register with the CDSCO. Manufacturers or importers need to submit an application along with the prescribed fees and necessary documents to obtain a cosmetic manufacturing license or an import registration certificate.
- *Product approval*: The CDSCO does not require product approval for most cosmetics, except for certain categories of products such as colorants, hair dyes, and sunscreens. These specific categories require product approval

from the CDSCO before they can be sold in India. The applicant needs to submit the necessary data and documentation to demonstrate the safety and efficacy of the product.

- *Safety and quality requirements*: All cosmetics products sold in India must comply with the safety and quality requirements specified under the Drugs and Cosmetics Act and Rules. This includes adherence to GMP, product labeling requirements, and restrictions on certain ingredients such as color additives.
- *Testing and analysis*: The CDSCO may conduct random inspections and sampling of cosmetics products to ensure compliance with safety and quality standards. Samples may be sent to government-approved laboratories for testing and analysis.
- *Labeling and packaging*: Cosmetics products must be labeled in compliance with the Drugs and Cosmetics Rules. The label should include information such as the name of the product, list of ingredients, manufacturing and expiry dates, directions for use, precautions, and contact details of the manufacturer or importer.
- *Advertising regulations*: Cosmetics advertising in India is subject to scrutiny by the Advertising Standards Council of India (ASCI) and the CDSCO. Advertisements should not make false or misleading claims, and they should not promote products that are prohibited or restricted under the regulatory framework.
- *Post-market surveillance*: The CDSCO carries out post-market surveillance activities to monitor the safety and quality of cosmetics products in the Indian market. This includes monitoring adverse events, consumer complaints, and conducting market inspections.

9.3.3 Process of Regulation and Licensing of Medical Devices

The Medical Devices and Diagnostics Division of CDSCO has established comprehensive regulations for medical devices known as the Indian Medical Device Rules (IMDR) [16,23–30]. These regulations were initially released in January 2017 and came into effect in January 2018. In February 2020, an amendment called the Medical Devices (Amendment) Rules, 2020, was introduced and implemented in April 2020. The 2020 amendment included the addition of "registration of certain medical devices" to the rules.

9.3.3.1 Medical Device Classification

One important aspect of these regulations is the classification of medical devices. Devices are categorized into different risk classes based on factors such as their intended use, duration of use, and level of invasiveness. The classification system, outlined in the Medical Device Rules, 2017, which falls under the purview of the D&C Act, 1940, determines the specific regulatory requirements applicable to each device. The Central Licensing Authority (CLA) of India assigns medical devices and In-Vitro Diagnostic Medical Devices (IVDMDs) into four risk classes based on their intended use, associated risk, and other parameters mentioned in the IMDR [24]:

Class A: Low-risk devices
Class B: Low to moderate-risk devices
Class C: Moderate-to-high-risk devices
Class D: High-risk devices.

9.3.3.2 Manufacturing License

Manufacturers of medical devices in India are required to obtain a manufacturing license from CDSCO. The process of development and approval/licensing of medical devices is regulated in several regulatory steps (Figure 9.2). This license is crucial for ensuring compliance with GMP and other quality standards. To apply for a manufacturing license, the manufacturer must submit an application to the CDSCO along with the necessary documents and fees.

For the manufacturing of Class A and Class B devices, the license or loan license is granted by the State Licensing Authority upon application. On the other hand, for manufacturing Class C and Class D devices, the license or loan license is granted by the CLA. These licenses are valid indefinitely, unless they are suspended or canceled. However, it is important to note that the license retention fee must be paid before the completion of 5 years from the date of issue to maintain the validity of the license.

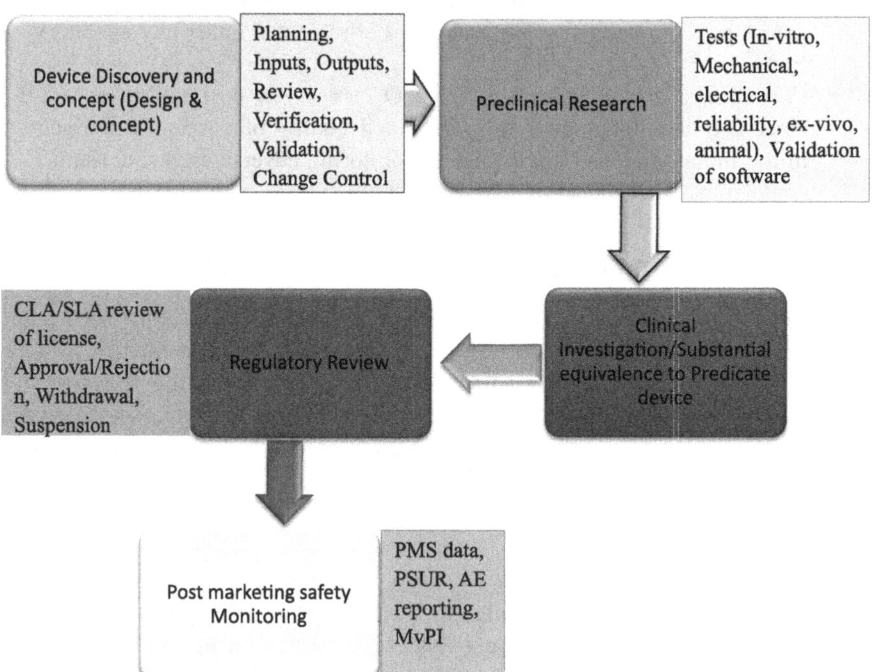

FIGURE 9.2 Medical Device Development and Approval Process. (CLA, Central Licensing Authority; MvPI, Materiovigilance Program of India; PMCI, Post-Marketing Clinical Investigation; PMS, Post-Marketing Surveillance; PSUR, Periodic Safety Update Report; SLA, State Licensing Authority.)

In certain cases, where a small quantity of medical devices is intended for purposes such as clinical investigations, tests, evaluation, examination, demonstration, or training, a specific license may be obtained. This license remains valid for a period of 3 years [24,25].

9.3.3.3 Import License

To import a medical device into India, it is necessary to obtain an import license. The importer must apply to the CDSCO for an import license by submitting the required application, documents, and fees. The import license is specific to the particular medical device being imported and remains valid for a specified period.

For the grant of an import license for medical devices from other countries, certain requirements must be fulfilled. In the case of Class C and Class D devices, a clinical investigation must be conducted in India to establish the safety and effectiveness of the device. For Class A and Class B devices, the import license can be granted if the safety and performance of the device have been established through published data or clinical investigation in the country of origin. Additionally, a free sale certificate from the country of origin must be provided.

Clinical investigation or clinical performance evaluation is an essential process step for certain medical devices. It involves conducting studies to assess the device's safety, efficacy, and performance. Permission to conduct such investigations is granted by the CDSCO based on specific conditions and requirements.

9.3.3.4 Clinical Investigation

Similar to drug approval, the evaluation of investigational medical devices in India requires conducting a clinical investigation involving human participants to assess the device's safety, performance, or effectiveness. For new IVDMDs, a clinical performance evaluation is conducted using specimens collected from human participants to assess its performance. These investigations are carried out following detailed protocols known as the clinical investigation plan or clinical performance evaluation plan [27].

Unlike the four-phase studies required for drug development according to Schedule Y, medical devices regulated under the IMDR undergo two-phase studies: a pilot (exploratory study) and a pivotal study. Upon completion or premature termination of a clinical investigation or clinical performance evaluation, a clinical investigation report or clinical performance evaluation report, respectively, must be submitted to the ethics committee, participating investigators, and the CLA [27,28].

In India, a clinical investigation is required for all Class B, Class C, and Class D medical devices if the device is an investigational medical device without a predicate device and is manufactured within the country. It is also required for new IVDMDs. However, for granting an import license, a clinical investigation is not mandatory if the device has been on the market for at least 2 years in Australia, Canada, Japan, Europe, or the United States, and the respective CLAs are satisfied with the available clinical evidence. In such cases, the CLA may request post-marketing investigations based on the review and recommendations of the Subject Expert Committee.

9.3.3.5 Post-Marketing Surveillance

After obtaining the registration or manufacturing license, it is the responsibility of the manufacturer or importer to ensure the quality, safety, and performance of the medical device [27,29,30]. Post-marketing surveillance is conducted to monitor the clinical safety of the device.

As part of post-marketing surveillance, a Periodic Safety Update Report (PSUR) is required for each medical device. The PSUR includes the reporting of relevant new information from reliable sources, the correlation of this data with patient exposure, a summary of the market authorization status in different countries, and any significant safety-related variations. The report also indicates whether any changes need to be made to the product information to enhance its use. Additionally, the PSUR captures significant changes to the reference safety information during the reporting period, such as contraindications, warnings, precautions, adverse events (AE), and important findings from ongoing and completed clinical investigations, as well as noteworthy non-clinical findings.

To minimize risks and maintain a favorable risk-benefit ratio, the Materiovigilance Program of India (MvPI) is operated by the Indian Pharmacopoeia Commission. Through continuous monitoring, MvPI assesses and detects adverse effects, malfunctions, and other issues related to use of medical devices that may lead to mortality or morbidity. Since its launch, MvPI has played a key role in keeping unsafe products out of the Indian market, resulting in the recall of 16 medical devices till date.

9.3.4 Process of Regulation and Licensing of Veterinary Products

- *Technical requirements*: Veterinary products must meet specific technical requirements set by CDSCO. These requirements include information on product composition, manufacturing process, stability studies, packaging, labeling, and storage conditions. The technical data should demonstrate the safety, efficacy, and quality of the product [16,31].
- *Product categories*: Veterinary products are categorized into different classes based on their nature and usage. These categories include veterinary drugs, vaccines, feed supplements, and diagnostics. Each category may have specific requirements for registration, licensing, and labeling.
- *Good manufacturing practices* (GMP): Manufacturers of veterinary products must adhere to GMP prescribed by the CDSCO. GMP guidelines ensure that products are consistently produced and controlled according to quality standards. Manufacturers are inspected by CDSCO for compliance with GMP requirements before granting a license.
- *Labeling and packaging*: Veterinary products must have appropriate labeling and packaging as per the guidelines specified by CDSCO. Labels should contain essential information such as product name, composition, directions for use, storage conditions, batch number, manufacturing and expiry dates, and cautionary statements.
- *Clinical trials and testing*: Veterinary drugs and vaccines may require clinical trials and testing to establish their safety and efficacy. Clinical trials are

conducted on animals, and the data generated from these trials are submitted to CDSCO for evaluation.
- *Post-marketing surveillance*: CDSCO conducts post-marketing surveillance to monitor the safety and quality of veterinary products in the market. Adverse events and quality issues should be reported to CDSCO by manufacturers, importers, or users of veterinary products.

9.4 CHALLENGES IN DRUG REGULATION IN INDIA

9.4.1 Enforcement of Laws and Regulations

Most drug regulations in India are based on the D&C of 1940 and the underlying regulations of 1945. In addition, public health is enshrined in the Constitution, so state governments are also involved in controlling drug regulations. This leads to confusion or lack of transparency in the distribution of powers and responsibilities between the states and the center, resulting in numerous problems related to drug regulation in India. In addition, India has various laws and regulations governing nutraceuticals, herbal medicines, drugs of other than chemical origin, control of psychoactive or narcotic drugs; moreover, several organizations are involved in the regulation of these substances, leading to undesirable confusion or complexity in the enforcement of regulations [17].

9.4.2 Regulatory Compliance by Stakeholders

The manufacturing of drugs or any process related to drugs in the market is governed by different sets of rules and requirements or the law created by the drug regulatory authorities. Adhering to these sets of drug regulatory guidelines, rules and law is known as drug regulatory compliance, which is necessary to achieve and maintain the optimum quality of drug products through its life in the market. Compliance is a two-way process, which requires active involvement of manufacturers/retailers and the regulators. Unfortunately, there is a huge gap in the number or strength of drugs inspectors/regulators in India (both Central and the states) with reference to the number of registered manufacturing units and retailers, resulting in an insufficient number of inspections for compliance to drug regulatory rules by manufacturers/retailers. Also, the related stakeholders are not properly aware about the current or updated rules applicable to their products, which often leads to the poor-quality products in market [17,20,32].

9.4.3 Administrative and Legal Disparities

From the beginning, the central and the state drug regulatory authorities have suffered from various administrative issues like shortage of technical personnel, lack of infrastructure and funding, and an absence of efficient management to control the whole drug regulation efficiently. Besides this the existing rules are outdated and complex in nature and understanding them is a Herculean task to most of the stakeholders [5,17].

9.4.4 Emerging Technological and Methodical Advancements

The advancement in technologies and various methods involved in drug development and manufacturing are evolving at a greater pace. These evolving technologies are much needed for the stakeholders at the present time to provide a quality drug efficiently and satisfy the needs of consumers' requirements. As the technologies evolve or adoption of new methods by the drug makers happens the regulators should also be trained parallelly to control or regulate this new development. But unfortunately, both the central and the state drugs regulatory authorities are not providing the enough training to its inspectors or personnel involved in the drug regulation which can be a great threat to controlling the quality of drugs in India [31,32].

9.5 Future Directions

Most of the Indian drug regulatory system is still based on classical and old traditional methods, and its update is very slow compared with the exponential growth of technology and globalization, especially in the pharmaceutical sector, resulting in delayed approval process/permitting for registration of new drugs.

This old system also causes an unnecessary workload in the workplace, which ultimately affects the end user of medicines in the country. To speed up this process and achieve the maximum benefit for the country's population, there is an urgent need to develop or modernize the drug regulatory system to match the pace of globalization. The implementation of GMP and other regulations such as Schedule M mentioned in the D&C Law and regulations can sometimes be very costly for companies, especially micro, small and medium enterprises, so the system should provide for easy provision of subsidies. In addition, the government should intervene and set the price of all medicines to minimize competition that directly or indirectly affects the quality of medicines in the country. Currently, it is quite a challenge to coordinate or communicate with the Indian Medicines Agency. A system should be created that allows as many stakeholders as possible to communicate and share their feedback. Regular and ongoing awareness programs should be organized for stakeholders to clarify their questions and issues and familiarize them with updated rules and guidelines, if any [33,34].

REFERENCES

[1] Ravishankar, B., & Shukla, V. (2008). Indian Systems of Medicine: A Brief Profile. *African Journal of Traditional, Complementary and Alternative Medicines*, *4*(3), 319. https://doi.org/10.4314/ajtcam.v4i3.31226

[2] Lele, R. D. (2021). *History of Medicine in India* (First, Vol. 1, pp. 5–20). National Centre of Indian Medical Heritage Central Council for Research in Ayurvedic Sciences (CCRAS) Ministry of AYUSH, Government of India Revenue Board Colony, Gaddiannaram Hyderabad- 500036. http://ccras.nic.in/sites/default/files/viewpdf/Publication/History_of_Medicine_in_India.pdf

[3] Jaiswal, Y. S., & Williams, L. L. (2017). A Glimpse of Ayurveda—The Forgotten History and Principles of Indian Traditional Medicine. *Journal of Traditional and Complementary Medicine*, *7*(1), 50–53. https://doi.org/10.1016/j.jtcme.2016.02.002

[4] Chowdhury, N., Joshi, P., Patnaik, A., & Saraswathy, B. (2015). *Administrative Structure and Functions of Drug Regulatory Authorities in India.* https://icricr.org/pdf/Working_Paper_309.pdf

[5] Bhattacharya, N. (2016). Between the Bazaar and the Bench: Making of the Drugs Trade in Colonial India, ca. 1900–1930. *Bulletin of the History of Medicine, 90*(1), 61–91. https://doi.org/10.1353/bhm.2016.0017

[6] The Drugs Enquiry Committee, India, 1930. (1930). *The Indian Medical Gazette, 65*(11), 640–642.

[7] Ravikumar, K. G. (2018). *Growth of Pharmacy Education in India from 1932 to 2007.* Pharmabiz.com. http://test.pharmabiz.com/special%20features/growth-of-pharmacy-education-in-india-from-1932-to-2007-44185

[8] Indian Pharmacopoeia. (2023, March 10). *About IP—Indian Pharmacopoeia Commission.* Ipc.gov.in. www.ipc.gov.in/mandates/indian-pharmacopoeia/about-ip.html#:~:text=IP%20is%20recognized%20as%20the

[9] Law, C. (2021, January 19). *India—Brief on the Drugs and Cosmetics Act, 1940.* Conventus Law. https://conventuslaw.com/report/india-brief-on-the-drugs-and-cosmetics-act-1940/

[10] Mahawar, S. (2022). *Drugs and Cosmetics Act, 1940.* IP-leaders. https://blog.ipleaders.in/drugs-and-cosmetics-act-1940/

[11] Bhatnagar, J., & Garg, V. (2007, December 13). *Patent Law in India—Intellectual Property—India.* www.mondaq.com. www.mondaq.com/india/patent/54494/patent-law-in-india

[12] Andrade, C., Shah, N., & Chandra, S. (2007). The new patent regime: Implications for patients in India. *Indian Journal of Psychiatry, 49*(1), 56. https://doi.org/10.4103/0019-5545.31520

[13] Ministry of Health and Family Welfare. (2013). *National Pharmaceutical Pricing Authority. Department of Pharmaceuticals.* Pharmaceuticals.gov.in. https://pharmaceuticals.gov.in/national-pharmaceutical-pricing-authority

[14] Singh, N., Madkaikar, N. J., Gokhale, P. M., & Parmar, D. V. (2020). New Drugs and Clinical Trials Rules 2019: Changes in Responsibilities of the Ethics Committee. *Perspectives in Clinical Research, 11*(1), 37–43. http://doi.org/10.4103/picr.PICR_208_19

[15] Rago, L., & Santoso, B. (2008). Drug Regulation: History, Present and Future 1. *Drug Benefits and Risks: International Textbook of Clinical Pharmacology, Revised 2nd Edition, 1*(1), 34–50.

[16] *Drugs and Cosmetics Act 1940, Rules 1945.* (2022, November 22). Cdsco.gov.in. https://cdsco.gov.in/opencms/opencms/system/modules/CDSCO.WEB/elements/download_file_division.jsp?num_id=OTIyNw==

[17] Agnihotri, S. (2019, September). *Thakur Foundation.* www.thakur-foundation.org/TFF%20State%20Drug%20Regulatory%20Authorities%20Capability%20Assessment%20Report.pdf

[18] Bhore Committee, 1946 | National Health Portal of India. Archived from the original on 9 October 2015 . https://en.wikipedia.org/wiki/Bhore_Committee [Last accessed on 2023 July 03].

[19] Pharmacy Council of India. (1991, January). *Pharmacy Council of India.* www.pci.nic.in/education_regulations_chapter1.html#:~:text=(2)%20They%20shall%20come%20into

[20] Prakash, J., Sachdeva, R., Shrivastava, T., Jayachandran, C., & Sahu, A. (2021). Adverse Event Reporting Tools and Regulatory Measures in India Through Outcome of Pharmacovigilance Programme of India. *Indian Journal of Pharmacology, 53*(2), 143. https://doi.org/10.4103/ijp.ijp_901_20

[21] Taparia, M., & Jain, M. (2022, January 1). *Procedure—Drugs & Cosmetic License Application in India.* Lawrbit. www.lawrbit.com/article/procedure-for-applying-drugs-and-cosmetic-license-in-india/

[22] Mayashree Acharya. (2022, April 29). *How to Get Cosmetic Registration in India*? Cleartax. https://cleartax.in/s/cosmetic-registration-in-india

[23] CDSCO. (n.d.-b). *Vaccines*. Cdsco.gov.in [Last accessed on 2023 July 06] https://cdsco.gov.in/opencms/opencms/en/biologicals/Vaccines/

[24] *Deloitte, NATHEALTH Medical Devices Making in India-a Leap for Indian Healthcare* (2016) [Last accessed on 2023 July 03]. https://www2.deloitte.com/content/dam/Deloitte/in/Documents/life-sciences-health-care/in-lshc-medical-devices-making-in-india-noexp.pdf

[25] *India—Overview of Medical Device Industry and Healthcare Statistics. Available via EMERGO* (2016 July) [Last accessed on 2023 July 03]. www.emergobyul.com/resources/market-india

[26] Markan, S., & Verma, Y. (2017). Indian Medical Device Sector: Insights from Patent Filing Trends. *BMJ Innovations*, *3*, 167–175.

[27] *Medical Device Rules, 2017: Ministry of Health and Family Welfare, Government of India. Available via CDSCO* [Last accessed on 2023 July 06]. https://cdsco.gov.in/opencms/opencms/en/Medical-Device-Diagnostics/Medical-Device-Diagnostics/

[28] *Union Budget of India 2020–21, Rebuilding Momentum. Available via Pricewaterhouse Coopers Private Limited* (2020 Feb) [Last accessed on 2023 July 05]. www.pwc.in/assets/pdfs/budget/2020/pwc-union-budget-analysis.pdf

[29] Radhadevi, N., Balamuralidhara, V., Kumar, T. M., & Ravi, V. (2012). Regulatory Guidelines for Medical Devices in India: An Overview. *Asian Journal of Pharmaceutics (AJP)*, *6*(1).

[30] Shukla, S., Gupta, M., Pandit, S., Thomson, M., Shivhare, A., Kalaiselvan, V., et al. (2020). Implementation of Adverse Event Reporting for Medical Devices, India. *Bulletin of the World Health Organization*, *98*, 206.

[31] Singh, R. (2023, January 18). *How to Get Veterinary Drug License for Veterinary Medicine Shop in India | Pashudhan Praharee*. Pashudhanpraharee. www.pashudhanpraharee.com/how-to-get-veterinary-drug-license-for-veterinary-medicine-shop-in-india/#:~:text=In%20India%2C%20Drug%20for%20Humans

[32] Team, C. (2023, February 25). *Drug Regulation in India*. ClearIAS. www.clearias.com/drug-regulation-india/

[33] Parvatam, S., Bharadwaj, S., Radha, V. et al. (2020). The Need to Develop a Framework for Human-Relevant Research in India: Towards Better Disease Models and Drug Discovery. *Journal of Biosciences*, *45*, 144. https://doi.org/10.1007/s12038-020-00112-8

[34] ET Health World (2023, June 20). *India's Thriving Pharmaceutical Landscape: Need for Enhanced Drug Regulation in India—ET HealthWorld | Pharma*. ETHealthworld.com | Pharma. https://health.economictimes.indiatimes.com/news/pharma/policy-regulations/indias-thriving-pharmaceutical-landscape-need-for-enhanced-drug-regulation-in-india/101111144

10 Regulations in Japan

Faraat Ali, Anam Ilyas, and Shaima Ahmadeen

10.1 INTRODUCTION TO DRUG REGULATION IN JAPAN

In Japan, the realm of drug regulation stands as a critical pillar within the broader landscape of healthcare governance. It represents an intricate web of protocols, institutions, and standards meticulously crafted to ensure the safety, efficacy, and quality of pharmaceutical products that reach the market. The stringent oversight of drug regulation in Japan is primarily orchestrated by the Pharmaceuticals and Medical Devices Agency (PMDA), an esteemed authority entrusted with the responsibility of safeguarding public health through the meticulous evaluation and supervision of pharmaceuticals [1,4].

At the heart of Japan's drug regulation lies a profound commitment to protect patients and consumers while fostering innovation in the pharmaceutical industry. The rigorous evaluation processes established by the PMDA serve as a robust gateway for pharmaceutical products seeking approval for market entry. This intricate journey commences with extensive clinical trials designed to assess the safety and efficacy profiles of potential drugs meticulously. These trials adhere to stringent guidelines set forth by the PMDA, emphasizing the need for comprehensive data and evidence to support the claims of safety and effectiveness for any pharmaceutical product seeking approval [2,3].

The PMDA's regulatory framework classifies drugs based on various criteria, including their intended use, pharmacological effects, and potential risks. This classification system delineates the distinct pathways and requirements for approval, guiding manufacturers, and developers through the complex process of bringing new drugs to market. The commitment to thoroughness and precision at every stage of drug evaluation ensures that only pharmaceuticals meeting the highest standards of safety and efficacy are granted approval for distribution and use within Japan. However, the role of drug regulation in Japan extends far beyond the initial approval stage. Post-marketing surveillance and pharmacovigilance form integral components of the regulatory landscape, emphasizing continuous monitoring, evaluation, and reporting of adverse effects or safety concerns associated with marketed drugs. This diligent oversight underscores Japan's commitment to ensuring ongoing safety and efficacy even after a drug has reached the market, thereby reinforcing consumer confidence and upholding the highest standards of healthcare delivery [2,4].

It is worth noting that the PMDA's regulatory science research activities are carried out within a unique, three-pillar system. This system involves the PMDA's collaboration with academia and industry, as well as its engagement with international regulatory authorities and organizations. Through this collaborative approach, the PMDA fosters innovation, promotes best practices, and maintains harmonization with international standards in regulatory science research. Japan's regulatory framework

DOI: 10.1201/9781003296492-11

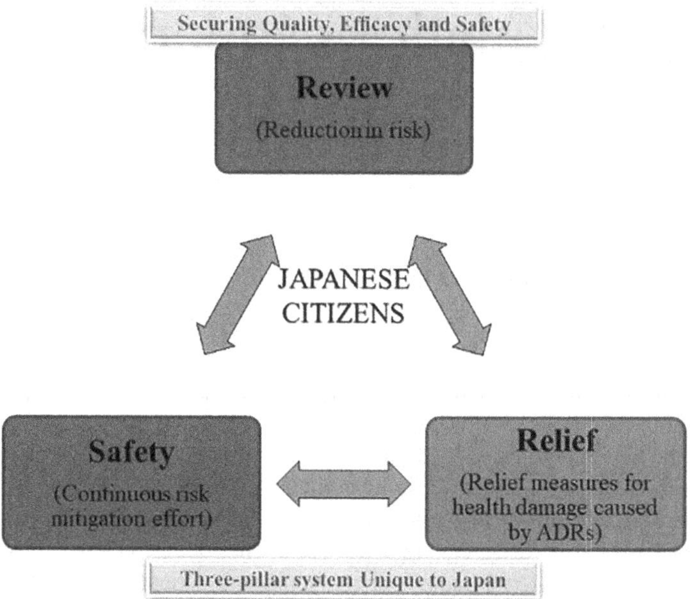

FIGURE 10.1 Safety Triangle: Comprehensive Risk Management Through the Three Functions.

for drugs embodies a delicate balance between protecting public health and fostering innovation [5]. The evolving landscape of drug regulation in Japan reflects not only the nation's commitment to its citizens' well-being but also its adaptability to the dynamic global pharmaceutical environment. Challenges persist, including navigating the complexities of international collaboration, adapting to rapid advancements in medical technology, and addressing the needs of an ageing population with diverse healthcare requirements. However, these challenges also present opportunities for innovation, collaboration, and continued enhancement of drug regulatory mechanisms to ensure the highest standards of healthcare delivery in Japan and beyond (Figure 10.1).

10.2 MINISTRY OF HEALTH, LABOUR, AND WELFARE (MHLW)

MHLW stands for the Ministry of Health, Labour, and Welfare in Japan. It is a government body responsible for overseeing various aspects related to public health, labour issues, and social welfare within Japan. The ministry plays a central role in formulating and implementing policies, regulations, and guidelines concerning healthcare, pharmaceuticals, medical devices, labour standards, pensions, and social welfare programs. MHLW works to ensure the well-being and safety of citizens by promoting public health initiatives, regulating healthcare services and products, addressing labour-related matters, and managing social welfare systems to support vulnerable populations [6]. MHLW plays a vital role in drug regulation in Japan through its partnership with the PMDA. This collaboration ensures the safety, efficacy, and quality of drugs available in the Japanese market. The MHLW, as a government agency, is responsible for establishing and enforcing regulations related to healthcare and pharmaceuticals. Its primary objective is to protect and promote the health of the Japanese population. The MHLW formulates policies, sets guidelines, and implements regulatory frameworks for drug approval and monitoring [7].

The MHLW works closely with the PMDA, an independent regulatory authority established in 2004. The PMDA operates under the supervision of the MHLW and is responsible for evaluating the safety and efficacy of drugs and medical devices before they can be marketed in Japan. The agency has a robust system in place to ensure that only safe and effective drugs are made available to the public. The MHLW and the PMDA collaborate throughout the drug development and approval process. They work together to establish guidelines for clinical trials, assess the quality and safety of drugs, review applications for drug approval, and monitor post-marketing safety. One of the key roles of the MHLW and the PMDA is to conduct thorough evaluations of drug applications and ensure that they meet stringent regulatory requirements. This involves assessing data from preclinical and clinical studies, considering the overall risk-benefit profile of the drug, and evaluating the manufacturing processes to ensure quality control. By performing these comprehensive evaluations, the MHLW and the PMDA help safeguard the Japanese population's health and well-being [6,8]. Furthermore, the MHLW and the PMDA actively contribute to international harmonization efforts in drug regulation. They participate in conferences, seminars, and other initiatives to exchange information and align their regulatory processes with international standards. This collaboration facilitates the timely availability of innovative drugs in Japan while ensuring patient safety [9]. In conclusion, the MHLW and the PMDA play critical roles in drug regulation in Japan. Through their partnership, they ensure the safety, efficacy, and quality of drugs available in the Japanese market, contributing to the overall health and well-being of the population. Their commitment to international harmonization further enhances their ability to provide timely access to innovative therapies while maintaining the highest standards of patient safety [1,7].

10.3 PHARMACEUTICALS AND MEDICAL DEVICES AGENCY (PMDA): THE REGULATORY BODY

The PMDA stands as the preeminent regulatory body in Japan, wielding significant influence in the meticulous evaluation, approval, and oversight of pharmaceuticals and medical devices. Founded in 2004, the PMDA embodies Japan's commitment to upholding the highest standards of safety, efficacy, and quality in healthcare products available to its populace. At its core, the PMDA operates with a multifaceted mandate encompassing regulatory reviews, post-marketing surveillance, and the facilitation of innovation within Japan's pharmaceutical and medical device industries. Empowered by a dedicated team of experts spanning various scientific disciplines—ranging from pharmacology to biostatistics—PMDA employs a rigorous and comprehensive approach to assessing the safety and efficacy of drugs seeking approval for market entry [7,10].

Central to the functions of PMDA is the meticulous evaluation process of pharmaceuticals seeking regulatory approval. This process commences with sponsors, typically pharmaceutical companies, submitting extensive data derived from preclinical and clinical trials conducted under the agency's stringent guidelines. These trials serve as the cornerstone for establishing the safety and efficacy profiles of the drugs under review. The PMDA's evaluators meticulously scrutinize this data, employing a risk-based approach to ensure that potential benefits outweigh any associated risks for patients and consumers. The PMDA operates within a regulatory framework that categorizes drugs based on their intended use, pharmacological effects, and risk profiles. This classification system delineates distinct pathways for approval, guiding manufacturers, and developers through the intricacies of Japan's regulatory landscape. The agency's commitment to transparency and communication is evident in its interaction with applicants, where it provides guidance and support throughout the approval process, fostering a collaborative environment aimed at achieving regulatory compliance [11].

Furthermore, the responsibilities of PMDA extend well beyond the initial approval stage. Post-marketing surveillance and pharmacovigilance mechanisms constitute integral components of its oversight functions. The agency continually monitors the safety profiles of drugs already in circulation, working in tandem with healthcare professionals and the pharmaceutical industry to detect and assess any adverse effects or safety concerns. This vigilant surveillance ensures timely intervention and appropriate measures to address emerging risks, upholding Japan's commitment to consumer safety and confidence in healthcare products. The role of PMDA as a regulatory body is not confined to pharmaceuticals alone. It also encompasses medical devices, including a wide array of products ranging from diagnostic tools to advanced medical equipment. Like its oversight of pharmaceuticals, the agency rigorously evaluates the safety and effectiveness of medical devices before granting market access, thereby ensuring the highest standards of quality and patient safety across the healthcare spectrum [12]. In essence, the PMDA epitomizes Japan's dedication to maintaining a robust regulatory framework that prioritizes the well-being of its citizens. Its commitment to stringent evaluation processes, post-market surveillance, and fostering innovation underscores its pivotal role in ensuring the availability of safe and efficacious pharmaceuticals and medical devices in Japan's healthcare landscape (Figure 10.2).

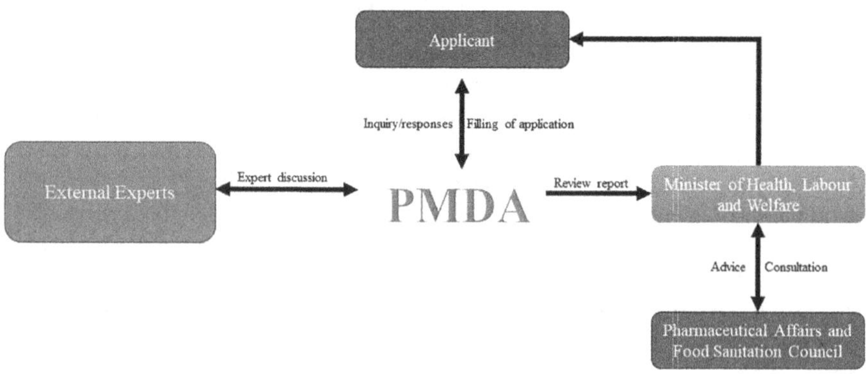

FIGURE 10.2 Regulatory Approval Process for Medical Products.

10.4 NINE FUNCTIONS AND RESPONSIBILITIES

The PMDA in Japan embodies a multifaceted role dedicated to ensuring the safety, efficacy, and quality of pharmaceuticals and medical devices within the country. Through rigorous regulatory evaluations, it meticulously assesses data from preclinical and clinical trials, defining distinct approval pathways based on intended use, pharmacological effects, and risk profiles. Throughout this process, the PMDA collaborates closely with sponsors, providing guidance and support while leveraging its scientific expertise to ensure compliance with stringent regulatory standards. Once products enter the market, the agency's responsibilities extend into robust post-marketing surveillance, monitoring for adverse effects and promptly addressing safety concerns through vigilant pharmacovigilance systems [7,12]. Upholding quality control standards, the PMDA oversees adherence to good manufacturing practices (GMP), ensuring the reliability and consistency of available healthcare products. Furthermore, the agency actively engages in international collaboration efforts, aligning regulatory practices and promoting global standards, while also fostering transparency through open communication, and disseminating regulatory information and guidelines to stakeholders. Collectively, these interconnected functions and responsibilities of the PMDA underscore its pivotal role in safeguarding public health, fostering innovation, and maintaining the highest standards of pharmaceutical and medical device regulation in Japan.

Primary functions and responsibilities of the PMDA include the following:

1. *Regulatory evaluation*: The PMDA conducts rigorous assessments and reviews of pharmaceuticals and medical devices seeking approval for market entry in Japan. It meticulously evaluates data from preclinical and clinical trials to determine the safety, efficacy, and quality of these products.
2. *Approval process*: It establishes guidelines and criteria for the approval of drugs and medical devices, providing guidance and support to sponsors (pharmaceutical companies or manufacturers) throughout the application process. The PMDA categorizes products based on intended use, pharmacological effects, and risk profiles, defining distinct pathways for approval.
3. *Post-marketing surveillance*: The agency implements robust surveillance mechanisms to monitor the safety and efficacy of pharmaceuticals and medical devices already on the market. This continuous monitoring involves collaborating with healthcare professionals, industry stakeholders, and using pharmacovigilance systems to detect and assess any adverse effects or safety concerns that may arise.
4. *Quality control*: Ensuring the quality and reliability of healthcare products remains a cornerstone of the PMDA's responsibilities. It oversees adherence to GMP and other quality standards, maintaining the integrity and consistency of pharmaceuticals and medical devices available in Japan.
5. *Scientific expertise and guidance*: The PMDA harnesses the expertise of a diverse team of scientific professionals spanning various disciplines. It

provides guidance and recommendations to sponsors during the development and regulatory submission phases, fostering collaboration and compliance with regulatory standards.

6. *International collaboration*: Actively engaging in international collaboration and harmonization efforts, the PMDA collaborates with global regulatory bodies and participates in initiatives aimed at aligning regulatory practices, sharing information, and promoting global standards of pharmaceutical and medical device regulation.
7. *Communication and transparency*: The agency promotes transparency by disseminating regulatory information, guidelines, and updates to stakeholders. It communicates openly with applicants, healthcare professionals, and the public, fostering an environment of trust and understanding regarding regulatory processes and decisions.

10.5 APPROVAL PROCESS FOR PHARMACEUTICALS

The approval process for pharmaceuticals in Japan is a rigorous and meticulous series of steps that is overseen by the PMDA. The primary goal of this process is to ensure the safety, efficacy, and quality of drugs before they are granted market access. Japan's strict regulations and comprehensive evaluation procedures make their approval process one of the most stringent in the world [13]. The first step in the approval process is the submission of a New Drug Application (NDA) to the PMDA. This application includes detailed information on the drug's composition, manufacturing process, safety data, and clinical trial results. The PMDA then conducts a thorough review of the NDA, scrutinizing every aspect of the drug's development and testing. Next, the PMDA consults with external experts through its Expert Advisory Council, seeking their input and expertise in the evaluation of the drug [14]. This council comprises physicians, scientists, and other professionals who provide valuable insight and recommendations on the drug's safety and efficacy. After the review and consultation process, the PMDA decides on whether to approve the drug. If approved, the drug is granted market access in Japan. However, the process does not end there. Post-marketing surveillance and monitoring are crucial components of the approval process. The PMDA closely monitors the safety and effectiveness of approved drugs, and manufacturers are required to regularly submit post-marketing safety reports [15]. Overall, the approval process for pharmaceuticals in Japan is a meticulously designed system that prioritizes ensuring the safety and effectiveness of drugs. Through the PMDA's comprehensive evaluation and monitoring procedures, Japan maintains high standards for pharmaceuticals, providing reassurance to both healthcare professionals and patients (Figure 10.3).

Important stages of drug approval in Japan include the following:

1. *Preclinical studies*: Before human trials, pharmaceutical companies conduct preclinical studies. These studies involve laboratory and animal testing to gather data on a drug's safety profile, pharmacokinetics, and potential efficacy. This phase typically takes 1 to 3 years.

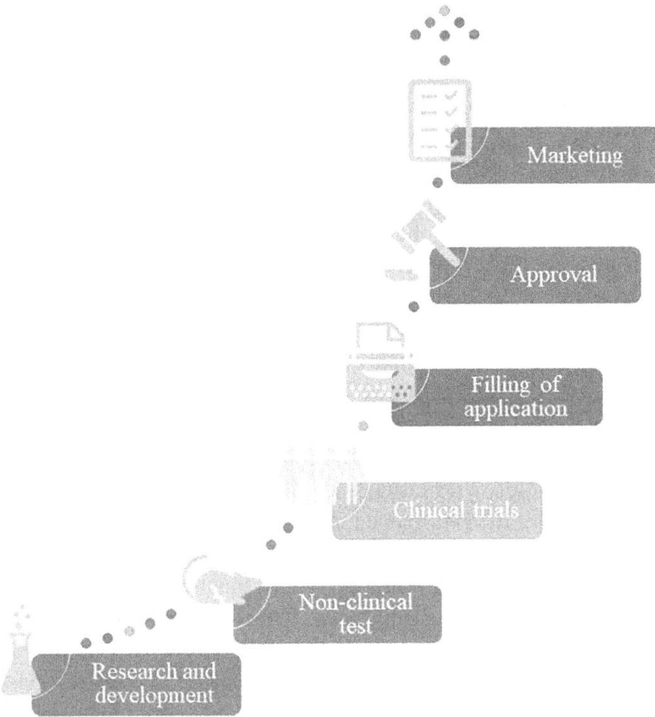

FIGURE 10.3 Drug Development Process in Japan.

2. *Clinical trials*: Clinical trials in Japan are divided into phases I, II, and III. Phase I focuses on safety in a small group of healthy volunteers. Phase II involves a larger group to assess efficacy and side effects. Phase III trials are extensive, involving thousands of patients to confirm efficacy, safety, and dosage. The overall duration of clinical trials can range from 3 to 7 years.
3. *New Drug Application (NDA) submission*: After completing clinical trials, the pharmaceutical company submits an NDA to the PMDA. This application includes comprehensive data on the drug's efficacy, safety, manufacturing methods, and quality control. The PMDA reviews the NDA dossier, a process that typically takes 1 to 2 years.
4. *PMDA review*: Upon receiving the NDA, the PMDA conducts a thorough review of the submitted data. This review involves assessing the drug's safety, efficacy, quality, and risk-benefit profile. The agency examines all aspects of the application to ensure compliance with regulatory standards. The review period usually spans 1 to 2 years.
5. *Approval decision*: Once the PMDA completes its review, it decides on the approval of the drug. The time taken for this decision can vary based on the complexity of the drug, the completeness of the submitted data, and any additional information requested during the review process.

6. *Post-approval phase*: After approval, the pharmaceutical company must continue to monitor the drug's safety and efficacy through post-marketing surveillance. This phase involves ongoing data collection and reporting of adverse events, ensuring continued safety in real-world usage.

It is important to acknowledge that the time frames provided are approximate and can vary considerably depending on several factors. These factors include the complexity of the drug under review, the adequacy of the submitted data, any regulatory changes that may arise during the evaluation process, and the responsiveness of the pharmaceutical company in addressing queries or providing additional information requested by the PMDA. The complexity of a drug can influence the length of time it takes for the PMDA to review and evaluate its safety and efficacy. Drugs with more intricate mechanisms of action or novel therapeutic targets may require more extensive scrutiny, leading to a longer review period. The adequacy of the submitted data is another critical factor. The PMDA relies on comprehensive data packages that demonstrate the safety and efficacy of the drug to make informed decisions. If the data submitted by the pharmaceutical company is incomplete or insufficient in supporting the drug's benefit-risk profile, it may prolong the review process as the PMDA requests additional information or clarifications. Regulatory changes can also impact the timeline for drug approvals. If there are new guidelines or regulations introduced during the review period, the PMDA may need to reassess certain aspects of the application, potentially leading to delays. Last, the responsiveness of the pharmaceutical company is crucial in ensuring a timely review process. If the company promptly addresses and provides satisfactory responses to the queries and requests for additional information from the PMDA, it can help expedite the overall evaluation process. In conclusion, the time frames for drug approvals set forth by the PMDA are approximate and subject to variation. The complexity of the drug, the adequacy of submitted data, regulatory changes, and the responsiveness of the pharmaceutical company all play significant roles in determining the duration of the evaluation process [16].

10.6 CLINICAL TRIALS REQUIREMENTS

Clinical trials conducted in Japan adhere to comprehensive and rigorous requirements stipulated by the PMDA. These stringent requirements are strategically developed to ensure the utmost patient safety, uphold data integrity, and facilitate thorough evaluations of a drug's safety and efficacy [17,18].

Some significant aspects of clinical trials include the following:

1. *Regulatory approval*: Before initiating clinical trials, sponsors (pharmaceutical companies or researchers) must obtain approval from the PMDA or Institutional Review Board (IRB) for each trial phase.
2. *Ethical considerations*: Trials must adhere to strict ethical guidelines, ensuring informed consent from participants, protecting their rights, and maintaining confidentiality of personal data.

3. *Trial design*: The trial design should be scientifically sound and robust, with clearly defined objectives, inclusion and exclusion criteria for participants, and a well-structured protocol outlining procedures, endpoints, and statistical analysis plans.
4. *Phases of clinical trials*: Trials typically progress through phases I, II, and III. Phase I assesses safety in a small group of often healthy volunteers. Phase II expands to a larger group to evaluate efficacy and side effects. Phase III involves a larger population to confirm efficacy, safety, and dosage.
5. *Data collection and reporting*: Trials require meticulous data collection, ensuring accuracy and consistency. Adverse events and outcomes must be reported promptly and comprehensively to the PMDA.
6. *Good clinical practice*: Adherence to GCP guidelines is mandatory. These guidelines ensure that trials are conducted ethically, and scientifically sound, and that the data collected is reliable and credible.
7. *Quality assurance and control*: Trials must implement quality control measures to ensure the accuracy and reliability of data. This includes proper documentation, monitoring, and auditing throughout the trial.
8. *Post-trial reporting*: After trial completion, sponsors are required to submit detailed reports of the trial results, including any adverse events or findings, to the PMDA.

Compliance with these stringent requirements is essential for the successful conduct of clinical trials in Japan. Adhering to these guidelines ensures the reliability of trial results, ultimately contributing to the evaluation and approval process of pharmaceuticals in the country.

10.7 CLASSIFICATION OF DRUGS IN JAPAN

In Japan, drugs are classified into several categories based on various criteria, including their pharmacological effects, intended use, and associated risks. The classification system helps streamline the regulatory process, providing distinct pathways and requirements for approval, manufacturing, marketing, and distribution [19,20].

Drug classifications include the following:

1. *New drugs (Shin'yaku):* New drugs refer to pharmaceuticals that have not been previously marketed in Japan or contain new active ingredients. These undergo comprehensive evaluations and stringent approval processes by the PMDA.
2. *Generics (Igai Yakuhin)*: Generic drugs are equivalents of already approved brand-name drugs with identical active ingredients, dosage forms, and efficacy. They undergo a simplified approval process by demonstrating bioequivalence to the original drug.
3. *Over-the-counter (OTC) drugs (non-prescription drugs—OTC Kusuri)*: OTC drugs are available without a prescription for self-medication. These

drugs are considered safe and effective for use without the direct supervision of a healthcare professional.

4. *Ethical drugs (Yakkan)*: Ethical drugs are prescription medications requiring a doctor's prescription for dispensation. They include a wide range of pharmaceuticals, from common medications to specialized treatments, and often undergo rigorous clinical trials and evaluations.
5. *Orphan drugs*: These drugs target rare diseases and medical conditions that have limited treatment options. In Japan, orphan drugs receive special considerations, including expedited reviews and certain incentives to encourage their development and availability.
6. *Narcotics and controlled substances*: Drugs falling under this category have strict regulations because of their potential for abuse or addiction. They are tightly controlled, with specific protocols for prescription, dispensation, and storage.

Each drug classification in Japan carries its set of regulations and requirements, ensuring the safety, efficacy, and appropriate use of pharmaceuticals within the country's healthcare system. The categorization serves as a framework that guides manufacturers, healthcare professionals, and regulatory bodies through the processes involved in the development, approval, and distribution of various types of drugs [21].

10.8 DRUG APPROVALS ACCORDING TO THEIR CLASSIFICATIONS

In Japan, the approval process for drugs varies according to their classification. The general approval pathways based on different drug categories are as new drugs (*Shin'yaku*) undergo a comprehensive and rigorous approval process by the PMDA. The process includes preclinical studies, followed by phased clinical trials (Phase I, II, and III) to establish safety, efficacy, and dosage. The sponsor submits an NDA dossier containing extensive data for PMDA review. Upon successful review, the drug receives marketing approval. Generic drugs (*Igai Yakuhin*), being equivalents of already approved brand-name drugs, go through a simplified approval process. To gain approval, generic manufacturers must demonstrate bioequivalence to the original drug through comparative bioavailability studies. These studies show that the generic drug delivers the same amount of active ingredients in the body within an acceptable range as the brand-name drug. OTC drugs or non-prescription drugs (OTC *Kusuri*) are generally considered safe for self-medication and have a streamlined approval process. However, they still undergo evaluations and must meet specific safety and efficacy standards. Manufacturers submit data supporting the drug's safety profile, including evidence of its effectiveness and low risk when used as directed without medical supervision. Ethical drugs (*Yakkan*), requiring a doctor's prescription for dispensation, go through a thorough evaluation process like new drugs. They undergo extensive clinical trials to establish safety, efficacy, and dosage before submission of an NDA to the PMDA for review and approval. Drugs designated as orphan drugs for rare diseases have a specialized approval process that includes certain incentives to encourage their development. They may receive expedited reviews and specific regulatory advantages to address unmet medical needs in rare conditions. Drugs falling under the Narcotics and Controlled Substances category have stringent regulations because of their potential for abuse or addiction. Their approval involves a meticulous evaluation of the drug's medical benefits versus the risks of misuse or dependency. Specific protocols are in place for prescription, dispensation, and storage to prevent misuse. Each drug classification in Japan follows a distinct approval pathway, tailored to ensure the safety, efficacy, and appropriate use of the pharmaceutical within the context of its intended classification.

10.9 POST-MARKETING SURVEILLANCE AND PHARMACOVIGILANCE

Post-marketing surveillance (PMS): Post-marketing surveillance involves continuous monitoring of pharmaceuticals once they are available to the public. It aims to detect and evaluate adverse events, side effects, and other safety concerns that might not have been evident during pre-approval clinical trials. Various methods are employed to gather data, including spontaneous reporting, literature reviews, observational studies, and registries. The PMDA in Japan oversees PMS activities and collaborates with healthcare professionals, pharmaceutical companies, and consumers to collect and analyze data related to drug safety [22].

Pharmacovigilance: Pharmacovigilance refers to the science and activities related to the detection, assessment, understanding, and prevention of adverse effects or any other drug-related problems. It involves the collection and analysis of data to determine the risks associated with pharmaceuticals and to implement measures to mitigate these risks. The PMDA operates a pharmacovigilance system to receive, evaluate, and respond to reports of adverse events or suspected adverse reactions to pharmaceuticals in the Japanese market. Reporting adverse events to the PMDA is mandatory for healthcare professionals and pharmaceutical companies [23].

Monitoring drug safety: Continuous monitoring of drug safety is conducted through multiple channels. Healthcare professionals, including physicians and pharmacists, play a vital role in identifying and reporting adverse events associated with pharmaceuticals they prescribe or dispense. Consumers also contribute by reporting any adverse effects or unexpected reactions they experience while using medications. Additionally, pharmaceutical companies are responsible for conducting ongoing safety evaluations and reporting any identified risks to regulatory authorities like the PMDA [24].

Reporting systems: In Japan, reporting systems for adverse events or suspected adverse reactions to pharmaceuticals are established to ensure timely and comprehensive data collection. The PMDA operates the Adverse Drug Reaction Reporting System (YAKUGEN), a platform where healthcare professionals, pharmaceutical companies, and consumers can report suspected adverse events related to medications. Reporting to YAKUGEN is mandatory for healthcare professionals and pharmaceutical companies, encouraging a proactive approach to drug safety monitoring [24].

10.10 CHALLENGES AND FUTURE TRENDS

In Japan's pharmaceutical and healthcare landscape, several challenges and future trends shape the trajectory of the industry [26]. Japan faces the challenge of an increasingly ageing population, leading to a higher prevalence of chronic diseases and complex healthcare needs. Addressing these needs requires innovative approaches, including personalized medicine, geriatric care advancements, and tailored healthcare solutions for the elderly demographic. With an ageing population and advanced healthcare technologies, managing healthcare costs becomes a significant concern. Balancing the need for innovative treatments with cost-effectiveness poses a challenge, prompting efforts to optimize healthcare spending without compromising quality [25]. As medical technology advances, regulatory frameworks must adapt swiftly to accommodate emerging therapies, such as regenerative medicine, gene therapy, and advanced medical devices. Ensuring safety and efficacy while expediting the approval of breakthrough treatments remains a critical balancing act for regulatory bodies. The integration of digital health technologies, telemedicine, and artificial intelligence presents both opportunities and challenges. Enhancing regulatory frameworks to ensure the safety, security, and effectiveness of digital health solutions while promoting their adoption within Japan's healthcare system is a key focus. Japan's pharmaceutical market seeks increased collaboration with international partners to access a broader range of innovative treatments. Harmonizing regulatory practices, fostering international partnerships, and navigating global market access remains essential for Japan's pharmaceutical industry. There is a growing emphasis on patient-centric healthcare models, tailoring treatments, and services to individual patient needs. This shift toward personalized medicine requires advancements in diagnostics, treatment modalities, and data-driven healthcare delivery. With an increased global focus on sustainability, Japan's healthcare sector aims to reduce its environmental footprint. Efforts include green manufacturing practices, waste reduction, and sustainable healthcare infrastructure development [27].

10.11 REGULATORY CHANGES

Regulatory changes in Japan's pharmaceutical and healthcare landscape often aim to enhance patient safety, streamline processes, and adapt to evolving scientific and technological advancements. Japan frequently aligns its regulations with global standards set by organizations like the International Council for Harmonisation of Technical Requirements for Pharmaceuticals for Human Use (ICH). This alignment facilitates smoother international collaborations and ensures Japan's regulatory practices are in line with global best practices. PMDA periodically revises approval pathways to expedite the review and approval of innovative drugs addressing unmet medical needs. These pathways include schemes such as Sakigake Designation and Priority Review programs, which provide faster access to critical medicines. Japan encourages innovation in healthcare by implementing policies that support research and development, especially in areas like regenerative medicine, orphan drugs, and advanced therapies. Regulatory frameworks are updated to accommodate breakthrough treatments, fostering an environment conducive to innovation. Continuous improvement in pharmacovigilance systems ensures robust monitoring of drug safety post-approval. The PMDA introduces updated reporting mechanisms, evaluates safety data comprehensively, and implements measures to address emerging risks promptly. To maintain high quality standards, revisions in manufacturing and quality control guidelines are periodically introduced. These changes align with international quality standards, ensuring consistency and reliability in pharmaceutical manufacturing processes. The integration of digital health technologies and telemedicine has prompted regulatory adjustments to accommodate these advancements. Frameworks are updated to regulate and ensure the safety and efficacy of health-related digital products and services. Japan continues to focus on enhancing transparency in regulatory processes. Efforts to engage stakeholders, seek public input, and provide clear guidelines contribute to a more transparent and collaborative regulatory environment.

10.12 INTERNATIONAL COLLABORATION

International collaboration plays a pivotal role in Japan's pharmaceutical and healthcare sectors, fostering innovation, knowledge exchange, and advancements in medical research. Collaborations with global research institutions, universities, and pharmaceutical companies enable Japan to participate in cutting-edge research projects. These partnerships facilitate the exchange of scientific knowledge, expertise, and resources, accelerating discoveries and innovations in drug development and healthcare. Aligning regulatory practices with international standards, especially through initiatives like the ICH, promotes consistency in drug development processes. Harmonized regulations streamline approval pathways and facilitate the global acceptance of pharmaceuticals developed in Japan. International collaborations facilitate market access for Japanese pharmaceuticals and medical devices in foreign markets. Trade agreements, partnerships, and regulatory collaborations create avenues for Japanese products to reach a wider global audience, contributing to the growth of the pharmaceutical industry. Collaborative clinical trials conducted across borders provide diverse patient populations for research studies. Shared data and insights derived from multinational trials enhance the understanding of disease mechanisms, treatment efficacy, and safety profiles, benefiting global healthcare advancements. International collaborations enable the exchange of best practices, expertise, and training opportunities among healthcare professionals, researchers, and regulatory authorities. This knowledge-sharing enhances skill, fosters innovation, and strengthens capabilities within Japan's healthcare ecosystem. Participation in global health initiatives and partnerships allows Japan to contribute to addressing global health challenges. Collaborations in areas such as infectious diseases, vaccination programs, and public health interventions demonstrate Japan's commitment to global health security and well-being.

REFERENCES

[1] Tejima, Y. (2022). Drug Regulation in Japan. In *Competition Law and Policy in the Japanese Pharmaceutical Sector* (pp. 35–47). Singapore: Springer Nature Singapore.

[2] Kuribayashi, R., Matsuhama, M., & Mikami, K. (2015). Regulation of Generic Drugs in Japan: The Current Situation and Future Prospects. *The AAPS Journal*, *17*, 1312–1316.

[3] Bareilles, M., Gagnon, S., Kimura, M., Naito, H., & Wakita, H. (2011). Japanese Regulations. In *Global Clinical Trials* (pp. 63–85). Academic Press.

[4] Labbé, E. (2010). Japanese Regulations. *Principles and Practice of Pharmaceutical Medicine*, 509–527.

[5] Jawahar, N., & Datchayani, B. (2018). Comparison of Generic Drug Application and Their Approval Process in US, Europe and Japan. *Journal of Pharmaceutical Sciences and Research*, *10*(3), 523–527.

[6] Ono, S. (2007). Ministry of Health, Labour and Welfare (MHLW, Japan). *Wiley Encyclopedia of Clinical Trials*, 1–8.

[7] pmda.go.jp. PMDA Profile of Services (cite 04 Dec. 2023). Available from www.pmda.go.jp/files/000241469.pdf.

[8] Mori, K., & Toyoshima, S. (2009). Recent Approaches by the PMDA to Promoting New Drug Development: Change in the Status of the PMDA in Relation to New Drug Development Over the Last Five Years. *Drug Information Journal*, *43*(1), 47–55.

[9] Tamura, A., & Matsukawa, K. (2022). Japan: Medical Device Regulatory System. In *Medical Regulatory Affairs* (pp. 491–534). Jenny Stanford Publishing.

[10] Asahina, Y., Tanaka, A., Uyama, Y., Kuramochi, K., & Maruyama, H. (2013). The Roles of Regulatory Science Research in Drug Development at the Pharmaceuticals and Medical Devices Agency of Japan. *Therapeutic Innovation & regulatory Science*, *47*(1), 19–22. https://doi.org/10.1177/2168479012469950

[11] Uyama, Y. (2019). The Importance of a Regulatory Science Approach for Better Pharmaceutical Regulation. *Translational and Regulatory Sciences*, *1*(1), 8–11. https://doi.org/10.33611/trs.1_8

[12] Pharmaceutical Regulations in Japan: Chapter 1 Organization and Function of the Ministry of Health, Labour and Welfare (cite 07 Dec. 2023). Available from www.jpma.or.jp/english/about/parj/eki4g6000000784o-att/2020e_ch01.pdf

[13] Kusakabe, T. (2015). Regulatory Perspectives of Japan. *Biologicals*, *43*(5), 422–424.

[14] Oye, K. A., Eichler, H. G., Hoos, A., Mori, Y., Mullin, T. M., & Pearson, M. (2016). Pharmaceuticals Licensing and Reimbursement in the European Union, United States, and Japan. *Clinical Pharmacology & Therapeutics*, *100*(6), 626–632.

[15] Tsuji, K., & Tsutani, K. (2010). Approval of New Drugs 1999–2007: Comparison of the US, the EU and Japan Situations. *Journal of Clinical Pharmacy and Therapeutics*, *35*(3), 289–301.

[16] Ono, S., Yoshioka, C., Asaka, O., Tamura, K., Shibata, T., & Saito, K. (2005). New Drug Approval Times and Clinical Evidence in Japan. *Contemporary Clinical Trials*, *26*(6), 660–672.

[17] pmda.go.jp. Regulation of Clinical Trials in Japan (cite 07 Dec. 2023). Available from www.pmda.go.jp/files/000221892.pdf

[18] Asano, K., Tanaka, A., Sato, T., & Uyama, Y. (2013). Regulatory Challenges in the Review of Data from Global Clinical Trials: The PMDA Perspective. *Clinical Pharmacology & Therapeutics*, *94*(2), 195–198.

[19] Pharmaceutical Regulations in Japan: Chapter 2 Pharmaceutical Laws and Regulations. Available from www.jpma.or.jp/english/about/parj/eki4g6000000784o-att/2020e_ch02.pdf

[20] Pharmaceutical Regulations in Japan: Chapter 3 Drug Development (cite 07 Dec. 2023). Available from www.jpma.or.jp/english/about/parj/eki4g6000000784o-att/2020e_ch03.pdf

[21] Credevo.com. The Drug Approval Process in Japan (cite 07 Dec. 2023). Available from https://credevo.com/articles/2020/04/15/the-drug-approval-process-in-japan/

[22] Maeda, K., Katashima, R., Ishizawa, K., & Yanagawa, H. (2015). Japanese Physicians' Views on Drug Post-Marketing Surveillance. *Journal of Clinical Medicine Research*, *7*(12), 956.

[23] Kawahara, A. (2009). Future Perspectives for Pharmacovigilance in Japan. *Journal of Health Science*, *55*(4), 593–600.

[24] Tanaka, K., Morita, Y., Kawabe, E., & Kubota, K. (2001). Drug Use Investigation (DUI) and Prescription-Event Monitoring in Japan (J-PEM). *Pharmacoepidemiology and Drug Safety*, *10*(7), 653–658.

[25] Nakatani, H. (2019). Population Ageing in Japan: Policy Transformation, Sustainable Development Goals, Universal Health Coverage, and Social Determinates of Health. *Global Health & Medicine*, *1*(1), 3–10. https://doi.org/10.35772/ghm.2019.01011

[26] Maeda, H. (2022). The Current Status and Future Direction of Clinical Research in Japan from a Regulatory Perspective. *Frontiers in Medicine*, *8*, 816921.

[27] DIA 2015. New Regulation in Japan and Future Direction of PMDA (cite 07 Dec. 2023). Available from www.pmda.go.jp/files/000205834.pdf

11 Regulations in the African Union/Southern African Region (SADC Region/West African Region)

Faraat Ali, Evans Sagwa, and Colin Shamhuyarira

11.1 BACKGROUND

Regulatory approaches and processes for the registering and marketing approval of medicines on the African content, including within the Southern African Development Community (SADC) region, have been fragmented, inconsistent, and disparate across national medicines regulatory authorities (NMRAs) of numerous countries (Magubane & Robles, 2017). Besides, not all NMRAs have the same regulatory capacity maturity levels, with some relying more heavily on others (Moran et al., 2011). In some countries in the SADC, independent regulatory institutions are nonexistent and regulatory functions are very basic, being carried out by an entity within the Ministry of Health.

In 2021, health ministers in Africa agreed to the establish the African Medicines Agency (AMA) to help build and strengthen capacity of regional and national regulatory systems on the continent (Zarocostas, 2018), to increase the continent's access to high-quality, secure, and effective medical products (AMA Treaty). It is anticipated that the AMA would support the creation of an atmosphere that will facilitate improved coordination among various partners and stakeholders involved in the continent's efforts to enhance and harmonize medicine regulations. (African RH).

SADC is a regional monetary community. The 16 nations that are members of SADC are Angola, Botswana, Comoros, Democratic Republic of the Congo, Eswatini, Lesotho, Madagascar, Malawi, Mauritius, Mozambique, Namibia, Seychelles, South Africa, United Republic of Tanzania, Zambia, and Zimbabwe.

Within the SADC region, NMRAs have varying regulatory capacities, with 11 countries having actively issued marketing authorizations as at 2017. In 1999, the SADC Ministers of Health issued a directive on harmonisation of registration of medicines. This ushered in foundational work that began with the development of core technical guidelines. At the individual country level, NMRAs, counting the South African Health Products Regulatory Authority (SAHPRA), are re-designing their regulatory systems and re-engineering processes for better efficiency in service delivery and to be more adaptive to the current national, regional, and global

 DOI: 10.1201/9781003296492-12

regulatory environments for improved regulatory effectiveness (Keyter, Salek, Banoo et al., 2020a). NMRAs conduct scientific reviews and assessment of product dossiers and decide whether to register or record a drug based on their evaluation of the health aids and menaces of the product to its intended users (Keyter, Salek, Banoo et al., 2020a).

11.2 STATUS OF MEDICINES REGISTRATION IN SADC

11.2.1 Interventions (CTD, MRH, Collaboration, Process Streamlining, and Use of Electronic Tools)

11.2.1.1 Creation of ZAZIBONA

Regulatory convergence, reliance, and recognition among NMRAs within SADC are essential harmonizing regulatory processes and eliminate unnecessary replication of governing efforts to lessen the regulatory problem on the regulatory bodies and the pharmaceutical industry (Keyter, Salek, Banoo et al., 2020a).

One of the regulatory functions that was prioritized for harmonization and convergence is product registration and marketing authorization. The SADC cooperative drugs authorization campaign (ZAZIBONA) was established in 2013 (Sithole et al., 2022) and approved by SADC Ministers of Health overseeing HIV and AIDS in January 2015.

The ZAZIBONA initiative seeks to enhance cooperation in the evaluation of documentation and regulatory inspections for the registration of medicines. Its goals include alleviating workload, expediting medicine registration timelines, fostering mutual trust in regulatory collaboration, establishing a platform for training and collaboration across various regulatory domains, and facilitating the adoption of the Common Technical Document (CTD) in the SADC region.

The CTD for pharmaceutical product registration unifies and harmonizes technical information and documentation required for the authorization of a human therapeutic invention (Jordan, 2014). This guidance document was developed by the International Conference on Harmonisation (ICH), with the first set of ICH CTD guidelines being published in 2002 (Guy, 2014). The CTD format ensures that the information submitted to the national regulatory authority is unambiguous, systematic, and transparent. It has become a key tool for promoting regulatory harmonization of pharmaceutical product registration and market authorization process across countries.

11.2.1.2 SADC Dossier Submission and Joint Review Process

Central or Common submission of an application dossier, along with Manufacturer's Consent for the regulatory authorities to work together and share dossier information including Chemistry, Manufacturing and Control Data..

One Primary Assessment by a lead country and five other countries, generating through consensus a Consolidated Assessment Report (CAR) and Consolidated List of Questions to the candidate (CLoQ).

Concatenation

- *Day 0 of the ZAZIBONA process*: Initial Meeting: Consensus is reached on selecting a Rapporteur, with the understanding that country screenings are acceptable.
- *Day 75*: The Rapporteur distributes the Initial Assessment Report (AR1) to ZAZIBONA National Regulatory Authorities (NRAs) and the reviewer. The reviewer evaluates both the AR1 and LoQ1.
- *Day 90 (Second Meeting)*: Deliberations and establishment of a shared stance on compliance and inspection triggers.
- *Day 105*: LoQ1 sent to the applicant, with a response deadline of 45 days (not exceeding 90 days).
- *Day 150*: The Rapporteur receives Responses1 from the applicant and commences the evaluation process.
- *Day 165*: The Rapporteur shares Assessment Report 2 (AR2) and Limits of Quantification 2 (LoQ2) with ZAZIBONA NRAs and the reviewer. The reviewer evaluates both AR2 and LoQ2.
- *Day 180 (Third Meeting)*: Discussion and establishment of a unified stance.
- *Day 195*: LoQ2 sent to the applicant, with a response period of 45 days (maximum 90 days).
- *Day 240*: The Rapporteur receives Responses2 from the applicant and initiates the evaluation process.
- *Day 255*: The Rapporteur distributes Assessment Report 3 (AR3) and a suggested position on registration to ZAZIBONA NRAs and the reviewer. The reviewer assesses AR3 and the proposed position.
- *Day 270 (Fourth Meeting)*: Deliberation and consensus on the recommendation or non-recommendation of registration.
- *Day 285*: The Rapporteur disseminates the final ZAZIBONA position.
- *Day 330*: Countries are to make decisions on registration, either rejecting or approving.
- *Day 360 (Fifth Meeting)*: Compilation of information regarding national registrations, noting differences and dates.

Despite the implementation of the ZAZIBONA collaboration, some NMRAs such as SAHPRA are still experiencing long delays in the registration of medicines, partly because of resource shortages, ineffective operating procedures, and a rise in the number of applications for registration of medicines (Keyter, Salek, Gouws et al., 2020b). Use of electronic tools and digital documents could facilitate faster reviews, sharing, and management of dossiers.

11.3 PROGRESS (WHAT HAS WORKED AND WHAT HAS NOT WORKED?)

The SADC nations may now work together to undertake joint evaluations of applications because the standards for the registration of medicines have been harmonized through the use of the CTD format. The ZAZIBONA initiative, established

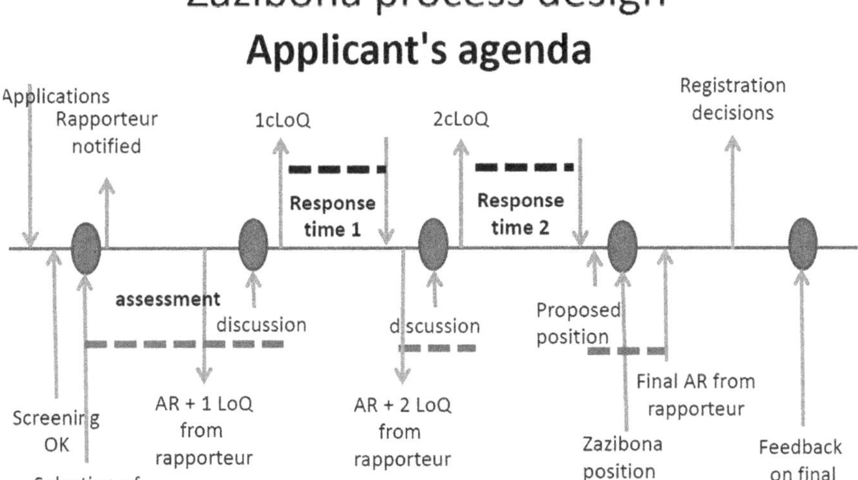

FIGURE 11.1 ZAZIBONA Registration Process.

Source: Selelo (2017), https://rr-africa.woah.org/wp-content/uploads/2000/11/selelo.pdf

in 2013, has continued to gain traction and has attracted more membership than the initial founders. Sithole and associates recently carried out a study in collaboration with a total of nine ZAZIBONA member regulatory bodies to assess the efficacy and efficiency of the ZAZIBONA initiative's present functioning model, taking into account the obstacles it faces and identifying areas for betterment from the candidates' point of view. (the pharmaceutical industry; Sithole et al., 2022). In this study, pharmaceutical sector reports suggest, the ZAZIBONA project has shortened the time it takes for medical approval, increasing the amount of high-quality medications that patients in the SADC region can get. Furthermore, the regulatory authorities' and the pharmaceutical industry's workloads have been lessened by the harmonization of registration requirements and cooperative reviews (Sithole et al., 2022).

11.4 PROCESS OF REGULATORY REVIEW

The laws and requirements of the medications Act, particularly regulations and established recommendations, control the authorization of medications in South Africa. Statutory structures necessitate the NRA to examine medications, especially New Chemical Entities (NCEs), multisource/generic pharmaceuticals, biological pharmaceuticals, supplementary drugs, and medicines for animals, ahead of advertising for the product. Scientific paperwork must be submitted by candidates to establish the efficacy, safety, and quality of such medications proposed for commercialization in South Africa. The 34th section of the Medicines Act, which governs the upkeep of secret, governs the anonymity details given to the NRA. The NRA evaluated pharmaceutical application for registration using both domestic and foreign expertise (Keyter et al., 2018).

The expert panels looked at an exhaustive examination of data, in addition to the evaluations that were generated by the respondents, and made suggestions on the acceptance of the commercial name of the good, granting of a planning a status for the active substance, and a review of the GMP practices of the submitter, the producer of the active drugs component, and the supplier of the finished product. The Medicines Control Council (MCC) made the ultimate conclusion on permission or denial.

11.5 GOVERNMENT BODIES OVERSEEING REGULATIONS IN SPECIFIC NATIONS

11.5.1 Zimbabwe

The legislative authority in Zimbabwe tasked with safeguarding both human and animal health is the Medicines Control Authority of Zimbabwe (MCAZ). The Drugs and Allied Substances Control Act, a parliamentary act, created it on September 1, 1969. The Drugs Control Council and the Zimbabwe Regional Drug Control Laboratory have been replaced by the MCAZ (Sithole et al., 2021). The World Health Organization (WHO) developed a worldwide network of sites known as Vaccine Safety Net, of which the MCAZ has been an affiliate since 2020. The MCAZ employs 101 to 250 people as of 2021.

11.5.2 Tanzania

An Executive Department under the Ministry of Health, Community Development, Elderly and Children is Tanzania Medicines and Medical Devices Authority (TMDA). The TMDA is in charge of policing the efficacy, safety, and quality of medications, medical equipment, and diagnostics. The Health Policy of 2007 outlines the primary role of the TMDA, while its mission is delineated in the Tanzania Food, Drugs and Cosmetics Act cap. 219, as modified by the Financial Services Act of 2019. The legislation outlines effective and thorough regulations for quality control measures for medications, medical equipment, and diagnostics throughout Tanzania's mainland (Fimbo et al., 2022). The Executive Agencies Act, cap. 245 as revised in 2009 governs how TMDA is operated as a federal agency with the goal of enhancing the provision of public services.

11.5.3 Egypt

All medications, medical equipment, their accessories, and in vitro diagnostics (IVDs) sold in Egypt are subject to control by the Egyptian Drug Authority (EDA). The Ministry of Health and Population Affairs oversees it. The registration, manufacturing, transportation, shipment, distribution, and usage of medicines and medical supplies in Egypt are all under the control and supervision of the EDA (Abd El-Rady et al., 2023).

11.5.4 South Africa

Protecting the wellness and welfare of humans and animals is the main goal of the South African government's establishment of the SAHPRA, which functions as a section of the National Department of Health (NDoH). As a public institution under Schedule 3A, SAHPRA is responsible for the following:

- Supervising the control of medicinal goods intended for ingestion by humans and animals.
- Granting licenses to companies that produce, distribute, and wholesale pharmaceuticals, medical equipment, radiation-emitting devices, and radioactive nuclides.
- Following the national pharmaceuticals policy while conducting clinical studies.

SAHPRA took over the responsibilities of the NDoH's MCC and Directorate of Radiation Control. After this, SAHPRA was established as a separate organization under the board of which reports to the National Minister of Health (Dureja & Dhiman, 2021).

All health goods must be regulated (monitored, evaluated, investigated, inspected, and registered) by SAHPRA. This covers the use of IVDs, medical equipment, alternative and complementary healthcare, and research studies. SAHPRA also has the additional duty of managing radiation control in South Africa. The Hazardous Substances Act (Act No. 15 of 1973) and the Medicines and Related Substances Act (Act No. 101 of 1965 as modified) also specify SAHPRA's jurisdiction.

11.6 CHALLENGES (WHAT ARE THE HURDLES AND BOTTLENECKS?)

Regulatory agencies in Africa and in SADC continue to experience human, technical, financial, and other resource shortages, which impair their capacity to efficiently and effectively perform registration and marketing authorization and other core regulatory functions recommended by the WHO (Moran et al., 2011). In addition, absence of proper laws, guidelines, and weak governing systems, a nonexistence of skilled regulatory specialists and unproductive regional associations amongst NMRAs have continued to hamper patients' avail to reasonably priced, high-quality, safe, and effective medical items in Africa (Ncube et al., 2021). Balancing interests between promoting national economic and industrial growth on the one hand and regulatory control to safeguard public health continues to be a thin line to walk. At other times, concerns for national sovereignty have posed a challenge in some countries collaborating with on medicines regulation.

11.7 RESTRAINTS

The present research was confined to an evaluation of the South African regulatory framework; nevertheless, the template produced via this investigation offers an outline that other NRAs may use to improve regulatory efficiency. Given the parallels in the issues encountered by NRAs in developing nations, it is quite probable that this approach will be adopted by such NRAs in the African area and beyond.

It might be beneficial to investigate regulatory competence and prospects for improving local and continent collaboration activities in Africa. Addressing regulatory agencies who used an abbreviated review process to establish the parameters and existing procedures for adoption might be part of future studies. This data will shed light on the potential uses of Facilitated regulatory Pathways (FRPs) for enhancing work-sharing/joint assessments or the legislative function of the ZAZIBONA cooperative effort in the area of the SADC or on the African continent.

11.8 CONCLUSION AND RECOMMENDATIONS (HOW DO WE MOVE FORWARD?)

- Implementation of the recommendations identified by various regulatory system assessments and reviews in the SADC region will lead to enhanced regulatory performance.
- Risk-based regulatory approaches.
- Technology for efficiency gains.
- Reliance and work-sharing.

REFERENCES

Abd El-Rady, D., Sheded, S., Isamail, A., & El-Hosary, E. (2023). Regulatory Impact Analysis for the Risk Based Lot Release Policy for Biological Products in Egypt. *Journal of Regulatory Science*, *11*(1), 1–13.

Dureja, H., & Dhiman, S. (2021). SAHPRA-Relevance of the New South African Health Products Regulatory Authority and Opportunities Ahead. *Journal of Regulatory Science*, *9*(2), 1–14. https://doi.org/10.21423/JRS-V09I2DUREJA

Fimbo, A.M., Maganda, B.A., Mwamwitwa, K.W., Mwanga, I.E., Mbekenga, E.B., Kisenge, S., Mziray, S.A., Kulwa, G.S., Mwalwisi, Y.H., & Shewiyo, D.H. (2022). Post Marketing Surveillance of Selected Veterinary Medicines in Tanzania Mainland. *BMC Veterinary Research*, *18*(1), 216. https://doi.org/10.1186/s12917-022-03329-x

Guy, R. (2014). *International Conference on Harmonisation*. Retrieved July 23, 2023, from https://sciencedirect.com/science/article/pii/b9780123864543008617

Jordan, D. (2014). An Overview of the Common Technical Document (CTD) Regulatory Dossier. *Medical Writing*, *23*(2), 101–105. Retrieved July 23, 2023, from http://journal.emwa.org/regulatory-writing-basics/an-overview-of-the-common-technical-document-ctd-regulatory-dossier/article/1693/2047480614z2e000000000207.pdf

Keyter, A., Banoo, S., Salek, S., & Walker, S. (2018). The South African Regulatory System: Past, Present, and Future. *Frontiers in Pharmacology*, *9*, 1407. https://doi.org/10.3389/fphar.2018.01407

Keyter, A., Salek, S., Banoo, S., & Walker, S. (2020). A Proposed Regulatory Review Model to Support the South African Health Products Regulatory Authority to Become a More Efficient and Effective Agency. *International Journal of Health Policy and Management*, *1*. https://doi.org/10.34172/ijhpm.2020.213

Keyter, A., Salek, S., Banoo, S., & Walker, S. (2020a). Can Standardisation of the Public Assessment Report Improve Benefit-Risk Communication? *Frontiers in Pharmacology*, *11*, 855. https://doi.org/10.3389/fphar.2020.00855

Keyter, A., Salek, S., Gouws, J., Banoo, S., & Walker, S. (2020b). Evaluation of the Performance of the South Africa Regulatory Agency: Recommendations for Improved Patients' Access to Medicines. *Therapeutic Innovation & Regulatory Science*, *54*(4), 878–887. https://doi.org/10.1007/s43441-019-00013-5

Moran, M., Strub-Wourgaft, N., Guzman, J., Boulet, P., Wu, L., & Pécoul, B. (2011). Registering New Drugs for Low-Income Countries: The African Challenge. *PLoS Medicine*, *8*(2). Retrieved July 23, 2023, from https://doi.org/10.1371/journal.pmed.1000411

Ncube, B.M., Dube, A., & Ward, K. (2021). Establishment of the African Medicines Agency: Progress, Challenges and Regulatory Readiness. *Journal of Pharmaceutical Policy and Practice*, *14*(1), 29. https://doi.org/10.1186/s40545-020-00281-9

Sithole, T., Mahlangu, G., Salek, S., & Walker, S. (2021). Evaluation of the Regulatory Review Process in Zimbabwe: Challenges and Opportunities. *Therapeutic Innovation & Regulatory Science*, *55*, 474–489. https://doi.org/10.1007/s43441-020-00242-z

Sithole, T., Mahlangu, G., Walker, S., & Salek, S. (2022). Pharmaceutical Industry Evaluation of the Effectiveness and Efficiency of the ZaZiBoNa Collaborative Medicines Registration Initiative: The Way Forward. *Frontiers in Medicine*, *9*, 898725. https://doi.org/10.3389/fmed.2022.898725

Zarocostas, J. (2018). Health Ministers Adopt African Medicines Agency Treaty. *The Lancet*, *391*(10137), 2310–2310. Retrieved July 23, 2023, from https://thelancet.com/journals/lancet/article/piis0140-6736(18)31313-8/fulltext

12 Regulations in Latin American Countries

Tausif Alam and Irfan Ansari

12.1 TERMINOLOGY

Pharmaceutical raw materials: Those substances or raw materials that we use in manufacturing drugs and medicines [1].

Health product and medical devices: Devices, apparatus and instruments that assist healthcare providers to diagnose and treat the patients. These devices are available in hospitals and image diagnostic centres [1].

New product: A product containing active pharmaceutical ingredients (synthetic or semisynthetic) in different dosage forms, different strengths, different routes of administration and different therapeutic indications by a pharmaceutical company that is not the registered holder of products formulated with that active pharmaceutical ingredient.

A new product can also be defined as new salts, isomers of already approved salt, or an agent modifying pharmacokinetic property of an already approved salt.

Innovative medicinal product: A medicinal product approved for marketing in Brazil, formulated with at least one active ingredient that has been patented (expired or not) in the country of origin. Generally, it is considered as the Reference Medicinal Product by ANVISA [2].

Generic product: A consumer product without a widely recognized name or logo because it usually is not advertised. A product that is similar to the reference product. Generic drugs are allowed for sale after the patents on the original drugs expire or refuse to extend protection. A generic drug is a pharmaceutical drug that contains the same chemical substance as a drug that was originally protected by chemical patents. A company can only market a generic medicine once the ten-year exclusivity period for the original medicine has expired. When efficacy, quality and safety has been scientifically proven, its name is given in accordance with the Common Brazilian Name Listing (DCB) or the Common International Name Listing (DCI) [1].

Similar product: A product that contains same active ingredient of an innovative medicinal product. in physicochemical, in vitro and in vivo biological characteristics, and clinical data showing similarity in efficacy, safety, and immunogenicity. It needs to be advertised or marketed inside the equal energy, dosage form, dosage regimen, path of management, healing indication, analysis and prevention symptoms and for the same as that of the reference medicinal product already accepted for marketing via the ANVISA and also approved for the same indications as for an Afecta Licensed Product after Effective Date.

DOI: 10.1201/9781003296492-13

The main difference between the similar medicinal product and reference medicinal products is about its size, layout, expiry period and packaging excipients. Its efficacy, quality and safety has been proved. Products like this should have some commercial name or brand name [2].

Clone product: An identical product, so its generic product is already approved or vice versa. In this case it is compulsory to submit a clone application even by the registered innovator drug applicant who wants to approve its generic product or similar product [1].

12.2 INTRODUCTION

Latin America (LA) consists of 20 countries. Each country has its own rules and regulations for the registration of medicinal products. Unlike European Medicines Evaluation Agency (EMEA) for all European countries, there is no centralized regulatory authority for LA. Brazil is the biggest pharmaceutical market of Latin America and also has the strongest regulation. Brazil is followed by Mexico, Colombia and Argentina. Some countries have weak regulations that enable the registration of unsafe and ineffective drug simply on the basis of bioequivalence study [3]. Out of 20 countries of LA, 7 countries (Bolivia, Brazil, Chile, Cuba, Honduras, Nicaragua and Venezuela) do not accept regulatory reliance of national regulatory authorities like the US Food and Drug Administration (FDA), EMEA or Health Canada to approve new medicinal products [4]. The main regulatory authorities of LA are summarized in Table 12.1.

TABLE 12.1
Regulatory Authority of Latin American Countries with Average Approval Timelines of Drug Products

S. No.	Countries	Regulatory Authority	Average Approval Timelines	Reference
1.	Brazil	National Health Surveillance Agency (ANVISA)	6–8 months	[5]
2.	Argentina	National Administration of Drug Products, Food and Medical Technology (ANMAT)	12 to 18 months for small molecules, 24 months for vaccines and biologicals. Variation of 12 for small molecules and 6 to 18 months for vaccines and biologicals	[6]
3.	Costa Rica	Costa Rica Ministry of Health	12 to 15 months	[5]
4.	Chile	Public Health Institute (ANAMED—ISP)	6 to 10 months	[7]
5.	Cuba	Center for State Control of Medicines, Equipment and Medical Devices (CECMED)	3 months	[8]
6.	Colombia	National Institute for Food and Medicine Surveillance (INVIMA)	2.5 years or 1.5 years with on-site CMC dossier review (small molecular products) with variation of 12 to 18 months	[6]

(Continued)

TABLE 12.1 (Continued)
Regulatory Authority of Latin American Countries with Average Approval Timelines of Drug Products

S. No.	Countries	Regulatory Authority	Average Approval Timelines	Reference
7.	Mexico	Federal Commission for Protection against Health Risks (COFEPRIS)	12 to 18 months with variation of 12 to 24 months	[6]
8.	Peru	General Directorate of Medicines, Supplies and Drugs (DIGEMID)	12 to 18 months with variation of 3 to 6 months	[6]
9.	Bolivia	Medicines and Health Technology Unit (UNIMED)	10 to 30 days	[9]
10.	Venezuela	National Institute of Hygiene Rafael Rangel (INH-RR)	6 months	[10]
11.	Paraguay	National Directorate of Health Surveillance	—	
12.	El Salvador	Directorate of Medicines and Health Products (DIRMED)	3 to 6 months	[11]
13.	Ecuador	National Health Regulation, Control, and Surveillance Agency (ARCSA)	2 to 6 months	[12]
14.	Dominican Republic	National Directorate for Drug Control (DNDC)	3 months	[13]
15.	Guatemala	Department of Regulation and Control of Pharmaceutical and Related Products	12 to 15 months	[5]
16.	Panama	National Directorate of Pharmacy and Drugs	2 years	[5]
17.	Honduras	Sanitary regulatory agency (ARSA)	12 to 15 months	[3]
18.	Nicaragua	Ministry of Health	8 to 12 months	[14]
19.	Uruguay	National Drug Board (JND)	10 to 12 months	[15,16]
20.	CRS	Caribbean Public Health Agency (CARPHA)	6 months	[17]

The Pan American Health Organization (PAHO) evaluates the National Regulatory Authorities (NRA) for Drug Products, based on recommendations of the World Health Organization (WHO) for strengthening regulatory bodies [18].

For the registration of drugs in America there are some document requirements, prepared by Pan American Network on Drug Regulatory Harmonization (PANDRH). Document must be in the language of that country where application is submitted for drug registration [19].

Documents generally consists of four modules and two annexes.

Module 1: Administrative and legal information
Module 2: Quality information
Module 3: Nonclinical reports
Module 4: Clinical reports
Annex 1: Summary of Product Characteristics (SPC)
Annex 2: Information on labeling and package inserts.

12.2.1 Module 1: Administrative and Legal Information

Each country has its own format but at minimum the application should contain the following information;

1 ***Table of contents***

2 ***Characteristics of products***

   2.1 API name as per International Non-proprietary Names System (INN) and the Anatomical Therapeutic Chemical Classification System (ATC).
   2.2 Brand name (not indicating therapeutic use or inducing consumption).
   2.3 Composition: Name and quantity of each ingredient in conventional units recognized internationally.
   2.4 Dosage form.
   2.5 Route of administration.
   2.6 Packaging: Specify type of primary and secondary package and the content of medicine into it. Specifies whether distributed as single unit or multiple unit pack. Any additional accessory like transfer device should be indicated.
   2.7 Description of lot and batch number: For easy identification during manufacturing and distribution.
   2.8 Expiry date: For both reconstituted and non-reconstituted product.
   2.9 Dispensing requirement: Must specify one of the following:

      i. Classified as narcotic and psychotropic medicines;
      ii. Dispensing without prescription;
      iii. Dispensing with prescription;
      iv. Restriction on use: Exclusively used in clinics or hospitals.

   2.10 Storage condition: Packing should include condition to store a product indicating temperature, humidity, light or other conditions.
   2.11 Conditions for handling.

3 ***Legal documentation***

   3.1 Technical director/health professional responsible: The following information must be submitted for technical director/health professional responsible for product in the country of registration:
   - Their name, address, telephone number, fax number, e-mail address, licensing number, degree;
   - Document issued by the competent health authority authorizing the director.

   3.2 Market authorization holder (MAH): State full name, address, phone number, fax number and e-mail address of market authorization holder. The information on MAH should be submitted first time when registration of product is being done. There is no need to submit such information again upon variation in the registered product in America.
   3.3 Legal representative in the country: This refers to the country that will hold market authorization in the America. Full name, address, telephone number, fax number, and e-mail address must be provided apart from the following information:

- Document from the MAH of product in the country of origin authorizing the company to hold MAH in America;
- This information is essential to furnish for the registering product for the first time. If there are some changes involved, then there is no need to furnish such information again.

3.4 Manufacturer of the Active Pharmaceutical Ingredient: Specify the names, addresses, telephone numbers, fax numbers, and e-mail addresses of the laboratories that manufacture API.

3.5 Manufacturer of the finished product: Specify the name, addresses, telephone numbers, fax numbers, and e-mail addresses of all laboratories that manufacture the final product and submit the following information:

- If there is more than one manufacturer, then specify main manufacturer and steps at which other manufacturers were involved;
- If manufacturer is not the MAH, then a legal document is submitted indicating association between two;
- Certificate of GMP: Submit GMP certificate of excipients manufacturer, labs, labeling and packaging unit. Certificate of GMP indicates areas in which plant is authorized to function;
- Product that needs reconstitution name, address, telephone number, fax number, and e-mail address of the manufacturer of the diluent must be provided, confirming that it is included in final packaging.

4 *Information on the medicine regulatory status in other countries, for imported products*

Certificate of Pharmaceutical Product: It is the certificate issued in the format recommended by WHO that identifies the status of pharmaceutical product and the applicant in the country where product is to be registered. If the country of the applicant is not a member of the WHO certification scheme, then the following must be submitted:

- Certificate of Free Sale;
- Certificate of Good Manufacturing Practices;
- Evidence of registration of product in the country of origin;
- Evidence of marketing of product in the country of origin.

5 *Product technical information*

5.1 Summary of Product Characteristics (SPC).

5.2 Labeling and package information: Text for the label on primary and secondary container and packaging insert should be included.

5.3 Samples for evaluation: Two samples for evaluation should be submitted for each dosage form.

6 *Environmental risk assessment*

Detail on the product like hormones, antineoplastic agents, radiopharmaceuticals that can cause problem to environment and living beings should be included in packaging insert.

12.2.2 Module 2: Quality Information

This module includes information on the Active Pharmaceutical Ingredients, excipients and finished product as given below.

2.1 ***Active Pharmaceutical Ingredients***

Nomenclature and properties of the Active Pharmaceutical Ingredients. The following must be submitted.

2.1.1 ***Nomenclature and properties of API***

- Name of the API as per INN and the ATC;
- Chemical name as per WHO and Pharmacopeial monograph;
- Chemical Abstract Service (CAS) or International Union of Pure and Applied Chemistry (IUPAC) number.

2.1.2 ***Chemical structure and molecular formula of API***

- Molecular formula;
- Chemical structure including its stereoisomeric form;
- Molecular weight and molecular mass.

2.1.3 ***Physicochemical characteristics of the API***

- Organoleptic property and physical property like appearance, color, and physical state;
- Solubility in common solvents;
- Partition coefficient;
- Distribution of particle size;
- Hygroscopic properties;
- Polymorphism: Presence or absence of polymorphic form, hydrates, solvates etc.

2.1.4 ***Synthesis of API***

a. List of all the equipment, raw materials, chemicals and solvents involved in the synthesis of API.
b. Flow chart of the synthesis of API:
    - Identification of critical points;
    - Process controls and acceptance limits;
    - A list of operational parameters;
    - Control of critical steps and intermediate products and their quality specifications;
    - Identification and method of analysis of polymorphs;
    - Content of the stereoisomers that can compromise safety and efficacy of the product.
c. Process validation of the critical steps of the manufacturing process.
d. If API is synthesized through fermentation, then specification is required for type of microorganism, composition of the medium, precursors and controls of reaction conditions.
e. If API is of vegetable origin, then the following information is included:
    - Biological classification, pa

rt of plant used and method of extraction;

- Geographical origin and season at which they were collected;
- Chemical fertilizers, pesticides, fungicides or any other agricultural defensives used.

2.2 Control of Active Pharmaceutical Ingredients

2.2.1 Quality specifications

a. Physical, chemical and microbiological specifications and acceptance limits (pharmacopeial reference or manufacturer's own reference);
b. If manufacturer's own reference is used as acceptance limit, then rationale for such selection needs to be justified.

2.2.2 Methods of analysis

a. Specific monograph when pharmacopeia is used as reference;
b. If manufacturer's own reference is used, then full description of the method of analysis is given.

2.2.3 Validation of the method of analysis

a. For API having specification of reference pharmacopeia, the following information is required:
   - Information on evaluation/feasibility of the method performance when using method validation as mentioned in pharmacopeia;
   - If there is slight modification of parameters of analytical method validation as mentioned in pharmacopeia; then full information on those parameters are provided.
b. Where manufacturer's own methods of analysis are involved, it is important to provide analytical method validation summaries representing data of each validation parameter.

2.2.4 Certificates of analysis

Certificates of analysis of the lot of the API to be registered is provided. For the combination product containing two or more API, certificates of analysis for each need to be provided.

2.2.5 Stability

Documents on stability study mentioning shelf-life under that storage and container-closure system is required for the new API, new salt, ester, complex or derivative.

2.3 Excipients

The following information is required:

a. Name, quality reference, quality specifications (indexes and acceptance limits) for each ingredient;
b. If excipient is not mentioned in pharmacopeia, then method analysis mentioning quality specifications is needed;
c. List of excipients whose source is animal or human and description on its safety;
d. For excipients whose source can cause transmission of bovine spongiform encephalopathy, then supporting document on non-transmission of such infection by appropriate authority is needed;

e. If any excipient is used for a new route of administration, then detailed document on its manufacturing, characterization, quality control and toxicology is needed.

2.4 Finished product

2.4.1 Pharmaceutical development

All studies to decide final dosage form, manufacturing process and container-closure system is submitted along with compatibility with other excipients and API or combination of API.

2.4.2 Finished product description and composition

a. Composition of each excipient and API should be in table format;
b. If product needs reconstitution, then description of diluent and container used for dilution must be included;
c. If the content of API in formulation is more than that mentioned on label, then quantity and percentage by which it increases should be specified with proper justification to include increased amount;
d. When API is in the form of salt, hydrates and solvates with dose strength referring to the base, then it is essential to indicate amount equivalent to the base. When this is not possible to determine the amount equivalent to the base in each lot because of the quantity of salt, hydrate or solvate varying in potency, then such product is exempted from documentation of amount equivalent.

2.4.3 Manufacture of the finished product

2.4.3.1 Lot formula

Qualitative and quantitative formula including list of components for the production lot must be included.

2.4.3.2 Description of the manufacturing process

The following information must be included:

a. Description of steps involved in the manufacturing from raw materials till packaging;
b. Flow chart of manufacturing indicating critical points, material input and process control;
c. Description of control of critical steps and main intermediate products;
d. If two or more manufacturers are involved, then a flow chart indicating how they relate with each other for the dosage formulation should be included;
e. Process validation;
f. Reprocessing should be justified and properly validated.

2.4.4 Control of the finished product

2.4.4.1 Quality specifications

a. Description of physical, chemical and microbiological properties including acceptance limits as per pharmacopeia or manufacturer's own reference;
b. Justification of exclusion of quality index recognized in the reference pharmacopoeias;
c. Time-release testing of modified release dosage form.

2.4.4.2 Methods of analysis

Provide the information of specific monograph of pharmacopeia utilised for method of analysis, and if not, then provide complete description of method of analysis.

2.4.4.3 Validation of methods of analysis

a. If standard pharmacopeia is used as reference, then the following information is needed:
    - Information on method performance;
    - Information on validation of any parameters when changes are made in pharmacopeial procedure.
b. If manufacturer's own method of analysis is involved, then full description of process validation including data is required.

2.4.4.4 Certificates of analysis

Description of quality specification of the product by manufacturer.

2.4.4.5 Reference standards and materials

Information on reference standards and materials used in quality control test.

2.4.5 Description of the container-closure system

Description of type and form of material used for container and closure with their quality reference and quality specifications (index and acceptance limits).

2.4.6 Stability studies of the finished product

Stability studies must be submitted as per climatic zone including the following information.

2.4.6.1 Protocols of stability study justifying shelf life

a. Study protocol;
b. Quality specifications and methods of analysis;
c. Detail of container-closure system in which study is carried out;
d. Storage condition (temperature, light, humidity);
e. Results from a minimum of three lots;
f. Proposed shelf life;
g. Sign of the quality head involved in this study;
h. If the product is for reconstitution, then stability study of API with reconstituting medium must be submitted;
i. If product is packed in two or more container, then stability study in each container must be submitted;
j. If product is packed in same containers of different volume, then stability study as per international regulation in force must be submitted;
k. Accelerated stability studies.

2.4.6.2 Post-marketing authorization stability studies programme

Once product is in market, after that there is need to submit stability study. Stability study should be done on approved lots for marketing and approved storage and container-closure system.

Case requiring submission of long-term stability study: To confirm or increase the provisional shelf-life of the formulation when accelerated stability study and shelf-life study was done on pilot batch.

2.4.6.3 Description of the procedures used to guarantee the cold chain

Product requiring refrigeration and freezing, detailed description of temperature and humidity conditions are required to be submitted from manufacturing point to selling point. Controls taken at different stages to maintain the temperature and humidity should be described.

2.4.7 Biopharmaceutical documentation

The following documents may be required:

a. Dissolution test
b. In vitro equivalence studies
c. In vivo equivalence studies (for new molecule).

12.2.3 Module 3: Nonclinical Reports

3.1 Table of contents

Table of contents of all documents submitted as per this module.

3.2 Nonclinical trials

3.2.1 For new API

3.2.1.1 Pharmacokinetic studies

3.2.1.2 Pharmacodynamic studies

3.2.1.3 Toxicology

a. General toxicology
    - Study design and its justification;
    - Animal model, age and size of group;
    - Dose, route of administration and duration of study;
    - Parameters calculated;
    - Local tolerance.
b. Special toxicology
    - Toxicity study in special population;
    - Genotoxicity and carcinogenicity;
    - Reproductive toxicity study.

3.2.2 For new combinations

Pharmacodynamic studies are required.

3.2.3 For new excipients added to the formulation, such as any additives or stabilizer, the respective toxicology study must be submitted.

12.2.4 Module 4: Clinical Reports

4.1 Table of contents

4.2 Clinical trials

4.2.1 Clinical trials of new API

4.2.1.1. Summary of clinical trials conducted

4.2.1.2 Phase I studies

Primarily done to find out safety, pharmacokinetics and bioavailability of new API.

a. This study includes healthy volunteers that is then grouped on the basis of intrinsic factors (age, sex, disease) and extrinsic factors (smokers, concomitant medicines, diet). Data submitted includes absorption, distribution, metabolism and excretion studies.
b. Studies in this phase have no therapeutic objectives. Studies in this phase can be open, single blind or double blind.

4.2.1.3 Phase II studies

a. This study is done on patients and therapeutic efficacy of new API is explored.
b. Safety and efficacy of the product is evaluated at this stage. Dose and dosage regimen is determined in this phase.
c. Initially dose escalation design is used to find dose-response relationship that is further confirmed by parallel dose-response designs. Dose used in phase II are generally higher than phase I but this is not always true.
d. Other objectives include potential end point of the trial, dosage regime and target population (mild vs. severe disease).

4.2.1.4 Phase III studies

a. Safety and efficacy of the product is further confirmed in this trial. Several thousands of patients are included in this trial
b. Phase III studies confirm all the description given for summary of product characteristics.
c. Short-term and long-term safety studies are included especially for medicines for chronic diseases.

4.2.1.5 Phase IV studies

Results of the study already conducted after the drug is in market is required to be submitted.

Description of studies on special populations as per indication of medicine.

4.2.2 Clinical trials of known API

If the registered API is combined with new API or a new salt, complex of same API, then clinical trial is needed by regulatory authority as per document of WHO and PANDRH. New route of administration, new dosage form and new complex of same drug also require submission of documents to regulatory authority.

12.3 REGULATION IN BRAZIL

Brazil is the eighth largest pharmaceutical market in the world and is the largest in LA. Registration of a new drug product and generic is highly regulated in Brazil. The regulatory authority of Brazil, Agencia Nacional de Vigilancia Sanitaria (ANVISA), was established in 1999. Documents for product registration and market authorization should be presented in Portuguese to the ANVISA [20]. ANVISA was formed for the regulation of all those products that affect health such as food, drug, cosmetics, disinfectants and other health products [21]. ANVISA became the member of the International Council for Harmonization of Technical Requirements for Pharmaceuticals for Human Use (ICH) in November 1996. Brazil was the first country of LA to become an ICH member, after which Brazil had to adopt the ICH guidelines as given in Table 12.2.

12.4 DOSSIER FORMAT AND ORGANIZATION

Dossier submissions to ANVISA are always accepted in Portuguese only and generally in paper form (non-electronic submission). The format of the dossier submission to ANVISA deviates from the format of common technical dossier of ICH. To get market authorization of a product in Brazil, specific dossier format is required to be followed. The Brazilian dossier consists of five different modules like the ICH Common Technical Dossier (CTD). The organization of the dossier is given in Figure 12.1. An overall quality summary (part of module 2 of ICH) is not required by ANVISA [2].

The dossier is broadly divided into two parts, namely the administrative part consisting of module 1 and the technical part consisting of Modules 2, 3, 4 and 5 as described below.

12.4.1 Administrative Information

Module 1 is region specific, which means each country has its own requirement according to which documents (administrative information) are required to be submitted. The administrative data generally include:

1. Certificate of Pharmaceutical Product issued by Brazil;
2. Proof of payments;
3. Proof of the registration of product in the country of origin;
4. Certificate of Good Manufacturing Practice issued by ANVISA;
5. Repetition of product labeling for imported products once it has received market authorization.

12.4.2 Technical Information

The various information required is mentioned in Table 12.3.

Modules 2, 4 and *5* consist of safety and efficacy reports on non-clinical and clinical studies. Data required here is as per ICH CTD. Modules 2 and 4 is required when a dossier is prepared for new chemical entity; for generic and similar drugs, modules 2 and 4 are not required [22]. Module 5 consists of biopharmaceutics, pharmacokinetic and pharmacodynamic studies including post-marketing experience and patient case report forms. All these studies except bioequivalence studies are done for new chemical entities, whereas later study is done for generics and biosimilar products.

Module 3 consists of a quality report on Active Pharmaceutical Ingredients (API), excipients, packaging material, formulations and stability as described below [2].

I. Active Pharmaceutical Ingredient
   - DMF is submitted to ANVISA

TABLE 12.2
Implementation Plan for the ICH Guidelines in Brazil

Level	Timeline	ICH Code	ICH Guideline Title
1.	Immediate implementation	Q1	Guidelines for Stability Testing
		Q7	Good Manufacturing Practices Guide for Active Pharmaceutical Ingredients
		E6	Guidelines for Good Clinical Practice
2.	Implementation within 5 years (until November 2021)	E2A	Clinical Safety Data Management
		E2B	Data Elements for Transmission of Individual Security Reports
		E2D	Post-approval Security Data Management: Definitions and Standards for Expedited Reports
		M4	Common Technical Documents for the Registration of Medicinal Products for Human Use
		M1	Medical Dictionary for Regulatory Activities (MedDRA)
3.	Long-term implementation	—	Adoption of the Remaining the ICH Guidelines

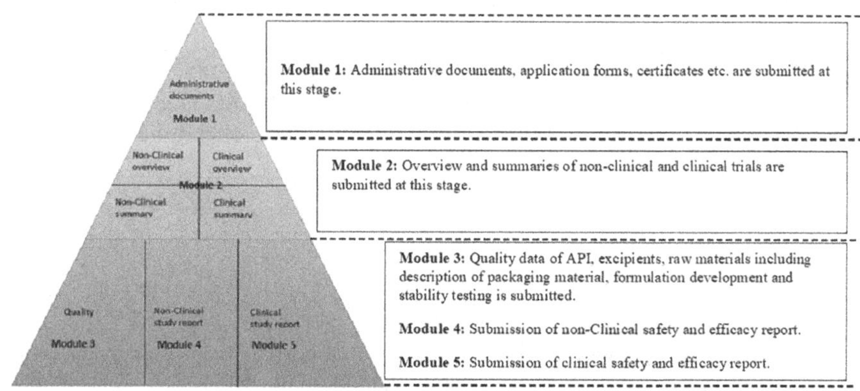

FIGURE 12.1 Technical Document Structure of Brazil.

- API quality control studies
- Certificate of analysis
- Analytical methods and validation
- Justification and references to describe the specification adopted by the manufacturer of finished product.

II. Excipient

- Documents containing the specifications
- Analytical methods and validation
- Copy of the pharmacopoeia used as reference
- Description of all tests done on the excipients as per monograph;
- Certificate of analysis.

III. Packaging material information
- Description of materials and quality control tests information of primary, secondary and tertiary containers
- Certificate of analysis.

IV. Formulation development
- Qualitative and quantitative details of ingredients, bioequivalence, stability and other tests detail
- Documents on characterization of the API and excipients, mainly indicating their physicochemical properties and impact of such properties on safety and efficacy
- Documents on compatibility study of API with excipients and primary packaging material
- Details on degradation profile and dissolution study.

V. Manufacturing report
- Batch formula record
- Certification of analysis
- Process validation.

VI. Finished product
- Specifications and their justification

TABLE 12.3
Technical Information for a New Chemical Entity and a Generic Product

S. No.	Data Required	New Chemical Entity	Generic
1.	Product information: • Labeling • Packaging insert	Required	Required
2.	Manufacturing report	Required	Required
3.	Quality control	Required	Required for API, excipients, finished product
4,	Packaging specifications	Required	Required
5.	Stability studies	Required	Required
6.	Price report	Required	Not required
7.	Non-clinical studies	Required	Not required
8.	Clinical studies	Required	Not required
9.	API information	Required (pharmacokinetic, pharmacodynamic, and toxicity data)	Not required
10.	Bioequivalence study	Not Required	Required

- Technical references used in support
- Rationale of not conducting residual solvent test
- Analytical methods and their validation
- Dissolution profile
- Certification of analysis.

VII. Stability studies (as per zone IVb)

- Protocols and reports on accelerated and long-term stability studies on three batches
- Protocols and reports on photostability study on three batches
- Intermediate stability study data is not required while filing DMF.

12.5 ANVISA STABILITY GUIDELINES

Stability documents required to be submitted to ANVISA deviates from ICH stability testing guidelines (ICH Q1).

12.6 PHOTOSTABILITY TEST/STRESS TEST

Photostability test is required to be performed on three batches, unlike ICH guideline where testing is done on one batch only. Stress testing is required for all the strength of medicinal product by ANVISA [2].

12.7 OTHER REGULATORY REQUIREMENTS

Microbiological tests must be routinely carried out and their absence must be justified. Sterility test of sample and hardness is carried out at the beginning and at the end of the stability studies. Other tests like dissolution test for solids, pH, sedimentation rate and clarity tests for liquids including phase separation study for emulsions and creams are required to be done at each stability test point [2].

The API used for formulation development must be ANVISA certified. If any polymorphic form of API is used, then the API and finished product x-ray diffraction pattern is required. Analytical method validation of API and finished product should be done at the manufacturing site only. For the registration of a generic drug, a sample is required to be submitted to Brazilian authority for the testing of its pharmaceutical equivalency. Analytical testing and dissolution profile of test product is required to be compared with Brazilian reference product in a Brazilian lab certified by ANVISA [1].

12.8 STORAGE CONDITIONS

ANVISA requires annual follow-up stability study. If a medicinal product is imported, then an additional stability study is to be carried out in Brazil [2].

12.9 STABILITY COMMITMENT

If the shelf-life of a product is 24 months and stability data is available for 12 months, then data can be submitted but the commitment is made that data of remaining 12 months will be submitted once available [2].

12.10 REGISTRATION OF DRUG AND ITS PRODUCT FOR MARKET AUTHORIZATION

ANVISA inspection of a manufacturer takes place 6 months after submitting the request. A GMP certificate is issued to the manufacturer 45 to 60 days after inspection (Figure 12.2).

12.11 COMMON REGULATORY REQUIREMENTS OF THE COUNTRIES OF LATIN AMERICA

For getting marketing approval of a drug, a common technical dossier is filed for the countries of LA (Argentina, Mexico and Brazil) [23]. Brazil has its own country-specific requirements (Figure 12.3).

12.11.1 Requirement of GMP Certification for Product Registration

If a pharmaceutical company of any other country wants market authorization in LA, that company must have GMP certificate. Bolivia, Chile, Costa Rica, the Dominican Republic, Guatemala, Nicaragua, Panama, Peru, Puerto Rico and Venezuela accept foreign GMP certificates. For market authorization in Brazil, a company must have Brazilian GMP certificates. Argentina, Colombia and Mexico accept GMP certificates of countries like the United States and regions such as Europe. Countries of LA that accept certificates of foreign regulatory authority are shown in Figure 12.4. Timelines for the approval of new products also vary from country to country.

12.12 STABILITY REQUIREMENT ACROSS THE COUNTRIES OF LATIN AMERICA

LA comes under three climatic zones as shown in Table 12.5 [25]. Table 12.6 represents climatic zone and stability study conditions as per ICH Guidelines. Stability study ensures that patients receives safe and effective medicine throughout its shelf life [26].

Apart from common requirements some country-specific requirements also need to be considered while filing registration of generic drugs. The following sections summarize country-specific requirements that are taken into consideration during regulatory submission.

12.13 REGULATION IN VARIOUS LATIN AMERICAN COUNTRIES

12.13.1 Regulation in Argentina

National administration of drug, food and medical technology (ANMAT) is the regulatory authority of Argentina that deals with regulation of drugs. Registration of drugs in Argentina depends upon in which country drug is being marketed. All the information of drug and its products is required to be given in CTD format. Drug registration and market authorization takes 180 days. Drug registration is required to be renewed every 5 years and the application for renewal is required to be submitted

30 days before [27]. For the registration of drug or its product first batch verification takes place. ANMAT either visits the manufacturing site or review the manufacturing records at last [28]. GMP inspection of a pharmaceutical company by ANMAT requires following documents [29];

- Written request
- Copy of ANMAT authorization to requestor
- Information on manufacturer(s)
- Site Master File
- Site authorization from Health Authority in country in which it is located
- List of pharmaceutical forms manufactured on site
- List of drug substances manipulated on site
- List of pharmaceutical forms by drug substances to import
- Information and documents on third parties involved in manufacturing or control
- Fee.

12.13.2 Regulation in Mexico

For the registration of generics in Mexico, a dossier is submitted to COFEPRIS. The dossier is then reviewed by COFEPRIS, and if there is any problem in the contents, then a deficiency letter is issued to the firm that submitted the dossier, the answer of which should be submitted within 6 months. To perform the quick revision of dossier third party called consultant can do pre-evaluation thereby decreasing the burden and

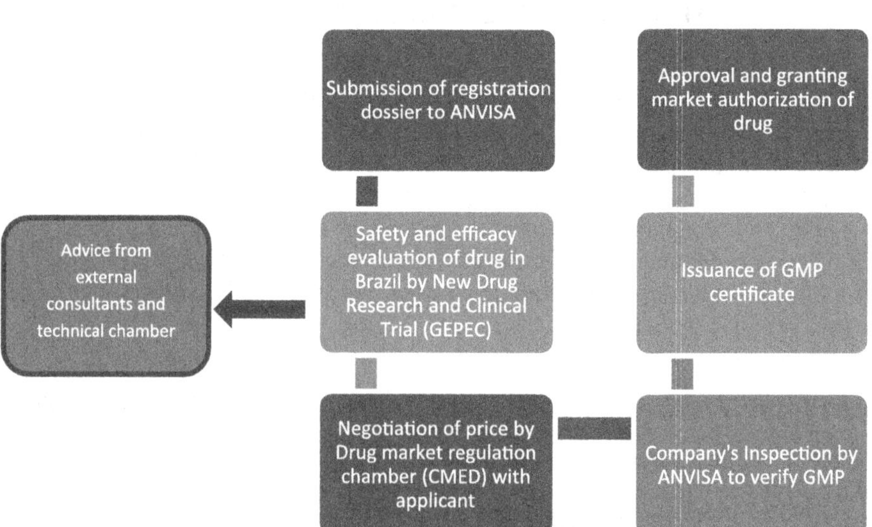

FIGURE 12.2 Steps of Registration of Drugs and its Product for Market Authorization in Brazil.

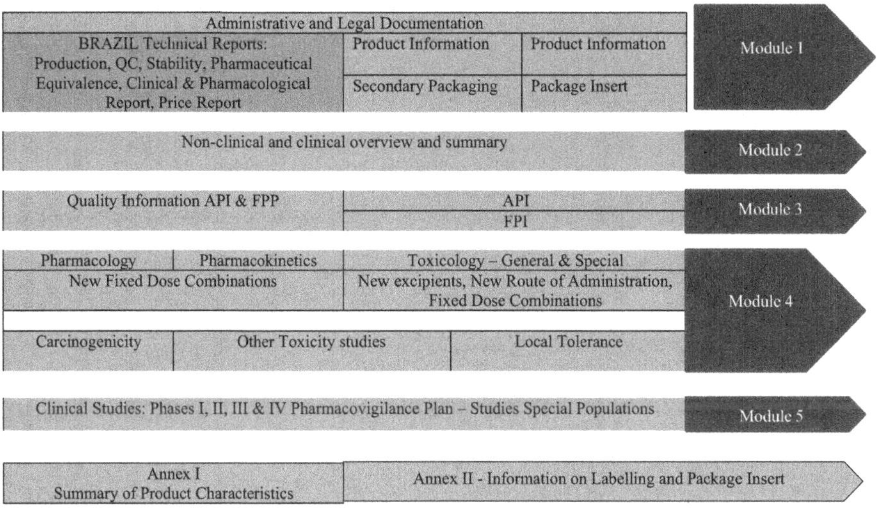

Administrative and Legal Documentation
BRAZIL Technical Reports: Production, QC, Stability, Pharmaceutical Equivalence, Clinical & Pharmacological Report, Price Report
Product Information | Product Information
Secondary Packaging | Package Insert
Module 1

Non-clinical and clinical overview and summary
Module 2

Quality Information API & FPP
API
FPI
Module 3

Pharmacology | Pharmacokinetics | Toxicology – General & Special
New Fixed Dose Combinations | New excipients, New Route of Administration, Fixed Dose Combinations
Carcinogenicity | Other Toxicity studies | Local Tolerance
Module 4

Clinical Studies: Phases I, II, III & IV Pharmacovigilance Plan – Studies Special Populations
Module 5

Annex I Summary of Product Characteristics
Annex II - Information on Labelling and Package Insert

FIGURE 12.3 Roadmap of Document Requirement During Dossier Submission [23].

time of health authority to evaluate the dossier. Documents required for drug registration are as follows [3];

- Fee
- Sanitary license
- Maquila agreement
- Packaging and its distributor information
- Insert
- Prescribing information
- Certification of GMP
- Bioequivalent test
- Complete information of drug like information on its structure, molecular formula, molecular name, synthesis etc.
- COA
- Analytical method and its validation
- Stability studies.

If a drug is manufactured outside Mexico, then there is additional requirement of the following:

- Certificate of Pharmaceutical Product
- Clinical trial documents in the Mexican population
- Brand name
- Letter of Patent
- Letter describing the activity to prevent risk of product

Regulatory authorities recognized as trusted regulators by LAC countries (n = 17)	Countries/regulators that recognize or abbreviate the marketing authorization issued by a foreign regulatory authority (n = 13)												
	Paraguay	Colombia	Guatemala	Dominican Republic	Ecuador**	El Salvador	Uruguay	Caribbean Regulatory System***	Peru	Panama	Argentina	Costa Rica	Mexico
EMA	•	•	•	•	•	•	•	•	•	•	•	•	•
FDA	•	•	•	•	•	•	•	•	•	•	•	•	•
Canada	•	•	•	•	•	•	•	•	•	•	•	•	•
Japan	•	•	•	•	•	•			•	•	•	•	
Switzerland	•	•	•	•		•			•	•	•	•	•
Australia	•	•	•	•	•	•			•	•		•	•
Brazil	•	•	•	•	•	•	•	•					
Argentina	•	•	•	•	•	•	•	•					
Chile	•	•	•	•	•	•	•	•					
Mexico	•	•	•	•	•	•	•	•					
Cuba	•		•	•	•	•	•	•					
Colombia	•		•	•	•	•	•	•					
Uruguay	•												
Israel	•	•									•		
New Zealand	•	•								•			
Republic of Korea		•			•				•				
Turkey		•											
Total	15	14	12	12	12	12	9	9	7	7	6	6	5

FIGURE 12.4 Reference (trusted) regulatory authorities for Latin American and Caribbean countries* (EMA, European Medicines Agency; FDA, US Food and Drug Administration

Notes:

* Bolivia, Brazil, Chile, Cuba, Honduras, Nicaragua, and Venezuela do not accept any form of medicine agency reliance.

** Ecuadorian legislation does not accept reliance on a marketing authorization if the drug is not included in the national list of essential medicines and if it has been approved under a fast-track process in the trusted regulator.

*** The Caribbean Regulatory System (CRS) is a collaborative initiative acting as regulatory unit for 15 Member States of the Caribbean Community and Common Market (CARICOM), including Antigua and Barbuda, Bahamas, Barbados, Belize, Dominica, Grenada, Guyana, Haiti, Jamaica, Montserrat, Saint Kitts and Nevis, Saint Lucia, Saint Vincent and the Grenadines, Suriname, and Trinidad and Tobago. The CRS registers a drug if has been approved by the designated trusted authority, and only if the product is named in the most recent update of the WHO Model List of Essential Medicines or in the PAHO Strategic Fund list.

Source: Duran et al., 2021 [24]

TABLE 12.5
Countries and Climatic Zones for Stability Studies

Climatic Zone	Country
II	Argentina, Mexico, Uruguay
IVA	Bahamas, Belize, Canada, Chile, Costa Rica, Dominica, Dominican Republic, Ecuador, El Salvador, Grenada, Guatemala, Haiti, Honduras, Jamaica, Nicaragua, Paraguay, Saint Kitts and Nevis, Trinidad and Tobago
IVB	Antigua and Barbuda, Barbados, Bolivia, Brazil, Colombia, Cuba, Guyana, Panama, Peru, Saint Lucia, Saint Vincent and the Grenadines, Suriname, Venezuela

TABLE 12.6
Temperature and Humidity Requirements for Conducting Stability Studies

Climatic Zone	Types of Climates/Storage Area	Temperature and Humidity	Duration
I	Temperate	21°C ± 2°C 45% RH ± 5% RH	12 months[L]
II	Subtropical and Mediterranean	25°C ± 2°C 60% RH ± 5% RH	12 months[L]
III	Hot and dry	30°C ± 2°C 35% RH ± 5% RH	12 months[L]
IVA	Hot and humid	30°C ± 2°C 65% RH ± 5 %RH	12 months[L]
IVB	Hot and very humid	30°C ± 2°C 75% RH ± 5% RH	12 months[L]
—	—	30°C ± 2°C 65% RH ± 5% RH	6 months[I]
—	—	40°C ± 2°C 75% RH ± 5% RH	6 months[A]
—	Refrigerator	5°C ± 3°C	12 months[L]
—	Refrigerator	25°C ± 2°C 60% RH ± 5% RH	6 months[A]
—	Freezer	−15°C ± 5°C No humidity	12 months[L]
—	Freezer	5°C ± 3°C No humidity	6 months[A]

Note: The superscripts L, I, and A refer to long-term, intermediate, and accelerated stability testing, respectively.

- Document certifying legal representative in Mexico
- Manufacturing license
- Conclusions of new molecule committee meeting
- Agreement for quality control test with a firm in Mexico.

12.13.3 Regulation in Colombia

There is no need to conduct clinical and non-clinical tests again if a drug is to be registered in Colombia. If plant is GMP certified from reference countries, then there is no need of GMP inspection by INVIMA of that plant again. If a manufacturer has authorized any company to be the market authorization holder in Colombia, then also drug can be registered at INVIMA. Product monograph can be used only from United States (USP), British (BP), French Codex, German (DAB), European and International (WHO), or the one in force for the European Union. Only a certificate of pharmaceutical product (CPP) or free sale certificate (FSC) needs to be notarized or attested at INVIMA. Drug registration application can be submitted online and offline both [30].

Documents required to be submitted to INVIMA for registration of drug:

- Name of the product, brand and manufacturer name;
- Statement that legal and technical information provided is accurate;
- GMP certificate;
- Certificate of existence of manufacturer, importer and packager issued in last 3 months;
- Power of attorney where representative is authorized to submit documents to get market authorization;
- Certificate as obtained patent and trademark office of Colombia stating that trade name is registered in the name of solicitor or is under the process of registration. If owner of trade name is not solicitor, then authorization letter for use from owner must be attached;
- Proof of the application fee;
- Certificate of pharmaceutical product;
- Quantitative formula of API and excipients;
- Structural and chemical formula of API;
- Batch formula record;
- Detailed description of manufacturing process;
- Analytical method reports as per pharmacopeia or proper validation report for non-pharmacopeial method;
- Pharmacological information;
- Stability studies;
- Report of bioavailability and bioequivalence study;
- Quality specification of raw materials, semi-finished and finished product;
- Information on all labeling materials (packaging, label, leaflets etc.).

12.13.4 Regulation in Peru

In Peru, drugs are regulated by General Directorate of Medicines, Supplies and Drugs (DIGEMID) [25]. DIGEMID classifies medicines as pharmaceutical specialties, diagnostic agents, radiopharmaceuticals and medical gases. Pharmaceutical products are further divided into three categories: API in the national formulary of

Peru (category I), API in other countries with high health monitoring standards (category II) and API not in category I or II (category III) [5].

12.13.5 Regulation in Costa Rica

In Costa Rica the following documents are required for the registration of generic drugs [5];

- COPP
- CoA of raw material and finished products
- Qualitative-quantitative formula
- Analytical method validation
- Generic letter
- Stability testing
- Product monograph
- Sample
- Working standard
- Safety data
- Power of attorney.

12.13.6 Regulation in El Salvador and Guatemala

Documents requirement for registration of drugs in El Salvador and Guatemala is similar to Costa Rica. Legal documents are required for drug registration in Guatemala.

- All documents submitted should be original and stamped/signed
- All percentages should be precise without any range
- Certificate of free sale should be notarized.

12.13.7 Regulation in Panama

The National Directorate of Pharmacy and Drugs regulates the drug registration process in Panama and requires following documents to be submitted for drug registration in the country [3]:

- Generic name of product
- Name and address of manufacturer
- Dosage form and its route of administration
- Details of therapeutic class of drug
- Sample
- Complete formula of finished product
- Indications
- Contraindications
- Warning and precautions
- Dose, frequency and range
- Pharmacological data

- Summary of clinical trials
- Data on adverse reactions and drug interactions
- Details of packaging copy and packaging insert (pharmaceutical companies are not bound to inform regulatory body of changes done in labeling of registered product). Package label must contain labeling information in Spanish.

12.13.8 Regulation in Honduras

The following are the document requirements by the Sanitary Regulatory Agency (ARSA):

- Free sale certificate
- Manufacturing good manner certificate
- Qualitative-quantitative formula
- Finished product analysis method
- Stability data
- Packaging information
- Working standard
- Monograph of generic
- Chromatograms and absorption spectra of generic
- Drug prescribing information
- Packaging information.

12.13.9 Regulation in Nicaragua

Documents required for the registration of generic drugs are similar to that of Honduras.

12.13.10 Regulation in Uruguay

Manufacturers or importers must obtain the authorization of the National Drug Board (JND) to market drug in Uruguay. Information required to be submitted to JND to take market authorization are [32]:

- Power of attorney granted to importer by foreign manufacturer to sale drug in Uruguay;
- GMP certificate as evidence that manufacturer is authorized to market drug in its own country;
- Name of API;
- API and raw materials monograph;
- Qualitative—quantitative formula;
- Analytical methods of finished product;
- Pharmaceutical form;
- Stability studies;
- Pharmacological studies;
- Labeling information.

12.13.11 Regulation in Chile

The regulatory authority of Chile is the Public Health Institute (ISP), which is directed by Ministry of Health. The various documents required to be submitted are [19]:

- Information on API, raw materials, semi-finished and finished product;
- Administrative and legal information;
- Bioequivalence study for generic;
- COPP;
- Certificate of free sale;
- GMP certificate;
- Evidence of marketing authorization of drug in country of origin;
- Summary of product characteristics;
- Labeling and packaging information;
- Stability studies.

12.13.12 Drug Registration in Caribbean Countries

When CARPHA reviews and accept the files of applicant for the registration of drug, after that the file is distributed among the government body and is published on a web page that can be accessed by the general public. Government makes decision on market authorization within 60 days provided three basic requirements are satisfied [33]:

1. Payment of fees
2. Administrative information
3. Identifiable importer.

There are some eligibility criteria that an applicant must fulfil when a document is submitted to CARPHA:

1. Submission should be on an essential medicine as listed in WHO essential medicines list. An unlisted medicine can only be submitted if health need of that medicine is justified.
2. The product is under market authorization in Argentina, Brazil, Canada, Chile, Colombia, Cuba, the European Union, Mexico, the United Kingdom, or the United States.
3. The product should be on the WHO prequalification list.

All the documents to CARPHA should be submitted in English. Documents required to be submitted are:

1. A cover letter containing the following information:
   - Statement that information furnished in application is true;

- Statement that the finished product with intention to market will have the same composition, strength, production process, packaging etc. as produced to CARPHA;
- Statement that the product is already marketed in the country of origin.

2. Overview of market authorization status:
   - Recent copy of market authorization of product to ensure that product is already registered in country of origin as per regulatory requirement;
   - List of countries where product has been granted market authorization;
   - List of countries where product has been rejected from market authorization and indicating reason for such rejection. If product has not been rejected from any country, then a statement is submitted indicating that no rejection of product has ever happened in past.
3. Latest version of summary of product characteristics (SmPC) and patient leaflet approved by RA. Link of the website should be provided where SmPC is published.
4. GMP certificates and inspection report.
5. Name, address of all sites involved in manufacturing API and finished product.
6. Certificate of analysis of recent batch of product.
7. Stabilities studies.
8. Picture of finished product (including primary and secondary packaging) as it will be marketed in CARICOM.
9. Bioequivalence and bioavailability study (if API is a new molecular entity, then clinical data is submitted as per ICH CTD module 2).

Additional information required to be submitted to CARPHA are:

1. Production
   - Product specific guidelines related to production, quality, safety, efficacy and potency adopted by the RA or WHO;
   - Notifiable changes in the product should be informed to CARPHA if done and approval letter from corresponding RA should be submitted once available.
2. Marketing authorization
   Products submitted to CARPHA should be manufactured as mentioned in documents and as per current market authorization of country of origin. Any rejection of market authorization should be immediately informed to CARPHA.
3. Labeling
   - Product label should be as per WHO prequalification requirements.
   - Label should be in English.
   - Re-labeling, over-labeling, and contents like "donation" or "free medicine" is not acceptable.
4. Adverse events and substandard and falsified medicines
   Any adverse event or substandard medicine related to the product should be reported to CARPHA.

5. Testing
   Products are subject to random quality control test by CARPHA. Product non-conforming to quality test is rejected, and applicant is asked to produce additional sample for quality test. Decision of lab conducting this test is considered final.
6. Right to share information with CARPHA/CRS member states
   Dossier submitted by applicant can be shared by CARPHA at its sole discretion with NRA from CARICOM.
7. Language
   All documents must be submitted in English

Documents are submitted to CARPHA in electronic form. Documents submitted should be as per checklist. Documents may be submitted as WHO prequalification requirement or as per ICH CTD format.

12.13.13 Requirements for the Registration of Medicines

- Specification on API and finished product and analytical techniques involved therein;
- Flow diagram and validation of manufacturing process;
- Technical documents that include MFR (Master Formula Record), BMR (Batch Manufacturing Record), BPR (Batch Packaging Record) and Raw Material Specification;
- Legal documents like manufacturing license and certificate of free sale with GMP;
- Good Manufacturing Process;
- Stabilities studies;
- Drafts of packing labels;
- Bioequivalence studies;
- Studies supporting safety and efficacy studies;
- Risk planning management;
- Certificate of pharmaceutical product if medicine is manufactured in other country [5,31].

12.14 CONCLUSION

Most of the countries of Latin America are not as much regulated as the FDA, EMEA, or Health Canada. These countries accept data of the developed country because of unavailability of resources and provide market authorization of product to foreign manufacturers. These countries follow CTD modules but there are other requirements also that is not the part of these modules. Regulation varies among LA on the basis of maturity of the regulatory system. There is greater need of harmonization for better regulatory framework and to decrease the challenges in getting market authorization in LA thus decreasing the time and cost of countries in getting market authorization. These countries are constantly changing their regulatory structure to provide safe and effective medication to their citizens.

REFERENCES

[1] V. Mohak, K. Charmy, and S. Manan, "Regulatory Technicalities for Drug Product Registration in Brazil," *International Journal of Drug Regulatory Affairs*, vol. 5, no. 4, pp. 18–25, 2017.

[2] *Critical Assessment—Implementation of ICH Guidelines in Brazil*, 2018. Academic Press.

[3] M. Sravani, M. Kusuma, A. Prabhahar, and R. Nadendla, "Registration of Generic Drugs in Central America and Mexico," *International Journal of Pharma and Chemical Research*, vol. 3, no. 3, pp. 635–650, 2017.

[4] C. E. Duran, et al., "Regulatory Reliance to Approve New Medicinal Products in Latin American and Caribbean Countries," *Revista Panamericana de Salud Publica*, vol. 45, p. e10, 2021.

[5] Mohit A. Deep, G. Khurana, J. Kumar, and A. Monga, "Comparison of Basic Regulatory Requirements for Generic Drug Products Registration in CIS and Latin American Countries," *Applied Clinical Research, Clinical Trials and Regulatory Affairs*, vol. 7, no. 2, pp. 117–125, 2020.

[6] J. Chapman, *Getting Drugs Approved in Mexico, Argentina, Colombia, and Peru*; 2022, 20 March. Available: https://redica.com/pharma-getting-drugs-approved-in-mexico-argentina-colombia-and-peru/

[7] Ministry of External Affairs, *Chile Pharmaceutical Market Legal Framework*; 2020.

[8] M. Cipriano, *Cuba: A Pharmaceutical Regulatory Snapshot*; 2016, 15 March. Springer. Available: https://pink.pharmaintelligence.informa.com/PS119282/Cuba-A-Pharmaceutical-Regulatory-Snapshot

[9] P. Gupta, *Bolivia Pharma Market*; 2018, 4 April. Available: www.linkedin.com/pulse/bolivia-pharma-market-dr-palak-gupta/

[10] W. A. Kaplan and R. Laing, "Paying for Pharmaceutical Registration in Developing Countries," *Health Policy Plan*, vol. 18, no. 3, pp. 237–248, Sep 2003.

[11] *Requirements for Registering Pharmaceutical Products EL SALVADOR 2014*; 2014, 5 April. Available: http://files.export.gov/x_6879464.pdf

[12] Arazy Group, *Medical Device Registration and Approval in Ecuador*; 2022, 16 Feb, 21 March. Available: https://arazygroup.com/medical-device-registration-ecuador/

[13] WDA, *Pharmaceutical Products Registration in Dominican Republic*; 2022, 18 March, 21 March. Available: https://wdalaw.com/publications/articles/natural-products-registration-in-dominican-republic.php

[14] B. Bendaña, *Requirements for Pharmaceutical Regulatory Affairs in Nicaragua*; 2019, 4 April. Available: https://pharmaboardroom.com/legal-articles/requirements-for-pharmaceutical-regulatory-affairs-in-nicaragua/

[15] *Evaluation Report on Drug Policies*; 2019. Academic Press.

[16] *Things You Should Know Before Registering Your Medical Devices in Uruguay*; 2019, 4 April. Available: www.regdesk.co/md-uruguay/

[17] *Requirements for Verification Review of Medicines and Vaccines*, C. P. H. A. (CARPHA); 2020. Academic Press.

[18] O. Pan Americal Health, *System for Evaluation of the National Regulatory Authorities for Medicines*; 4 April. Available: https://www3.paho.org/hq/index.php?option=com_content&view=article&id=1615:2009-sistema-evaluacion-autoridades-reguladoras-nacionales-medicamentos&Itemid=0&lang=en

[19] PANDRH, *Requirement of Medicines Registration in the America*; 2013. Springer.

[20] G. G. Vignesh and N. Sruthi, "Regulatory Requirement for Registration of Drugs in Brazil," *Journal of Critical Reviews*, vol. 7, no. 19, pp. 5290–5295, 2020.

[21] A. C. Carvalho, L. S. Ramalho, R. F. Marques, and J. P. Perfeito, "Regulation of Herbal Medicines in Brazil," *Journal of Ethnopharmacology*, vol. 158 Pt B, pp. 503–506, Dec 2 2014.

[22] *Reformating Your CTD Information for Your Brazilian Registration Dossier*; 2014, 4 April. Regulatory Agency. Available: file:///E:/Regulatory%20Latin%20America/File/Registration%20dossier%20of%20Brazil.pdf

[23] F. F. Silvia Bendiner, *Pharma Strategies in Latin America Keys to Success*; 2016, 4 April. Available: www.fdanews.com/ext/resources/Webinar-Presentations/2016/Presentation-PharmaStrategiesinLatinAmericaPart1-3-15-16.pdf

[24] C. E. Durán, et al., "Regulatory Reliance to Approve New Medicinal Products in Latin American and Caribbean Countries," *Revista Panamericana de Salud Pública*, vol. 45, p. e10, 2021.

[25] "Reformatting Your CTD Information for Your Brazilian Registration Dossier," ANVISA Web.

[26] CS, *Climatic Zone and Stability Study Conditions as Per ICH Guidelines*; 2020, 4 April. Available: https://pharmanhealth.com/2020/09/16/climatic-zone-and-stability-test-condition-as-per-ich/

[27] *Regulatory Affairs in Latin America*; 2013, 4 April. Available: https://latampharmara.com/argentina/drug-product-certificate-renewal-in-argentina/

[28] *First Batch Verification*; 2013, 4 April. Available: https://latampharmara.com/argentina/first-batch-verification/

[29] *GMP Inspections: Regulatory Aspects*; October, 4 April. Available: https://latampharmara.com/argentina/gmp-inspections-regulatory-aspects/

[30] *Invima Marketing Authorization Application (MAA) of Pharmaceutical Drugs in Colombia*; 4 April. Available: www.bioaccessla.com/invima-requirements-for-registration-of-drugs-in-colombia

[31] *An Overview of Regulation on Review and Authorization of Pharmaceutical Products and Medical Devices in Peru*, DIGEMID; 2021.

[32] *Legal & Regulatory > Uruguay > Regulatory, Pricing and Reimbursement*; 2018, 4 April. Available: https://pharmaboardroom.com/legal-articles/regulatory-pricing-and-reimbursement-uruguay/

[33] CARPHA, *Requirements for the Preparation of a Dossier for Medicines Recommendation for Marketing Authorization/Import Permit in CARICOM States*; 2017. Available: https://carpha.org/Portals/0/Documents/CRS_ReqsDS003.pdf

13 Regulations in ASEAN Countries

Manisha Trivedi, Faraat Ali, Kumari Neha, Neelam Singh, and Anam Ilyas

13.1 INTRODUCTION

For the registration of pharmaceutical goods, the Association of Southeast Asian Nations (ASEAN) has a variety of rules and regulations. For instance, with global harmonizing attempts, the legislative procedure for acquiring Marketing Authorizations (MAs) for pharmaceuticals in the ASEAN area remains mostly nation specific [1]. Examiners' complicated and changing irregular requirements need to be promptly handled to prevent costly postponements in product availability and licensing. Whereas the majority of ASEAN nations follow the rules set out by the European Medicines Agency (EMA) and the International Council for Harmonization (ICH), there are still criteria unique to each nation that must be met in order for Health Authorities (HA) to successfully approve MAs. The Common Technical Document (CTD) is not always necessary in its entirety, even though it might be a useful resource for the majority of regional MA applicants. Nonetheless, it is necessary to guarantee adherence to national stability requirements, regional managerial information, regulatory data, and item marking. Effective strategy is therefore required for rapid and efficient device licensing.

Numerous pharmaceutical firms are concentrating on economies in the ASEAN countries because of intense price rivalry in developed nations and the expansion of the generic medication industry. Pre-emptive awareness and intelligence of ASEAN nation-specific prerequisites and hygiene standards will aid the healthcare industry in enhancing MA application scheduling, optimizing and controlling internal demands, and above all facilitating expedited patient usage of treatments.

13.2 THE ASEAN REGION

Ten nations make up the ASEAN region: Brunei, Cambodia, Indonesia, Laos, Malaysia, Myanmar, the Philippines, Singapore, Thailand, and Vietnam [2]. By removing restrictions on trade, all ten of these nations aim to strengthen their international competitiveness via economic growth. Many ASEAN laws and regulations have been aligned with EU and ICH standards to achieve that. Nonetheless, nation-specific specifications continue to exist, with ASEAN countries that join the Pharmaceutical Inspection Co-operation Scheme (PIC/S) facilitating data exchange, mutual acceptance, and endorsement of current good manufacturing practices (cGMPs).

DOI: 10.1201/9781003296492-14

The ASEAN organization was founded in Bangkok, Thailand, on August 8, 1967. Five nations initially took part in the initiative: Indonesia, Malaysia, the Philippines, Singapore, and Thailand.

Afterwards, Brunei, Cambodia, Laos, Myanmar, Vietnam, and ASEAN were included [3]. By removing trade obstacles, the ASEAN Free Trade Area (AFTA) was established in 1992 as the group's first trade effort with the goal of enhancing competitiveness and fostering economic growth. The Pharmaceutical Product Working Group (PPWG) was established in 1999 as a follow-up to the first effort, with the goal of developing regional standards and harmonizing them with ICH recommendations [4].

The idea of generic medications has drawn greater scrutiny in the pharmaceutical sector because of its increased price and accessible to provide the majority of patients with high-quality, safe, and effective pharmaceuticals. Additionally, it has been noted that whereas generic pharmaceuticals account for just 18% of the overall margin, they make up half of the medications that are already on the market. In 1967, the area known as the Association of Southeast Asian Nations (ASEAN) was established. The ten nations that make up the ASEAN area share identical drug laws, known as ASEAN rules, which went into effect in 2008. As of right now, the ASEAN nations have made great strides toward the WHO's planned Universal Health Coverage (UHC) (see Figure 13.1 and Table 13.1) [5,6].

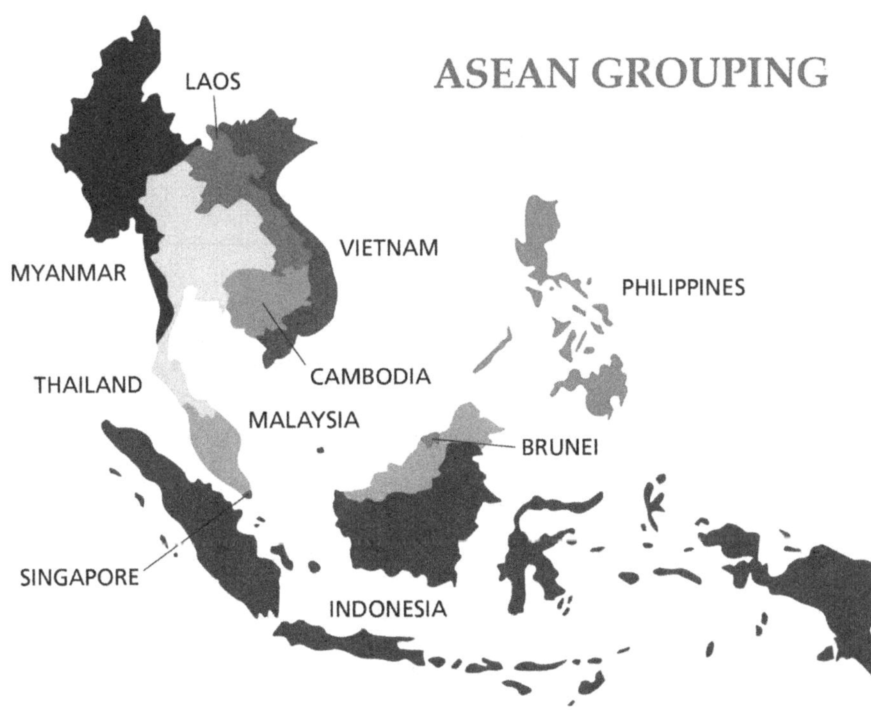

FIGURE 13.1 Representation of ASEAN Countries Based on Region.

TABLE 13.1
Regulatory Framework in ASEAN

Region/ Country	Drug Regulatory Authority	Medical Devices Regulatory Authority	Ministry of Health	Regional Affiliations
Brunei			Ministry of Health	AHWP, APEC, ASEAN
Cambodia	Department of Drugs and Food	Department of Drugs and Food	Ministry of Health	AHWP, ASEAN
Indonesia	National Agency of Drug and Food Control	Ministry of Health	Ministry of Health	AHWP, APEC, ASEAN
Laos	Food and Drug Department	Food and Drug Department	Ministry of Health	AHWP, ASEAN
Malaysia	National Pharmaceutical Regulatory Agency (NPRA)	Medical Device Authority (MDA)	Ministry of Health	AHWP, APEC, ASEAN
Myanmar	Food and Drug Administration	Food and Drug Administration	Ministry of Health and Sports	AHWP, ASEAN
Philippines	Food and Drug Administration	Food and Drug Administration	Department of Health	AHWP, APEC, ASEAN
Singapore	Health Sciences Authority	Health Sciences Authority	Ministry of Health	AHWP, APEC, ASEAN
Thailand	Food and Drug Administration	Food and Drug Administration	Ministry of Public Health	AHWP, APEC, ASEAN
Vietnam	Drug Administration of Vietnam	Department of Medical Equipment and Health Works (DMEHW)	Ministry of Health	AHWP, APEC, ASEAN

TABLE 13.2
Harmonization of ASEAN Guidelines

ASEAN Guidelines	Leading Country	Harmonized with Guidelines	Status
Process Verification	Singapore	EU	Approved and Implemented
Validation via Analysis	Thailand	ICH	
Bioequivalency, Bioavailability, and Variations	Malaysia	EU	
Studies of Stability	Indonesia	ICH Q1A (R2), Q1B, Q1C, Q1D, Q1E, Q1F, EMA Guideline, WHO Guideline	
Safety Research	Philippines	ICH S1A, S1B, S1C(R), S2A, S2B, S3A, S3B, S4, S5(R2), S6, S7A, M3, without modification	Adopted
Studies on Efficacy	Thailand	ICH E1, E2A, E2C, E3, E4, E6, E7, E8, E9, E10, E11	

13.3 CTD AND ACTD

Every nation in the ASEAN area compiles and submits a dossier for generic medical items using the ASEAN Common Technical Dossier (ACTD). ICH-CTD is the standard format from which ACTD is often derived. "ACTD is a governmental record for the creation and consolidation of necessary CTD submissions for medicinal authorization for consumption by humans, which must be submitted to the relevant regulatory body in ASEAN." The ICH-CTD and ACTD are the same; however, they have different modules. CTD is often divided into five components. ACTD, on the other hand, only consists of four because the source requests that the ASEAN countries received were previously accepted in other globally governed nations (the EU, the United Kingdom, and the United States). The primary emphasis of this component inspection is on summarizes and descriptions [7,8].

To prepare a well-structured CTD application that will be presented to ASEAN regulatory organizations for the licensing of medications and biological materials for human use, a single framework has been agreed upon. This format is outlined in the ACTD.

A mandatory component of each registration request for authorization to market is the CTD, often known as the Product Dossier. Together with other necessary technical information and legitimate production permits, the application is presented to the Ministry of Health, the Food and Drug Authority, or any other comparable body in CTD, ACTD, or local national form. Dossier Compilation and writing as per the CTD format.

- Administration-Related Data (Module 1)
- CT Description (Module 2)
- Medicine and Product Part/CMC (Module 3)
- Non-Clinical (Module 4)
- Clinical (Module 5)

CTD format dossiers are extensively used in semi-regulated and regulated markets such as the Middle East, Canada, the Commonwealth of Independent States, the EU, Australia, and Japan. This guideline only provides a proper structure for reporting obtained data. Nevertheless, to aid in the comprehension and assessment of the findings after pharmacological registration, applicants may alter as necessary to offer the most efficient display of the technical data [9].

- Documents to be included in accordance with the ACTD format are the following:
  - Part I: Administrative records
  - Part II: Quality records
  - Part III: Non-clinical records
  - Part IV: Clinical records.

Asia has harmonized the ACTD layout, which is used in countries such as Vietnam, Thailand, Singapore, Malaysia, and other Asian nations.

13.3.1 ACTD General Structure

The four parts of the ACTD are described as follows.

13.3.1.1 Part I: Table of Contents, Administrative Information, and Product Details

The first portion of Part I includes the comprehensive Table of Contents for the whole ACTD, which essentially provides the material that may be perused. The Organizational Information is the subsequent content type, where necessary specialized documentation—such as registration forms, labels, and package inserts—are compiled in detail. The product data is the final portion in this part, and it contains each detail that is required, such as negative effects, method of action, and prescription data.

It is recommended to give a broad overview to the medicine, detailing its pharmacologic class and mechanism of action.

13.3.1.2 Part II: High-Quality Record

The Research Findings should come after the Overall Summary in Part II. All data should be included in the standard assurance document as is feasible.

13.3.1.3 Part III: Non-Clinical Record

The Nonclinical Summary, Nonclinical Written Summaries, and Nonclinical Tabulated Reviews should be included in Part III. For generic goods, some major variant goods, and minor modification products, this part's paperwork is not necessary. If the initial items were registered previously and given the go-ahead for approval for sale in a reference nation, then the Study Reports for NCEs, Scientific Products, and other Major Modification Products may not be necessary for ASEAN member nations. As a result, the authority requesting certain Study Reports must request the required paperwork [10].

13.3.1.4 Part IV: Clinical Documentation

The scientific synopsis and medical review should be included in Part IV. For generic goods, some major modification products, and minor modification products, this part's paperwork is not necessary. If the initial goods were registered previously and given the go-ahead for approval from the market in the standard countries, then the Study Reports for NCEs, Biological Technology Items, and other Major Variant Goods may not be necessary for ASEAN member nations. As a result, the authority requesting certain Study Reports have to request the required paperwork.

13.3.2 CTD General Structure

The four parts of the CTD are described as follows.

13.3.2.1 Part I: Table of Contents: Administrative Data and Prescription Details

Section A: Overview

Section B: Comprehensive ASEAN Standard Technical Document Table of Contents

Section C: Registration-related documents (such as application forms, labeling, PDS, and prescription information).

13.3.2.2 Part II: High-Quality Record

Section A: Table of Contents

Section B: General Quality Synopsis

Section C: Data Set.

13.3.2.3 Part III: Non-Clinical Record

Section A: Table of Contents

Section B: Synopsis of Nonclinical Record

1. A broad perspective
2. Content and arrangement of the body.

Section C: Non-Medical Composed and Tabulated Synopses

1. Table of Contents
2. Pharmacology
3. Pharmacokinetics
4. Intoxication.

Section D: Reports on Nonclinical Studies

1. Table of Contents
2. Pharmacology
3. Pharmacokinetics
4. Toxicology.

For generic goods, certain significant variation goods, and minor modification goods, this part's paperwork is not necessary. If the initial goods have been approved and granted market authorization in referring nations, then members of ASEAN may not need to submit the Study Summaries for NCE, Biotechnological Products, and other Major Alteration Products. As a result, the authority requesting Study Reports ought to request the relevant paperwork.

13.3.2.4 Part IV: Medical Records

Section A: Table of Contents

Section B: Synopsis of the Clinical Records

1. Justification for Product Development
2. Biopharmaceutics Overview
3. Clinical Pharmacology Outline
4. Performance Overview

5. Security Overview
6. Advantages and Dangers in Conclusion.

A comprehensive study of the clinical information contained in the ACTD is what the Clinical Perspective aims to give. Regulatory organizations looking to assess an advertising application's medical part are the main users of the Clinical Overview. For administrative agency personnel reviewing other parts of the commercial application, it should provide a helpful overview of the whole clinical information. The Clinical Review should analyze the advantages and disadvantages of the medication in its intended application, highlight the positive and negative characteristics of the manufacturing programme and research results, and explain how the research findings support important aspects of the prescription information [11].

To achieve these objectives, the Clinical Overview should:

- Outline and clarify the general strategy for a drug's clinical advancement, including important choices on trial design.
- Evaluate the effectiveness of the study's design and execution, and provide a comment on GCP adherence.
- Describe the clinical results in brief and highlight any significant limitations (e.g., lack of data regarding certain patient categories, key endpoints, or usage alongside treatment, or lack of comparability with an especially pertinent active comparator).
- Provide a benefit-risk assessment based on the outcomes of the pertinent clinical trials, explaining how both safety and effectiveness evidence supports the suggested dosage and target indications; you should also evaluate how other strategies, such as recommending data, will maximize benefits and minimize risks.
- Discuss specific safety or effectiveness concerns that arose during development and the ways in which they were assessed and fixed.
- Examine outstanding problems, clarify why they shouldn't be viewed as obstacles to approval, and outline strategies to address them.
- Give a justification for any significant or odd parts of the prescribed information.

Generally speaking, the Clinical Overview ought to be a 30-page paper. However, the length will vary based on how complicated the application itself is. For the sake of clarity and ease of comprehension, it is recommended that the text's body make use of brief tables and graphs. Cross-referencing with more comprehensive descriptions found in the Clinical Synopsis or Clinical Research Summaries is welcomed; it is not intended for information offered in full otherwise to be duplicated in the Clinical Overview.

Section C: Synopsis of the Clinical Case

1. Overview of Related Analytical Techniques and Biopharmaceutics
2. Synopsis of Research on the Clinical Pharmacology

3. Clinical Effectiveness Review
4. Clinical Safety Synopsis
5. Individual Study Synopses

For generic goods, certain significant variation goods, and small variation products, this part's paperwork is not necessary. If the Original Items have previously been registered and given the go-ahead for marketing in referring nations, then the Clinical Study Reports for NCEs, Biotechnological Items, and other Major Modification Products aren't necessarily necessary for ASEAN member nations. Consequently, further evidence should be requested by the authority requesting such Medical Study Summaries.

The goal of the Medical Description is to give a thorough, accurate description of all medical information found in the ACTD. Data from any systematic reviews or various cross-study studies for which complete reports have been included in Clinical Study Reports, as well as aftermarket data for goods that were distributed in other areas, are also included [12]. This document's comparison and analysis of study findings should center on precise findings. On the other hand, a critical examination of the clinical research program and its outcomes, together with an analysis and interpretation of the clinical results and a consideration of the test drug's position in the arsenal, should be included in the ACTD Clinical Review paper.

The Diagnostic Summary's size will vary significantly depending on the data that needs to be communicated, but it is expected to be between 50 and 400 pages long on average (not including the tables that are attached).

Section D: Entire Clinical Study Tabular Listing

All clinical trials should be listed in tabular form, along with any pertinent data. This tabular listing pertains to each research. If the applicant feels that more information would be helpful, it can be added to this table. The listing of the studies should be done in the order specified in E: Clinical Study Reports on Clinical Studies.

Section E: Clinical Study Reports on Clinical Studies

1. Biopharmaceutic Study Reports
2. Reports on Research with Human Biomaterials that is Relevant to Pharmacokinetics
3. Human Pharmacokinetic (PK) Study Reports
4. Reports of Human Pharmacodynamic (PD) Studies
5. Efficacy and Safety Study Reports
6. Post-Marketing Feedback Reports
7. Case Report Forms and Listings for Specific Patients.

If the goods were initially registered and given the go-ahead for distribution in the referring countries, then the Study Assessments for NCEs, Biotechnological Products, and other Major Variation Products may not be necessary for ASEAN member nations. As a result, the authority requesting certain Study Reports have to request the required paperwork. When registering a medicine for human use, the ACTD contains references, additional clinical data, and clinical trial results. The ICH E3 offers recommendations on how these elements should be arranged. The applicant will submit Sections A, B, C, D, and F in this scenario.

Section F: List of Important Literature References

A list of cited materials should be included, such as significant publications that have been published, formal meeting minutes, or other regulatory guidelines or recommendations. Every source referenced in the Medical Overview, as well as significant references mentioned in the Clinical Overview and in the specific technical reports included in the Clinical Research Reports, are included. Last, copies of the papers that are cited should be provided upon request.

13.4 ASEAN STANDARD NEED FOR THE QUALITY OF MEDICINAL PRODUCTS REGISTRATION

The following provides an overview on NCE and biologics demands, along with referrals to the pertinent ICH Guidelines:

[1] DRUG SUBSTANCE
[1.1] General Information
[1.1.1] Nomenclature

- International non-proprietary name (INN);
- Compendial name if relevant;
- Registry number of chemical abstract service (CAS);
- Laboratory code (if applicable);
- Chemical name(s).

[1.1.2] Structural formula NCE

It is necessary to supply the structure formula, the molecular structure, the corresponding molecular mass, and both absolute and comparative stereochemistry.

Biologics: Where applicable, the molecular mass ratio and graphic sequence of amino acids depicting glycosylation places or other modifications after translation should be supplied. For instance, a diagram of amino acid order, which shows the glycosylation sites or additional modifications and comparative molecular mass, is included in synthetic vaccines including polysaccharides or proteins.

[1.1.3] Generally Speaking

The physicochemical and other pertinent characteristics of the drug material, such as its biological activity in the case of biologics, should be included.

Biologics: Provide an overview of the item's viral safety for each biologically starting source that was used to extract or produce the active component (if available).

[1.2] Production
[1.2.1] Name and complete information of the manufacturer(s) of the substance that acts, specifying city and nation;
[1.2.2] Outlining Process Management and the Production Process

The applicant's devotion to producing drug substances is shown in the description of the production process [13]. To fully explain the manufacturing procedure and process oversight, the information that follows must be given:

NCE:

- It is necessary to submit an illustrated flow chart of the creative process(es) that lists solvents and their working parameters; molecular formulas, weights, and yields; and the molecular structures of the precursors, intermediary molecules, reagents, and drug substances that represent stereochemistry.
- A step-by-step operational account of the process of production that includes machinery, processes controls, and operational parameters like humidity, pressure, temperature, pH, and time, as well as amounts of ingredients, solvent, catalysts, as well and chemicals that correspond to the typical batch scale.
- The explanation and description of an alternative process have to be as thorough as that of the main process. Reusing procedures must to be defined and supported.

Pharmaceuticals:

- Details on the production procedure, which usually begins with a vial or vials containing the cell bank and covers cell culture, harvesting, purifying and modification response, filling, preservation, and transportation circumstances. Indicate the number of paragraphs if appropriate.
- *Industrial procedure flow chart*: Display every stage of the production process, even the intermediary ones.
- *The batch identifying system's summary*: Identify the lot at every stage of the procedure, particularly the creation of combinations. Provide details about the lot size and manufacture scale as well.
- The agents and techniques employed, the parameters managed, and, if relevant, the stage of manufacturing at which it is carried out.
- Outline an inactivation or detoxifying process, including the components and reagents used, the conditions of operation that are regulated, and the specifications.

- *Outline the entire purification procedure*: Requirements for membrane and chromatography column usage and re-use, together with the corresponding validating investigations.
- *Stabilization of active component*: Describe the actions taken, such as the inclusion of modifiers or other processes, if necessary, to stabilize the component that is active.
- *Reprocessing*: An explanation of the standards and rationale for repurposing the active component or any subsequent product.
- *Packing process during production controls*: Outline the active ingredient's manufacturing manipulate, in-process oversight, acceptance requirements, container closure systems type, actively ingredient storing vessel type of seal, and, if relevant, storing and transferring circumstances.

[1.2.3] Management of Substances

All components used in the production of the medication, such as catalysts, substances, solvents, initial supplies, and beginning materials, should be specified together with their respective processes. It is necessary to offer details regarding the material's durability and supervision. When applicable, data proving that products (including biologically derived materials, such as media parts, monoclonal antibodies, and enzymatic) fulfill requirements suitable for their intended application, particularly control or removal of adventitious representatives, should be supplied. Details on the origin, manufacturing process, and characterization of materials derived from biological sources can be included in this.

Biologics:

- The source and beginning material of biologic origin are controlled.
- The origin, evolution, and history of the cell substrates.

As stated in Q5B and Q5D, details on the origin of the cell substrates and an examination of the expression build that was used to genetically alter cells and integrated into the first cell clone employed to create the Universal Cell Bank should be supplied.

- Evaluation and assessing the cell banking system.
- The Q5B and Q5D guidelines ought to be followed when offering data on the cell banking framework, quality assurance procedures, and the cell line's viability throughout manufacturing and preservation (including the processes used to create the Master or Working Cell Bank(s).
- An assessment of viral safety.

For items derived from biological sources, summaries of virus safety information have to be supplied.

[1.2.4] Regulations of Crucial Phases and Intermediaries

Important actions: Trials or acceptance standards are carried out at crucial stages of the production procedure to provide process control. The reason for these tests and criteria includes quality requirements and information from experiments.

In-betweens: Details, including any necessary analytical methods, for metabolites that are separated during the process.

It is necessary to give the results of any virological testing carried out during the production process, such as cell the substrate, raw bulk, and post-viral elimination testing. Comprehensive details on infectious safety have to be given.

[1.2.5] Validation and/or Assessment of the Process

Studies that validate or assess aseptic processing and sterilizing procedures.

Biologics: Enough data on assessment and validation research to show that the production procedure (including post-processing stages) is appropriate for the intended use and to support the choice of crucial process regulates (operational variables and in-process testing) and their upper bounds for crucial production stages (such as cell culture, gathering, cleansing, and alteration).

Data should contain an explanation of the strategy for carrying out the investigation and the findings, evaluation, and recommendations from the investigations carried out. It is necessary to cross-reference or give the validation of related assay and analytical procedures to support the choice of crucial process parameters and limitations.

When it comes to manufacturing procedures meant to eliminate or render viral contamination dormant, the data from assessment research have to be supplied.

[1.2.6] Development of Manufacturing Processes NCE

Describe and talk about the major modifications made to the drug substance's manufacturing facility or process that were used to produce pilot, medical conditions, clinical size-up, and, if accessible, commercially viable batches.

It is necessary to give the manufacturing procedure's development history, as outlined in 1.2.2. The outline of any modification(s) made to the procedure or vital machinery used in the production of drug ingredient samples used for backing a marketing request (e.g., non-clinical or clinical trials). It is necessary to provide an explanation for the modification. It is also necessary to submit pertinent data on drug ingredient batches produced throughout development, including a batch number, manufacturing size, and usage (e.g., stability, non-clinical reference materials) in connection to the modification [14].

The possible influence of a modification on the purity of the medication (and/or intermediate, if applicable) should be used to determine how significant it is. Information from comparison tests on relevant medication batch should be submitted for manufacturing modifications deemed substantial. Enclosed analysis of the information, along with a rationale for the test's selection and an evaluation of the findings.

Clinical and non-clinical research from other submissions components may also be included in the testing to evaluate how production modifications affect the drug substance(s) and related drug product(s).

[1.3] Description

[1.3.1] Clarification of Structure and Typical NCE: Verification of structure by techniques like synthetic routes and spectral examination.

It is also important to consider the possibility of isomerism, stereochemistry detection, or polymorphism formation.

Biologics: Information on biological activity, innocence, and immunochemical characteristics; also includes details on the primary, secondary, and more complex structure (where applicable).

Generics: Manufacturer-provided similar data or compendial requirements.

[1.3.2] Contaminants

An overview of the contaminants that are tested for or seen both before and after drug substance production.

Generics and biologics: Manufacturer-provided comparable data or compendial requirement.

[1.4] Regulation of Drug Ingredient Identification and Rationale for Identification(s).

An overview of the analytical process and its confirmation.

[1.4.1] Details

It is necessary to offer a comprehensive specification, testing, and acceptance process for the drug substance.

Compendial specifications or relevant producer data apply to biologics.

Indicate the source, such as details such as the kind of microbe, and type of animal.

Generics: The specifications in compendia are sufficient. Make it clear if the drug item has been examined by the applicant or was acquired according to specifications and accompanied by an evidence of examination.

[1.4.2] Methods of Analysis

Enough information about the approach that was used to analyze the drug material should be supplied so that another testing facility can repeat the test.

[1.4.3] Analytical Method Validation

It is necessary to submit analytical validation information, which should include experimental results for the analytical method employed to evaluate the drug material. Specificity, accuracy (consistency, middle precision, and consistency), precision, linearity, range, boundary of measurement, limits of identification, durability, and system appropriateness are typical validating features to be considered.

[1.4.4] Analysis in Batch

The findings of batch investigations and an overview of the batches must be included.

[1.4.5] Rationale for the Specification

It is necessary to give an explanation for the drug's chemical description.

[1.5] Materials or Criteria of Reference

It is necessary to mention the standard of reference or the material used to test the drug. If appropriate, the compendial benchmark ought to be applied.

[1.6] NCE and Biologics in Box Closure Systems

Each key packaging component's materials of manufacture and specifications, as well as a description of the container closing methods, should be included. A description, identification, and, if necessary, key measurements with illustrations should all be included in the requirements. When applicable, non-compendial techniques (with validations) ought to be used.

Just an overview should be given for inactive secondary packaging elements (those that do not assist to convey the product or offer further protection). More information needs to be included for functioning additional packaging elements.

The appropriateness should be covered in relation to, among other things, material selection, protection against light and humidity, and building components' compliance with the medication ingredient, particularly sorption to containers and leaking.

[1.7] Consistency

[1.7.1] Consistency Synopsis and Resolution

A summary of the protocols followed, the kinds of experiments carried out, and the findings should be included. Findings from experiments on forced deterioration and stress settings, for instance, as well as findings about the state of storage, retest dates, and shelf lives, should all be included in the report.

[1.7.2] Stability Pledge and the Post-Approval Durability Regime

It is necessary to give a stable promise and the post-approval stabilization procedure.

[1.7.3] Data on Stability

The stability evaluation results (such as stressful circumstances and enforced deterioration tests) should be provided in a way that makes sense, such tabular, graphical, or narrative. Details should be presented on the analytical processes that were used to produce the information and the verification of these processes.

[2] MEDICATION PRODUCT
[2.1] Synopsis and Constituency

The drug item's composition and descriptions ought to be given. For instance, the data supplied ought to include:

- An explanation of the dose form;
- Composition, which is a list of every ingredient in its dosage form, together with their quantity per unit (which includes any overages), operation, and references to the purity standards (such as compendial brochures or manufacturer's requirements) of each ingredient;
- Type of vessel and seal used for the concentration form and, if appropriate, the corresponding reconstitution diluent;
- the details of the associated replenishment diluent(s).

[2.2] Development of Pharmaceuticals
[2.2.1] Details Regarding Development Research

NCE and Biologics: Data and information from research projects are presented in the Medicine Growing section to demonstrate that the dose form, manufacturing procedure of the formulation, box closure system, microbiological characteristics, and usage instructions are suitable for the intended use as stated in the application. The investigations presented here are not to be confused with standard control testing carried out in accordance with standards. Furthermore, the process and formulation features (clinical parameters) that might affect batch reproducibility, effectiveness, and drug quality of the product should be identified and described in this subsection. You may incorporate or attach supporting data and findings from certain research or published sources to the Pharmaceutical Innovation Part. The pertinent non-clinical portions of the proposal may contain references to other supporting information [15].

[2.2.2] Pharmaceutical Product Component
[2.2.2.1] Ingredients in Action Biologics and NCE

It is important to talk about how well the medicinal ingredients work with the excipients mentioned in 1.1. Important physicochemical properties of the therapeutic ingredient, such as its percentage of water, dissolution, distribution of particles by size, polymorphism or solid-state shape, that may affect how well the drug product works should also be covered.

Compatibility between the active components in combination products should be addressed.

[2.2.2.2] Recipients

It is important to talk about the excipients chosen in 2.1 in relation to their individual functions, taking into account their features and concentration, which affect the therapeutic product's performance.

[2.2.3] Final Good
[2.2.3.1] Formulation Creation

Considering the suggested mode of consumption and usage, a succinct synopsis of the medication product's creation should be given. It is important to talk about the variations between the ingredients (i.e., medical formulations) and 1.1 and 1.2 compositions. When relevant, results from comparable in vivo research (like bioequivalence) or comparable in vitro research (like dissolution) should be described.

[2.2.3.2] Overruns

Any deviations from the formulation(s) given in 1.1 ought to be explained.

[2.2.3.3] Characteristics of Physicochemical and Biological Systems

A number of factors that affect how well a therapeutic product works should be taken into consideration, including pH, ion concentration, solubility, dispersion, reconstruction, distribution of particle sizes, accumulation, polymorphism, rheological characteristics, biological function or potency, and immunologic function.

[2.2.4] Development of Manufacturing Processes

It is necessary to provide an explanation of the manufacturing procedure's refinement and selection procedure outlined in 2.3.2, especially its crucial elements. When applicable, a justification and explanation of the sterilizing process should be provided.

Disparities that may affect the effectiveness of the item between the production processes used to create pivotal research batches and the procedure outlined in 2.3.2 should be addressed.

[2.2.5] Closure System for Containers

When it comes to the storage, shipment, and usage of the medication, the appropriateness of the package's closing system should be examined. The selection of substances, assurance from exposure to light and humidity, integration of building components with dosage forms, such as sorption to containers and the leaching process safety of contraction substances, and efficiency, such as repeatability of dose delivery from the instrument when included in the medication, should all be taken into consideration in this discussion.

[2.2.6] Microbiological Characteristics

The rationale behind not conducting microbial boundaries analysis for non-sterile items, as well as the choice and efficacy of preservative procedures for products having anti-microbial preservation ingredients, should be included when discussing the microbiological characteristics of the dose.

[2.2.7] Harmony

To offer relevant and supporting data for the categorization, it is important to address the drug item's compliance with reconstituted diluent or dosage equipment, such as its solubility, sorption on injection vessels, and durability.

Generics: Acceptable literary data

[2.3] Production
[2.3.1] Producer

Name, address, and duties of all participating manufacturers, especially contracted suppliers for quality assurance and manufacturing.

[2.3.2] Combination Formula

Provided in the equation should contain the name and amounts of all constituents, both active and inert, as well as any substance(s) eliminated during manufacturing:

- It is necessary to provide the precise amounts of each item (g, kg, L, etc.).
- *Overage*: Enclosed will be the justification for the overage, as well as additional evidence.
- It is necessary to specify the total number of dose units in each batch.
- Every step of the dosage form's manufacturing process must be described.

[2.3.3] Control of Processes and Production Procedures

The phases of the process should be shown in a flow diagram, together with the locations of the materials' entry points. It is important to identify the crucial phases and moments during the process when controls, transitional testing, or final outcome controls are carried out.

- A thorough explanation of the manufacturing procedure, with enough specifics to address every important aspect of each step of the process;
- The specification of a sterile item includes components pre-treatment and disinfection (e.g., shipping containers, closures);

- The batch recognition system's specification specifies the lot during the stages of filling, packing, and freezing (if applicable) phases.

[2.3.4] Critical Step and Intermediate Controls

Crucial steps: To guarantee that the process is under management, assessments and approval requirements ought to be offered (with reason, including experimental data) at the crucial phases listed in 2.3.2 of the procedures for manufacturing.

Intermediates: Details on the monitoring and quality of precursors that are separated during this procedure has to be included.

The results of virological testing carried out during manufacture have to be disclosed. An extensive section on viral safety ought to be included in Annex A.1.

[2.3.5] Validation and/or Assessment of the Process

Crucial stages or crucial assays used in the production procedure should offer details, records, and results of the validation inquiries. (For instance, sterile filling or interpreting, or verification of the sterilizing procedure).

When relevant, information about the product's viral safety must also be included.

[2.4] Management of Ingredients
[2.4.1] Details

It is necessary to supply the excipient specifications.

[2.4.2] Methods of Analysis

Where applicable, the analytical method used to test the excipient ought to be disclosed. Where applicable (e.g., for internally tested techniques), analytical validated data, including results from experiments, for the analytical processes used for testing the excipients should be given.

When applicable, justification for the suggested excipient requirements (such as non-compendial parameters) should be given.

[2.4.3] Human and Animal Origin Additives

Documentation on adventitious substances (e.g., sources, guidelines, an overview of the tests conducted, viral risk data) should be supplied for excipients that are either animal or human origin. It is important to give comprehensive details on viral danger.

[2.4.4] New Ingredients

According to the drug substance format, complete information of production, characterization, and control systems, along with connections to additional safety information (clinical or nonclinical), should be supplied for any excipient(s) used in a medication for the first time or via a new route of dosage.

[2.5] Oversight of the Final Product

Impurity characterization, an overview of the analytical process and confirmation, and requirement justification are all included.

[2.5.1] Details

The final product's specification ought to be given.

[2.5.2] Methods of Analysis

It is necessary to give a thorough explanation of the analytical methods used to test the final product

[2.5.3] Analytical Procedure Validation

Data on analytical confirmation, such as outcomes from experiments for confirming the analytical processes used to evaluate the final product, should be provided.

[2.5.4] Batch Analyses

All pertinent batch (pre-clinical studies, clinical test, expansion, and, if accessible, production-scale portions) that are used to establish specifications and assess uniformity during production ought to be described, along with their size, source, and intended purpose, as well as the test results.

Biologics: A synopsis of the batch manufacturing procedure and the monitoring of three successive lots of the end result. The format that is now accessible and advised by the WHO for the specific criteria for the manufacturing and control of the particular biologics filed for approval for market should be followed by this procedure.

[2.5.5] Description of Contaminants

If it was not already mentioned in 2.3.2, details on the characteristics of impurities must be included. Compendial specifications or relevant data from the producer.

[2.5.6] Rationale for the Specification

An explanation for the suggested final product must be given. Compendial specifications or comparable data from the manufacturer.

[2.6] Resources or Standard Standards

Demand: the supplies used to test the medication, or the standard of comparison should be given, together with a table of the quality data. Mandatory documentation or comparable data from the producer. If appropriate, the compendial standard of reference ought to be applied.

[2.7] Vessel Closure Method

Each major and additional packing component's building supplies should be identified, together with each requirement, in the description of the box closed systems. A description, proof of identity, and, if necessary, key measurements with illustrations should all be part of the requirements. When applicable, non-compendial techniques (with validations) ought to be used.

Just an overview should be given for non-functional tertiary packaging elements (those that don't assist to convey the product or offer further protection). Additional details need to be included for functioning additional packaging elements.

[2.8] Stability of Product

Proof must show that the product remains stable, that it satisfies completed product criteria for the duration of its intended shelf life, that no appreciable amount of harmful breakdown products is formed during this time, and that potency, preventative efficacy, and so on remains intact.

[2.8.1] Overview and Conclusion of Stability NCE and Biologics: A volatility summary proving the product will remain stable for the duration of its suggested shelf life.
[2.8.2] Stability Guarantee and Post-Approval Process

It is necessary to give the stability assurance and the post-approval stabilization protocol.

The stability programme or stability promise to be implemented once the good is on the marketplace, particularly the amount of lots that will participate in the study each year and the tests to be conducted, is contained in the agreement on post-approval stabilization surveillance. If necessary, these findings should be supplied on a regular basis to update the data about the product's reliability.

[2.8.3] Data on Stability

The stability study results have to be displayed in a suitable manner (e.g., tabular, pictorial, narrative). Included should be details on the analytical processes that were used to produce the data and the verification of these processes.

[2.8.4] Describe the Steps Taken (if Relevant) to Ensure the Cold Chain

Provide a thorough explanation of the steps used to ensure that the finished product is shipped at an appropriate moisture and temperature level from the manufacturing location to the final retail location. Include all of the distribution and storage phases and list the monitoring procedures that were implemented at each one. The expert who is in charge of this summary has to sign it.

[2.9] Interchangeability of Products

The study report should include the kind of study that was done, the methodology that was employed, and the findings.

The kind of research that is done should be in accordance with the WHO Manual for Drug Control power, the ASEAN (proposed) Bioavailability and Bioequivalence requirement, or the Recommended Practice for Bioavailability and Bioequivalence Research.

[3] ANNEX

[3.1] Safety Assessment of Adventitious Agents (name, dose form, manufacturer)

The next section ought to offer facts evaluating the risk of possible adventitious agent infection.

For accidental agents that are not viruses: Comprehensive guidance must to be provided for the prevention and management of non-viral accidental agents, such as molds, bacteria, mycoplasma, and pathogens that cause passed on spongiform encephalopathy. For instance, accreditation, examination, and/or oversight of the manufacturing process, depending on the substance, method, and agent, might be included in this data.

Regarding viral spontaneous agents: This part ought to contain comprehensive data from studies that evaluate the safety of viral agents. Research on viral assessment should show that the production-related materials are deemed safe and that the methods employed to assess, test, and remove any possible hazards throughout the process of production are appropriate. For more information, the applicant should consult Q5A, Q5D, and Q6B.

Commodities with biological origin: It is necessary to offer information to assess the virological risk associated with materials originating from animals or humans, such as biologic fluids, tissues, organs, and cell lines. (Refer to the relevant details found in 1.2.3 and 2.4.3.) Details about the choice, examination, and safety evaluation of cell strains for possible infectious contamination of the cells, as well as the viral certification of tissue banks should be included. (Refer to the relevant details in 1.2.3).

Testing at the proper manufacturing phases: Justification must be provided for the choice of virological assays (e.g., the substrate, untreated bulk, or post-viral removal assays) that are carried out through the production process. It should include the test kind, its accuracy and specificity, if relevant, and how frequently it is conducted. Results of tests must be made available to verify that the good is free of viral contamination at the proper point in manufacturing. (Refer to the relevant details found in 1.2.4 and 2.3.4.)

Testing for viruses in unprocessed bulk: Results for virus screening of raw bulk should have been incorporated into compliance with Q5A and Q6B.

Virus elimination investigations: In compliance with Q5A, the justification, plan of practice, and findings and assessment of the viral elimination studies must be given. The results can show that the scaled-down model remains valid compared with the commercially viable process, that the methods for eliminating or deactivating viruses from production goods and machinery are adequate, and that the production stages are capable of doing so.

13.5 PHARMACOPOEIA ACCEPTABILITY

It should be taken into consideration throughout formulation/product preparation that APIs and additives need to adhere to the existing the pharmacist's manual.

Regional pharmaceutical manuals do not exist in Singapore or Malaysia. On the other hand, native pharmacopeia are in existence in Indonesia, Thailand, the Philippines, and Vietnam. In addition to regional pharmacopoeias, ASEAN nations broadly recognize international pharmaceutical standards, including the US Pharmacopoeia (USP)/National Formulary (NF), British Pharmacopoeia (BP), EU Pharmacopoeia, and Japanese Pharmacopoeia [16].

13.6 HALAL COMPLIANCE FOR MUSLIM PATIENT POPULATIONS

The medicinal product must comply with halal regulations, particularly in Indonesia and Malaysia, which demand halal compliance. The following Shariah legal requirements must be followed by halal medications [17,18].

They cannot include any components or by-products of non-halal species or animals that were not killed humanely.

- No *najs* (blood, urine, or feces) present;
- Safe for human use: intoxicating, non-poisonous, or not health-hazardous when taken as directed;
- Cannot be produced, processed, or prepared with machinery tainted by *najs*;
- The absence of any human components or non-halal derivatives;
- They ought to be kept physically apart from any non-halal goods and *najs* throughout the making, the process, using, packing, storing, and delivery phases.

The standard pre- and post-marketing procedures established by the appropriate national pharmacy regulatory bodies apply to halal medicines. Halal items need to be certified by appropriate Islamic organizations. The Ministry of Islamic Development Malaysia (Jabatan Kemajuan Islam Malaysia, or JAKIM) and the Lembaga Pengkajian Panjan Obat Obatan dan Kosmetika Majelis Ulama (LPPOM MUI) of Indonesia are the organizations that handle certification as halal. Multiple organizations with varying levels of shared acceptance can certify something as halal in other nations [19,20].

13.7 SCOPE OF THE GUIDELINE

The purpose of this chapter is to offer guidelines on the structure of an application for medicinal product registration with respect to the ASEAN CTR. NCEs (New Chemical Entities), Biologics (Biotechnological Goods and Vaccine), Major

Differences, Minor Differences, and Gs (Generics) may all use this format. Only the prerequisites for novel product licensing (NCE, biological products, and generic medication) are provided by the ACTR Standards. It is recommended to consult the ASEAN Variable recommendations on the criteria for variations in medicines. The guidelines issued by the WHO on Processes and Information Demands for modifications to Accepted Biotherapeutic Products (2017) and WHO Instructions on Methods and Data Specifications for alterations to authorized Vaccines (WHO TRS 993, Annex 4) should be consulted for information regarding the prerequisites for modifications to biotechnological products and vaccines, accordingly. The candidate ought to speak with the relevant National Regulation Agencies to ascertain if this design is acceptable for a certain kind of goods.

This guideline's "Framework of Data" just specifies the location of the data. This guideline fails to address the kind or volume of particular proof of validity, and either may rely on national guidelines and/or well-recognized leading worldwide standards (pharmacopoeias).

REFERENCES

[1] Narine, Shaun. "Forty years of ASEAN: A historical review." *The Pacific Review* 21.4 (2008): 411–429.

[2] Frankel, Jeffrey, and Shang-Jin Wei. "ASEAN in a regional perspective." *Macroeconomic issues facing ASEAN countries*, 1997. Academic Press.

[3] Jetschke, Anja. "Asean." *Routledge handbook of Asian regionalism*. Routledge, 2012, 340–350.

[4] Keling, Mohamad Faisol, et al. "The development of ASEAN from historical approach." *Asian Social Science* 7.7 (2011): 169–189.

[5] Albert, Eleanor, and Lindsay Maizland. "What is ASEAN." *Council on Foreign Relations, Backgrounder* (2019). Springer.

[6] Nesadurai, Helen ES. "The association of Southeast Asian nations (ASEAN)." *New Political Economy* 13.2 (2008): 225–239.

[7] Quet, Mathieu, et al. "Regulation multiple: Pharmaceutical trajectories and modes of control in the ASEAN." *Science, Technology and Society* 23.3 (2018): 485–503.

[8] Bhavana, J. Sai, et al. "Regulatory requirements for registration of drugs in ASEAN countries." (2019). Academic Press.

[9] Rani, V. Sudha, et al. "Regulatory requirements for the registration of drugs in ASEAN countries." (2021). Springer.

[10] Panchal, Vruddhi, et al. "Regulatory requirement for the approval of Generic Drug in Vietnam as per ASEAN Common Technical Dossier (ACTD)." *International Journal of Drug Regulatory Affairs* 10.3 (2022): 66–69.

[11] Dellepiane, Nora, Sonia Pagliusi, and Registration Experts Working Group. "Challenges for the registration of vaccines in emerging countries: Differences in dossier requirements, application and evaluation processes." *Vaccine* 36.24 (2018): 3389–3396.

[12] Achin, Jain, M. P. Venkatesh, and Kumar Pramod. "ACTD: Bridge between regulatory requirements of developed and developing countries." *International Journal of Drug Regulatory Affairs* 1.4 (2013): 1–11.

[13] Deep, Aakash, et al. "Comparison of regulatory requirements for registration of pharmaceutical drugs in ASEAN and GCC regions." *Applied Clinical Research, Clinical Trials and Regulatory Affairs* 6.1 (2019): 62–70.
[14] Godiyal, Shrikant. "Regulatory requirements for preparation of Dossier for registration of Pharmaceutical products in ACTD & CTD format." *International Journal of Drug Regulatory Affairs (IJDRA)* 7.2 (2019): 51–61.
[15] Sandeep, D. S., et al. "Generic drugs regulations and registration in Indonesia, Malaysia and Vietnam: A drug regulatory case study." *Journal of Young Pharmacists* 14.1 (2022): 33.
[16] Patel, Ravish, Amit Patel, and Tejasvini Gohil. "Regulatory requirement for the approval of generic drug in Cambodia as per ASEAN Common Technical Dossier (ACTD)." *International Journal of Drug Regulatory Affairs* 6.2 (2018): 67–71.
[17] Panchal, Vruddhi, et al. "Regulatory requirement for the approval of Generic Drug in Vietnam as per ASEAN Common Technical Dossier (ACTD)." *International Journal of Drug Regulatory Affairs* 10.3 (2022): 66–69.
[18] Lätzel, Ruth. "Development of the ASEAN pharmaceutical harmonisation scheme-an example of regional integration." Academic Press.
[19] Kohno, Ayako, et al. "Factors influencing healthcare-seeking behaviour among Muslims from Southeast Asian countries (Indonesia and Malaysia) living in Japan: An exploratory qualitative study." *BMJ Open* 12.10 (2022): e058718.
[20] Azizah, Siti Nur. "Protection of halal product guarantee for Muslim consumers in facing the ASEAN Economic Community (AEC)." *International Journal of Criminal Justice Sciences* 17.2 (2022): 153–166.

14 Regulations in Gulf Cooperation Council (GCC) Countries

Usama Ahmad, Anas Islam, and Vazahat Ali

14.1 INTRODUCTION

The Gulf Cooperation Council (GCC) is a regional intergovernmental, political and economic alliance that comprises six countries in the Middle East: Saudi Arabia, United Arab Emirates (UAE), Kuwait, Bahrain, Oman and Qatar. These countries have a combined population of over 50 million and a GDP of more than $1.5 trillion. Active Pharmaceutical Ingredients (APIs) are the chemical compounds that make up the active ingredient in a drug product. APIs are the substances responsible for the therapeutic effect of a drug and are typically produced through chemical synthesis or biological processes. They are used to manufacture finished dosage forms, such as tablets, capsules and injectables. The regulation of APIs is critical to ensure the safety, efficacy and quality of pharmaceutical products. According to the research results, the Gulf Cooperation Council (GCC) region is considered an emerging market for pharmaceutical exports and bilateral trade [1]. The pharmaceutical industry in the GCC countries started some 25 years ago with the main idea of decreasing the cost of medications, which was increasing rapidly. Some of the GCC countries have started manufacturing pharmaceutical products under the license of major pharmaceutical companies but soon discovered that generics saving and raw materials can be purchased much cheaper than from the major pharmaceutical companies they manufacture for. The GCC pharmaceutical plants practically kicked off their partners and moved into the line of generics, competing with the major companies. The GCC pharmaceutical companies got some success in reducing the prices of the raw materials but this was at the expense of the quality of their products [2–5].

The Gulf region is an important market for pharmaceuticals and the demand for high quality drugs is increasing rapidly. The GCC countries have recognized the importance of regulating APIs and have developed regulatory frameworks to ensure that pharmaceutical products meet the necessary standards. API regulations play a critical role in the healthcare systems of GCC countries. These regulations are designed to ensure that APIs used in the production of pharmaceuticals meet stringent quality standards. By enforcing these regulations, the GCC countries aim to prevent the entry of substandard or counterfeit APIs into their markets, safeguard public health and maintain consumer confidence in the pharmaceutical industry. The purpose of this chapter is to provide an overview of the regulatory framework for APIs in the GCC

DOI: 10.1201/9781003296492-15

TABLE 14.1
Demographic and Economic Structures of the Gulf Cooperation Council (GCC) Countries

GCC Member State	Total Area (km^2)	Total Population (millions)	Median Age (years)	Life Expectancy (years)	GDP (billion USD)	Pharmaceutical Market Size (billion USD)	Share of Pharmaceutical Market in GDP (%)
Bahrain	760	1.6	32.3	77.2	37.7	0.5	1.3
Kuwait	17,818	4.2	33.4	75.4	134.6	1.2	0.9
Oman	309,500	4.6	25.6	77.1	76.3	0.8	1.0
Qatar	11,586	2.6	31.9	80.1	175.8	1	0.6
Saudi Arabia	2,149,690	33	30	75	792.9	10.7	1.3
UAE	83,600	9.6	33.8	77.8	421	4.8	1.1

countries. It will explore the registration process for APIs, the approval process, post-approval requirements and monitoring. In addition, it will compare the API regulations in different GCC countries, identify challenges and issues in API regulations and discuss potential future developments. This chapter will be useful for pharmaceutical companies, regulatory authorities and anyone interested in understanding the regulatory landscape for APIs in the GCC countries. Demographic and economic structures of the Gulf Cooperation Council (GCC) countries are summarized in Table 14.1 [6,7].

14.2 REGULATORY FRAMEWORK FOR APIs IN GCC COUNTRIES

14.2.1 General Regulatory Landscape for APIs in GCC Countries

The regulatory framework for APIs in the Gulf Cooperation Council (GCC) countries is based on the principles of the GCC. The GCC was established in Riyadh, Saudi Arabia, in May 1981 with the purpose of achieving unity among its members based on their common objectives and their similar political and cultural identities, which are rooted in Arab and Islamic cultures [8–10].

One of the objectives of the GCC is to promote cooperation among its members in various fields, including health and pharmaceuticals. In this regard, the GCC has established several committees and initiatives to harmonize the standards and requirements for APIs among the GCC countries. These include:

- The Executive Board of Health Ministers' Council for GCC States, which is the supreme authority for health policies and programs in the GCC region;
- The Gulf Central Committee for Drug Registration (GCC-DR), which is composed of two members from each GCC country and is responsible for evaluating and approving applications for marketing authorization of pharmaceutical products, including APIs, in the GCC region [11];
- The Gulf Central Committee for Drug Pricing (GCC-DP), which is composed of two members from each GCC country and is responsible for setting and reviewing the prices of pharmaceutical products, including APIs, in the GCC region;
- The Gulf Health Council (GHC), which is an independent entity that provides technical and administrative support to the health ministries and committees of the GCC countries;
- The Gulf Pharmaceutical Inspection Convention and Cooperation Scheme (PIC/S), which is a regional agreement that aims to enhance cooperation and harmonization among the national drug regulatory authorities of the GCC countries in the field of GMP inspection and quality control of pharmaceutical products, including APIs [12,13].

14.2.2 Registration Process for APIs

The registration process for APIs in the GCC countries follows the guidelines and procedures of the GCC-DR, which was established in 1999 as a centralized system for drug registration in the GCC region. The GCC-DR evaluates and approves applications for marketing authorization of pharmaceutical products, including APIs, based on scientific criteria and international standards. The GCC-DR also issues certificates of registration that are valid for 5 years and are renewable upon request.

The registration process for APIs consists of several steps, as follows:

- The applicant submits an application form along with the required documents and fees to the GHC, which acts as the secretariat of the GCC-D;
- The GHC reviews the application for completeness and assigns it to one of the GCC countries as a reference member state (RMS) based on a rotation system;
- The RMS conducts a scientific assessment of the application within 120 days and prepares a draft assessment report that is circulated to other GCC countries as concerned member states (CMS) for comments;
- The CMS provide their comments within 60 days and either agree or disagree with the RMS's assessment report;
- The RMS consolidates the comments from the CMS and prepares a final assessment report that is submitted to the GHC;
- The GHC organizes a meeting of the GCC-DR to discuss and approve or reject the application based on consensus or majority vote;
- The GHC notifies the applicant of the decision of the GCC-DR within 15 days and issues a certificate of registration if approved [14,15].

14.2.3 Approval Process for APIs

The approval process for APIs in the GCC countries follows the same guidelines and procedures as the registration process described above. However, there are some differences depending on whether the API is a new chemical entity (NCE) or an existing chemical entity (ECE).

For NCEs, which are APIs that have not been previously approved or marketed in any country, the applicant must submit a full dossier that includes data on quality, safety, efficacy, stability, bioequivalence, pharmacokinetics, pharmacodynamics, clinical trials, risk management plan, labeling and packaging. The applicant must also provide evidence of patent protection or non-infringement of existing patents in each GCC country.

For ECEs, which are APIs that have been previously approved or marketed in one or more countries, the applicant must submit an abridged dossier that includes data on quality, stability, bioequivalence, pharmacokinetics, pharmacodynamics, risk management plan, labeling and packaging. The applicant must also provide evidence of marketing authorization or certificate of pharmaceutical product (CPP) from one or more reference countries that have similar regulatory standards as the GCC countries [16].

A general regulatory map of review processes is illustrated in Figure 14.1.

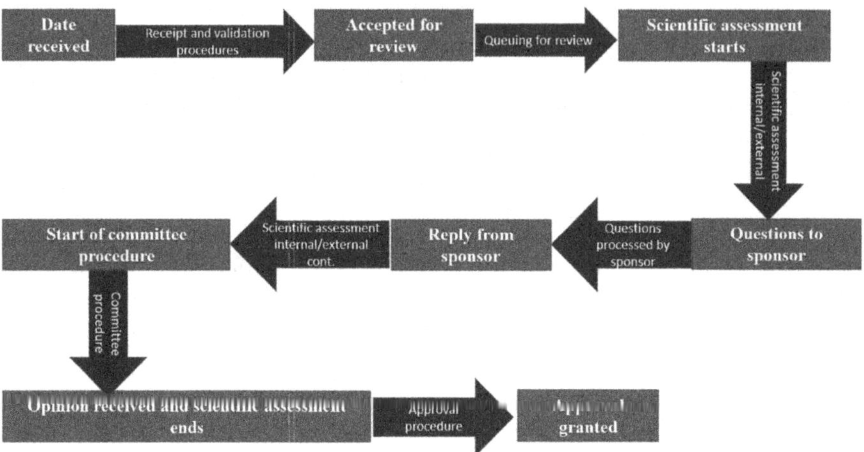

FIGURE 14.1 Overview Diagram Showing Evaluation and Endorsement Stages Shared by Established and Emerging Regulatory Bodies in GCC Entities.

14.2.4 Post-Approval Requirements and Monitoring

The post-approval requirements and monitoring for APIs in the GCC countries follow the guidelines and procedures of the PIC/S agreement, which was signed by all GCC countries in 2014 as a regional scheme for cooperation and harmonization in GMP inspection and quality control of pharmaceutical products. The PIC/S agreement aims to ensure that APIs are manufactured according to GMP standards and comply with their specifications throughout their shelf life [17].

The post-approval requirements and monitoring for APIs consist of several activities, as follows:

- The manufacturer must maintain a quality management system that covers all aspects of API production, testing, storage, distribution and recall.
- The manufacturer must conduct self-inspections at regular intervals to verify compliance with GMP standards and identify areas for improvement.
- The manufacturer must report any changes in API specifications, manufacturing process or quality system to the GHC within 30 days and obtain approval before implementing them.
- The manufacturer must report any adverse events or quality defects related to APIs to the GHC within 15 days and take corrective actions as required.
- The manufacturer must submit periodic safety update reports (PSURs) to the GHC every 6 months for NCEs or every year for ECEs that summarize all relevant safety information on APIs during a specified period.
- The manufacturer must comply with any requests from the GHC or any GCC country for samples or information on APIs as part of post-marketing surveillance activities [18].

14.3 COMPARISON OF API REGULATIONS IN GCC COUNTRIES

14.3.1 Saudi Arabia

Saudi Arabia is the largest market for pharmaceutical products in the GCC region, with a total value of about $8.5 billion in 2020. The main regulatory authority for APIs in Saudi Arabia is the Saudi Food and Drug Authority (SFDA), which was established in 2003 as an independent entity under the Council of Ministers. The SFDA is responsible for ensuring the quality, safety and efficacy of pharmaceutical products, including APIs, through registration, inspection, testing, monitoring and enforcement activities.

The SFDA follows the guidelines and procedures of the GCC-DR for the registration and approval of APIs in Saudi Arabia. The SFDA also adopts the PIC/S agreement for the GMP inspection and quality control of APIs in Saudi Arabia. The SFDA has issued several regulations and guidelines for APIs, such as the following:

- The Drug Law (2004), which sets the legal framework and general principles for regulating pharmaceutical products, including APIs, in Saudi Arabia [19];
- The Guidance for Registration of Active Pharmaceutical Ingredients (APIs) (2019), which specifies the requirements and procedures for submitting applications for marketing authorization of APIs in Saudi Arabia;
- The Guidance on Good Manufacturing Practice (GMP) Inspection of Active Pharmaceutical Ingredients (APIs) (2019), which outlines the criteria and process for conducting GMP inspections of API manufacturers in Saudi Arabia or abroad;
- The Guidance on Post-Marketing Surveillance (PMS) of Active Pharmaceutical Ingredients (APIs) (2019), which describes the responsibilities and obligations of API manufacturers and importers regarding PMS activities, such as reporting adverse events, quality defects, changes and PSURs.

14.3.2 United Arab Emirates (UAE)

The UAE is the second-largest market for pharmaceutical products in the GCC region, with a total value of about $4.2 billion in 2020. The main regulatory authority for APIs in the UAE is the Ministry of Health and Prevention (MOHAP), which was established in 1971 as the federal ministry responsible for overseeing the health sector in the UAE. The MOHAP regulates pharmaceutical products, including APIs, through its Drug Department, which consists of several sections, such as Registration and Drug Control Section, Inspection and Control Section, Pharmacovigilance Section and Drug Information Section [20].

The MOHAP follows the guidelines and procedures of the GCC-DR for the registration and approval of APIs in the UAE. The MOHAP also adopts the PIC/S agreement for the GMP inspection and quality control of APIs in the UAE. The MOHAP has issued several regulations and guidelines for APIs, such as:

- The Federal Law No. 4 of 1983 Concerning Pharmacy Profession and Pharmaceutical Institutions (1983), which sets the legal framework and general principles for regulating pharmaceutical products, including APIs, in the UAE [21];
- The Ministerial Decree No. 366 of 2010 Concerning Registration Requirements of Pharmaceutical Products (2010), which specifies the requirements and procedures for submitting applications for marketing authorization of pharmaceutical products, including APIs, in the UAE;
- The Ministerial Decree No. 550 of 2015 Concerning Good Manufacturing Practice Requirements for Pharmaceutical Products (2015), which outlines the criteria and process for conducting GMP inspections of pharmaceutical product manufacturers, including API manufacturers, in the UAE or abroad;
- The Ministerial Decree No. 551 of 2015 Concerning Post-Marketing Surveillance Requirements for Pharmaceutical Products (2015), which describes the responsibilities and obligations of pharmaceutical product manufacturers and importers regarding PMS activities, such as reporting adverse events, quality defects, changes and PSURs.

14.3.3 Kuwait

Kuwait is the third-largest market for pharmaceutical products in the GCC region, with a total value of about $1.4 billion in 2020. The main regulatory authority for APIs in Kuwait is the Ministry of Health (MOH), which was established in 1951 as the federal ministry responsible for overseeing the health sector in Kuwait. The MOH regulates pharmaceutical products, including APIs, through its Department of Pharmacy and Drug Control (PDC), which consists of several sections, such as the Registration Section, Inspection Section, Quality Control Section and Pharmacovigilance Section.

The MOH follows the guidelines and procedures of the GCC-DR for the registration and approval of APIs in Kuwait. The MOH also adopts the PIC/S agreement for the GMP inspection and quality control of APIs in Kuwait. The MOH has issued several regulations and guidelines for APIs, such as:

- The Law No. 28 of 1996 Concerning Pharmacy Profession Practice Regulation (1996), which sets the legal framework and general principles for regulating pharmaceutical products, including APIs, in Kuwait;
- The Ministerial Resolution No. 78/2007 Concerning Registration Requirements of Pharmaceutical Products (2007), which specifies the requirements and procedures for submitting applications for marketing authorization of pharmaceutical products, including APIs, in Kuwait;
- The Ministerial Resolution No. 79/2007 Concerning Good Manufacturing Practice Requirements for Pharmaceutical Products (2007), which outlines the criteria and process for conducting GMP inspections of pharmaceutical product manufacturers, including API manufacturers, in Kuwait or abroad;

- The Ministerial Resolution No. 80/2007 Concerning Post-Marketing Surveillance Requirements for Pharmaceutical Products (2007), which describes the responsibilities and obligations of pharmaceutical product manufacturers and importers regarding PMS activities, such as reporting adverse events, quality defects, changes and PSURs.

14.3.4 Bahrain

Bahrain is the fourth-largest market for pharmaceutical products in the GCC region, with a total value of about $0.8 billion in 2020. The main regulatory authority for APIs in Bahrain is the National Health Regulatory Authority (NHRA), which was established in 2010 as an independent entity under the Supreme Council of Health to regulate health services and products, including pharmaceutical products, in Bahrain. The NHRA regulates pharmaceutical products, including APIs, through its Directorate of Licensing and Registration, which consists of several units, such as Drug Registration Unit, Inspection Unit, Quality Control Unit and Pharmacovigilance Unit.

The NHRA follows the guidelines and procedures of the GCC-DR for the registration and approval of APIs in Bahrain. The NHRA also adopts the PIC/S agreement for the GMP inspection and quality control of APIs in Bahrain. The NHRA has issued several regulations and guidelines for APIs, such as:

- The Law No. 35 of 2012 Concerning Health Services Regulation (2012), which sets the legal framework and general principles for regulating health services and products, including pharmaceutical products, in Bahrain;
- The NHRA Guidelines on Registration Requirements of Pharmaceutical Products (2018), which specify the requirements and procedures for submitting applications for marketing authorization of pharmaceutical products, including APIs, in Bahrain;
- The NHRA Guidelines on Good Manufacturing Practice Requirements for Pharmaceutical Products (2018), which outline the criteria and process for conducting GMP inspections of pharmaceutical product manufacturers, including API manufacturers, in Bahrain or abroad;
- The NHRA Guidelines on Post-Marketing Surveillance Requirements for Pharmaceutical Products (2018), which describe the responsibilities and obligations of pharmaceutical product manufacturers and importers regarding PMS activities, such as reporting adverse events, quality defects, changes and PSURs.

14.3.5 Oman

Oman is the fifth-largest market for pharmaceutical products in the GCC region, with a total value of about $0.7 billion in 2020. The main regulatory authority for APIs in Oman is the Ministry of Health (MOH), which was established in 1971 as the federal ministry responsible for overseeing the health sector in Oman. The MOH regulates pharmaceutical products, including APIs, through its Directorate General of Pharmaceutical Affairs & Drug Control (DGPA&DC), which consists of several departments, such as Registration Department, Inspection Department, Quality Control Department and Pharmacovigilance Department.

The MOH follows the guidelines and procedures of the GCC-DR for the registration and approval of APIs in Oman. The MOH also adopts the PIC/S agreement for the GMP inspection and quality control of APIs in Oman. The MOH has issued several regulations and guidelines for APIs, such as:

- The Law No. 41/1996 Concerning Pharmacy Profession Regulation (1996), which sets the legal framework and general principles for regulating pharmaceutical products, including APIs, in Oman;
- The Ministerial Decision No. 145/2003 Concerning Registration Requirements of Pharmaceutical Products (2003), which specifies the requirements and procedures for submitting applications for marketing authorization of pharmaceutical products, including APIs, in Oman;
- The Ministerial Decision No. 146/2003 Concerning Good Manufacturing Practice Requirements for Pharmaceutical Products (2003), which outlines the criteria and process for conducting GMP inspections of pharmaceutical product manufacturers, including API manufacturers, in Oman or abroad;
- The Ministerial Decision No. 147/2003 Concerning Post-Marketing Surveillance Requirements for Pharmaceutical Products (2003), which describes the responsibilities and obligations of pharmaceutical product manufacturers and importers regarding PMS activities, such as reporting adverse events, quality defects, changes and PSURs.

14.3.6 Qatar

Qatar is the sixth-largest market for pharmaceutical products in the GCC region, with a total value of about $0.6 billion in 2020. The main regulatory authority for APIs in Qatar is the Ministry of Public Health (MOPH), which was established in 2013 as the federal ministry responsible for overseeing the health sector in Qatar. The MOPH regulates pharmaceutical products, including APIs, through its Department of Pharmacy and Drug Control (PDC), which consists of several sections, such as Registration Section, Inspection Section, Quality Control Section and Pharmacovigilance Section.

The MOPH follows the guidelines and procedures of the GCC-DR for the registration and approval of APIs in Qatar. The MOPH also adopts the PIC/S agreement for the GMP inspection and quality control of APIs in Qatar. The MOPH has issued several regulations and guidelines for APIs, such as:

- The Law No. 13 of 2002 Concerning Pharmacy Profession Regulation (2002), which sets the legal framework and general principles for regulating pharmaceutical products, including APIs, in Qatar;
- The Ministerial Decision No. 51 of 2011 Concerning Registration Requirements of Pharmaceutical Products (2011), which specifies the requirements and procedures for submitting applications for marketing authorization of pharmaceutical products, including APIs, in Qatar;

- The Ministerial Decision No. 52 of 2011 Concerning Good Manufacturing Practice Requirements for Pharmaceutical Products (2011), which outlines the criteria and process for conducting GMP inspections of pharmaceutical product manufacturers, including API manufacturers, in Qatar or abroad;
- The Ministerial Decision No. 53 of 2011 Concerning Post-Marketing Surveillance Requirements for Pharmaceutical Products (2011), which describes the responsibilities and obligations of pharmaceutical product manufacturers and importers regarding PMS activities, such as reporting adverse events, quality defects, changes and PSURs.

14.4 CHALLENGES AND ISSUES IN API REGULATIONS IN GCC COUNTRIES

14.4.1 Compliance Challenges

Compliance challenges refer to the difficulties and costs that API manufacturers and importers face in meeting the regulatory requirements and standards for APIs in the GCC countries. Some of the compliance challenges include:

- The lack of clarity and consistency in some of the regulatory guidelines and procedures for APIs, especially regarding the classification, evaluation and approval of different types of APIs (e.g., NCEs, ECEs, biologics, biosimilars);
- The variation and complexity of the registration and approval processes for APIs among the GCC countries, which may require different application forms, fees, timelines, documents and data for the same API;
- The duplication and redundancy of some of the regulatory requirements and activities for APIs among the GCC countries, such as GMP inspections, quality testing and PMS reporting, which may increase the administrative burden and operational costs for API manufacturers and importers;
- The lack of adequate infrastructure and resources for some of the regulatory authorities and agencies for APIs in the GCC countries, such as laboratories, equipment, personnel and training, which may affect their capacity and efficiency in performing their regulatory functions;
- The lack of sufficient incentives and support for local API manufacturers and innovators in the GCC countries, such as tax breaks, subsidies, grants and loans, which may limit their competitiveness and growth potential in the regional and global markets [23].

14.4.2 Quality Control

Quality control challenges refer to the risks and threats that may compromise the quality, safety and efficacy of APIs in the GCC countries. Some of the quality control challenges include:

- The increasing prevalence and sophistication of substandard or counterfeit APIs in the GCC markets, which may pose serious health hazards to consumers and undermine consumer confidence;
- The increasing complexity and diversity of APIs, especially biologics and biosimilars, which may require more advanced and specialized methods and techniques for quality testing and analysis;
- The increasing dependence on imported APIs from foreign sources, especially from China and India, which may raise concerns about their quality standards and compliance with the GCC regulations;
- The increasing vulnerability of APIs to environmental factors, such as temperature, humidity and light, which may affect their stability and potency during storage, transportation and distribution;
- The increasing occurrence of adverse events or quality defects related to APIs in the GCC markets, which may require prompt investigation, reporting and corrective actions by the regulatory authorities and stakeholders [24].

14.4.3 Intellectual Property Challenges

Intellectual property challenges refer to the issues and conflicts that may arise from the protection or infringement of intellectual property rights (IPRs) for APIs in the GCC countries. Some of the intellectual property challenges include:

- The lack of harmonization and alignment of the IPR regimes for APIs among the GCC countries, which may create legal uncertainty and inconsistency for API manufacturers and importers;
- The lack of adequate enforcement and deterrence of IPR violations for APIs in the GCC countries, which may encourage piracy and counterfeiting of APIs and discourage innovation and investment in API development;
- The lack of sufficient recognition and respect of IPRs for APIs in some of the GCC countries, which may result in unfair competition and market access barriers for API manufacturers and importers;
- The lack of effective mechanisms and platforms for resolving IPR disputes for APIs in the GCC countries, which may lead to prolonged litigation and arbitration costs and delays for API manufacturers and importers;
- The lack of adequate awareness and education of IPRs for APIs among the regulatory authorities, stakeholders and consumers in the GCC countries, which may affect their compliance and cooperation with IPR regulations and policies.

14.4.4 Harmonization Challenges

Harmonization challenges refer to the obstacles and barriers that may hinder or prevent the convergence and integration of the regulatory frameworks and systems for APIs among the GCC countries. Some of the harmonization challenges include:

- The diversity and complexity of the political, economic, social and cultural factors that influence the development and implementation of API regulations in each GCC country;
- The lack of sufficient coordination and collaboration among the regulatory authorities and agencies for APIs in each GCC country, as well as with other regional or international organizations or initiatives that aim to harmonize API regulations;
- The lack of common or compatible standards and criteria for evaluating and approving APIs among the GCC countries, which may create discrepancies or conflicts in their regulatory decisions or outcomes;
- The lack of mutual recognition or acceptance of API registrations or approvals among the GCC countries, which may require duplication or repetition of some regulatory requirements or activities for APIs;
- The lack of adequate incentives or benefits for harmonizing API regulations among the GCC countries, such as reduced costs, increased efficiency, improved quality or enhanced market access [25,26].

14.4.5 Future Trends

Future trends refer to the anticipated changes or developments that may affect or shape the regulatory landscape for APIs in the GCC countries. Some of the future trends include the following:

- The increasing adoption of digital technologies and solutions for API regulation in the GCC countries, such as e-submission, e-registration, e-inspection and e-monitoring, which may enhance transparency, speed, accuracy and convenience of regulatory processes and services;
- The increasing demand for personalized medicine and precision medicine in the GCC markets, which may require more customized and tailored APIs that meet specific patient needs or preferences;
- The increasing emergence of new types or categories of APIs, such as nanomedicines, cellular therapies and gene therapies, which may pose new challenges or opportunities for regulatory innovation and adaptation;
- The increasing participation or involvement of non-traditional players, such as tech companies, telecom companies and fintech companies, in providing or facilitating API-related services, such as data analytics, artificial intelligence and blockchain, which may create new competition or collaboration scenarios for existing stakeholders;
- The increasing integration or alignment of API regulations with other related regulations or policies in the GCC countries, such as data protection, cybersecurity and environmental protection, which may enhance coherence, consistency and comprehensiveness of regulatory governance [27].

14.5 CONCLUSION

This chapter has discussed the current status and challenges of API regulations in the GCC countries, which are Bahrain, Kuwait, Oman, Qatar, Saudi Arabia and the UAE. The chapter has covered the following aspects:

- The overview and definition of APIs and their importance for the pharmaceutical industry and public health;
- The regulatory framework and authorities for APIs in each GCC country and their alignment with the GCC-DR and PIC/S agreements;
- The registration and approval process for APIs in each GCC country and the differences and similarities among them;
- The post-approval requirements and monitoring for APIs in each GCC country and the compliance with GMP standards and PMS activities;
- The challenges and issues in API regulations in the GCC countries, such as compliance, quality control, intellectual property and harmonization challenges;
- The future trends in API regulations in the GCC countries, such as digitalization, personalization, innovation, diversification and integration.

API regulations are significant for the GCC countries for several reasons. First, API regulations ensure the quality, safety and efficacy of pharmaceutical products that are essential for the health and well-being of the population. Second, API regulations promote the development and growth of the local pharmaceutical industry that contributes to the economic diversification and competitiveness of the GCC countries. Third, API regulations facilitate the trade and cooperation of pharmaceutical products within the GCC region and with other countries that enhance the regional and global integration of the GCC countries.

The chapter has identified some potential areas for future developments in API regulations in the GCC countries. These include:

- Improving the clarity and consistency of the regulatory guidelines and procedures for APIs among the GCC countries to reduce ambiguity and complexity for API manufacturers and importers;
- Streamlining and simplifying the registration and approval processes for APIs among the GCC countries to reduce duplication and redundancy of regulatory requirements and activities for APIs;
- Enhancing the infrastructure and resources of the regulatory authorities and agencies for APIs in each GCC country to improve their capacity and efficiency in performing their regulatory functions;
- Providing adequate incentives and support for local API manufacturers and innovators in each GCC country to encourage their competitiveness and growth potential in the regional and global markets;
- Strengthening the enforcement and deterrence of IPR violations for APIs in each GCC country to protect innovation and investment in API development;

- Increasing the coordination and collaboration among the regulatory authorities and agencies for APIs in each GCC country, as well as with other regional or international organizations or initiatives that aim to harmonize API regulations;
- Adopting or adapting to new technologies and solutions for API regulation in each GCC country, such as e-submission, e-registration, e-inspection and e-monitoring, to leverage their benefits and opportunities for regulatory improvement and innovation.

REFERENCES

[1] Pateriya S, Janodia MD, Deshpande PB, Ligade VS, Talole KB, Kulshrestha T, Kamariya Y, Musmade PB, Udupa N. Regulatory Aspects of Pharmaceuticals' Exports in Gulf Cooperation Council Countries. *Journal of Young Pharmacists*. 2011;3(2):155–162.

[2] Alsaddique A. Future of the Pharmaceutical Industry in the GCC Countries. *Integrative Molecular Medicine*. 2017;4(4):1–3.

[3] Global Edge. Available from: https://globaledge.msu.edu/tradeblocs/gcc

[4] Secretariat General of the Gulf Cooperation Council (GCC). Available from: www.gcc-sg.org/enus/AboutGCC/pages/primarylaw.aspx

[5] Gulf Cooperation Council. Available from: www.mea.gov.in/portal/ForeignRelation/Gulf_Cooperation_Council_MEA_website.pdf

[6] The Gulf States Assessment and Experience with the Centralised Procedure. Available from: https://basicmedicalkey.com/thegulf-states-assessment-and-experience-with-the-centralised-procedure/

[7] The Gulf Central Committee for Drug Registration (GCC-DR). Available from: www.pharmalinkconsulting.com/blog/blog/the-gulfcommittee-for-drug-registration-gcc-dr/

[8] www.trade.gov/country-commercial-guides/saudi-arabia-healthcare

[9] www.globenewswire.com/news-release/2020/01/27/1975313/0/en/20-Billion-Pharmaceutical-Market-in-the-GCC-2020-2025-Saudi-Arabia-Dominates-with-50-Market-Share.html

[10] Regulatory Collaboration in Principles in GCC States (GCCDR). *Saleh Bawazir Vice-president for Drug Regulatory Affairs, Saudi Food and Drug Authority, Riyadh, Saudi Arabia*. ICDRA 2010 Singapore, 27 Nov-4 Dec. Available from: www.who.int/medicines/areas/quality safety/regulation legislation/PL2_2.pdf

[11] Europa.Eu. Available from: www.eeas.europa.eu/sites/default/files/documents/Regulatory%20Barriers%20to%20Bilateral%20EU-GCC%20Trade%20in%20services%20recommendations%20-%20report.pdf. Accessed May 28, 2023.

[12] Sravani M, Gowthami B, Prabhahar E, Rama Rao N. Regulatory Aspects of Pharmaceuticalsin Gulf Co-operation Council Countries. *International Journal of Pharma And Chemical Research*. 2017;3(3):397–414.

[13] www.api.org/-/media/apiwebsite/products-and-services/api-international-usage-and-deployment-report-2022.pdf

[14] www.biomapas.com/centralized-registration-procedure-gcc-region/

[15] Al-Essa R. *An Evaluation of the Regulatory Review Processes, the Quality of Decision Making and Strategic Planning in the Gulf Cooperation Council (GCC) States*. The Welsh School of Pharmacy, Cardiff University. Doctor of Philosophy thesis; 2011.

[16] Bujar M, McAuslane N. *The Impact of the Changing Regulatory Environment on the Approval of New Medicines Across Six Major Authorities 2004–2013 (R&D Briefing 55)*. Centre for Innovation in Regulatory Science (CISR); 2014. Available from: www.

fdanews.com/ext/resources/files/01-15/01-14-2015-International-Drug-Approvals.pdf?1421272458

[17] Khan S, U, Kamaraj R. A Review on the Centralised Registration Procedure in the Gulf Cooperation Council (GCC) Region. *Research Journal of Pharmacy and Technology*. 2018;11(12):5653–5668.

[18] https://picscheme.org/en/about-introduction

[19] https://lexmena.com/law/en_fed~1983-06-06_00004_2020-01-27/

[20] Saudi Food and Drug Authority (SFDA). *About SFDA* [Online]; 2013. Available from: www.sfda.gov.sa/en/about/Pages/overview.aspx

[21] www.doh.gov.ae/-/media/F84FA37968DA4B638D171481637F3E62.ashx

[22] CPhI. *Global API Industry Snapshot: Pharma Demands and Evolving Markets*; 2020 [online]. Available from: www.cphi.com/content/dam/Informa/cphi/europe/en/2020/pdf-files/API-CPhI_Zone_Article_0.pdf

[23] Lezotre PL. Value and Influencing Factors of the Cooperation, Convergence, and Harmonization in the Pharmaceutical Sector. In *International Cooperation, Convergence and Harmonization of Pharmaceutical Regulations*. 2014:171–219. Springer.

[24] www.wto.org/english/tratop_e/trips_e/trilatweb_e/ch4b_trilat_web_13_e.htm

[25] Lezotre PL. State of Play and Review of Major Cooperation Initiatives. In *International Cooperation, Convergence and Harmonization of Pharmaceutical Regulations*. 2014: 7–170. Academic Press.

[26] www.eeas.europa.eu/sites/default/files/documents/IPR%20regulatory%20frameworks%20in%20the%20GCC%20Report%202021%2004.pdf

[27] Singam SLSR, Yetukuri K, Nadendla RR. Drug Registration Requirements for Pharmaceuticals in Emerging Markets. *International Journal of Drug Regulatory Affairs*. 2020;8(4):73–82.

Section 2

Global Regulatory Perspectives of Food Products

15 Introduction, Challenges and Safety Issues of Food Regulation

Leo M.L. Nollet

15.1 CHALLENGES OF FOOD SAFETY

Since 2009, an annual 3-month international Intensive Training Program on Food Safety, Quality Assurance and Risk Analysis has been organized at Ghent University [1,2]. The trainees are asked to express their opinion on food safety concerns in their country and to select a case study to work on throughout the course. In Table 15.1 the topics that concern them are shown. This gives an idea of their concerns and the challenges they and we face.

The European Union and the Centers for Disease Control and Prevention (CDC) of the national public health agency of the United States bear responsibilities in food safety. CDC is a US federal agency under the Department of Health and Human Services.

Much of the text below is based on reference 3.

Major current and future challenges of food safety are the following [3–5]:

- Globalization of food chains combined with climate change may contribute to increased incidences of foodborne diseases and toxins in food, and increase the necessity of identifying emerging food safety issues and international cooperation;
- International trade agreements, new norms for standard setting and regulatory coherence are putting pressure on food safety policy;
- Foodborne pathogens such as *Salmonella* and Campylobacter are persistent and evolving, while at the same time new threats are emerging;
- Antimicrobial resistance (AMR) is perhaps the most daunting public health challenge of our time and is intrinsically related to food production systems. Addressing this challenge requires a broad-based strategy;
- Endocrine disruptors (ED) pose challenges to developing regulation, as traditional risk-based approaches cannot adequately assess the potential risk and illustrates the importance of the precautionary principle to deal with "scientific uncertainty";
- Nanotechnology also brings to question the adequacy of the current legislative framework on novel foods to deal with the complexity of issues like nanotechnology and animal cloning, and whether specific legislation on nanotechnology is necessary in light of this complexity.

DOI: 10.1201/9781003296492-17

TABLE 15.1

Case Studies on Food Safety Identified by International Participants (29 Countries) to the UGent VLIR-UOS Funded Intensive Training Program of Food Safety, Quality Assurance and Risk Assessment (2009–2015)

Food Safety Topics: Chemical Hazards (*n* = 38)	
Pesticide use and pesticide residues on banana and plantain production, cocoa or coffee beans, or at smallholder vegetable farmers and markets	10
Pesticide monitoring plans in fresh produce	1
Pesticide residues, mycotoxins, and prohibited food colorants in spices	2
Mycotoxins (e.g., aflatoxin) in nuts, seeds, coffee, corn, cereal flours, or sun-dried fruit and vegetables	10
Veterinary drugs (antibiotic) residues in fish, shrimp, and fishery products	2
Heavy metals in fresh fish and in fruits and vegetables and animal products due to use of (contaminated) river water	3
Nitrofuran, formalin, heavy metals, antibiotic residues in fish and shrimp	2
Chloropropanols, polycyclic aromatic hydrocarbons, and heterocyclic amines in processed foods	1
CFPA in baobab oil	1
Ethephon use and residues thereof in pineapple	1
The plasticizer DEHP in foodstuffs	1
TTX due to Japanese *fugu* fish (puffer fish)	1
Non-permitted food additives in fresh wheat noodles	1
Sudan IV dye adulteration of palm oil	1
Impact of harmful algal blooms and toxins on fish and fishery products	1
Food Safety Topics: Microbial Hazards (*n* = 38)	
Microbiological quality of milk and milk products, the issue of *Salmonella, Listeria monocytogenes*, and coagulase positive *Staphylococcus aureus* during cheese production	11
Microbial hazards (including histamine production) in fish and fishery products, traditional smoked fish	7
Slaughterhouse hygiene, sanitary quality of red meat and poultry processing and issues related to *Salmonella* and human pathogenic *Escherichia coli*	
Microbiological quality of street foods	7
Clostridium botulinum and botulinum toxin in home canned food	2

(Continued)

TABLE 15.1 (*CONTINUED*)

Bacterial load of vegetables irrigated with wastewater	1
Antibiotic resistance of *E. coli* isolates from poultry	1
Spore-forming bacteria and bacterial toxin production in cooked chilled foods	1
Parasitic infections (e.g., cysticercosis) in meat	1
Food Safety Topics: General Issues (*n* = 9)	
National food control systems and elaboration of an HACCP-based approach in small and medium processing companies	5
Food safety problems associated with food donations to avoid food waste	1
Food safety concerns in fried potato products	1
Food safety issues on functional foods	1
Food safety concerns in energy drinks	1

Note: CFPA, Cyclopropenoic fatty acid; DEHP, di-(2-ethylhexyl)phthalate; HACCP, hazard analysis and critical control points; TTX, tetrodotoxin; UOS, University Development Cooperation; VLIR, Flemish Interuniversity Council.

Challenges in food safety according CDC [5] are:

- Changes in our food production and supply, including more imported foods;
- Changes in the environment leading to food contamination;
- New and emerging bacteria, toxins, and antimicrobial resistance;
- Changes in consumer preferences and habits;
- Changes in the tests that diagnose foodborne illness.

15.2 GLOBALIZATION, CLIMATE CHANGE AND FREE TRADE AGREEMENTS

A first challenge of food safety is *globalization, climate change and free trade agreements*. The scope and speed of the global food trade has increased dramatically during the past 20 years. Food safety issues can have an international and even a global dimension, as international trade increases and emerging countries assume an increasing share of global GDP [6].

This interconnectedness allows contaminated food to be distributed far and wide, and makes tracing contamination increasingly difficult. At the same time, international cooperation and standard setting is increasing and private standards for food safety are gaining importance compared with public standards. Warmer climates, in combination with the globalization of food chains, may contribute to increased incidence of foodborne diseases and toxins in food. A number of food safety issues relating to climate change have been identified, such mycotoxins formed on plant products in the field or during storage, increased residues of pesticides in plant products affected by changes in pest pressure; and the presence of pathogenic bacteria in foods after more frequent extreme weather conditions, such as flooding and heat waves [7]. Climate change may affect zoonoses, diseases and infections that are naturally transmitted between vertebrate animals and humans (e.g., *Salmonella* and *Campylobacter*), by increasing the transmission cycle, range and prevalence of vectors of disease, and by increasing the animal host populations of disease. In some regions, climate change will contribute to the establishment of diseases not historically associated with the region [8]. Some more information on climate change and food safety may be found in references 9 and 10.

The spread of Bluetongue virus into Northern Europe is an alarming example of an "exotic" vector-borne livestock established within new geographical region, with little understanding of its origin, presenting a new and significant risk to livestock production. Both increased speed and scope of globalization of food trade and climate change will affect the vectors for food borne illness. Although the World Health Organization (WHO), the World Organization for Animal Health, and the European Commission and its agencies are already active in monitoring and evaluating some infections, there is much more to be done to fill gaps in the evidence base, build capacity within public health authorities and raise the political profile of the issue, and to examine the possible emergence of new threats and the expansion of diseases already present in Europe or the United States. See also references 11–13.

Because of globalization, climate change and new international agreements, more focus will need to be placed on identifying emerging food safety issues and international cooperation. One of the key tools to ensure the cross-border flow of information to swiftly react when risks to public health are detected in the food chain is RASFF (Rapid Alert System for Food and Feed). The legal basis of the RASFF was established Regulation (EC) No. 178/2002 [14]. The RASFF is one of the areas to be reviewed in an external study as part of the REFIT process. The purpose of the RASFF is to avert or mitigate food safety risks that cause harm to European consumers. Increasing globalization of food chains and emerging risks due to new vectors of disease exacerbated by climate change increases the reliance on early warning and alert systems like the RASSF increased international cooperation [15].

It is predicted at global level that the number of free trade agreements [16] and the number of countries involved in setting food safety standards and private food standards will increase [17]. The EU is negotiating a number of bilateral free trade agreements, most notably the free trade agreement with the United States, the Transatlantic Trade and Investment Partnership (TTIP) [18]. This process has been associated with a decline in the costs of cross-border trade in farm and other products [19].

Tariffs between the EU and United States are already low (about 4% on average). This means that the focus is on removing non-tariff barriers to trade such as sanitary and phytosanitary measures going beyond the World Trade Association Agreement on the Application of Sanitary and Phytosanitary Measures [20, 21].

In simple terms, this agreement allows countries to set their own standards to protect human, animal or plant health, but it requires that these standards should be based on science and should not unjustly discriminate between countries where there are identical or similar standards. Harmonizing regulation and standards on food safety poses a variety of challenges to current food safety approach, which is based on the farm-to-fork approach and the precautionary principle. In the current

TTIP negotiation, for instance, the principle has been criticized by food industry groups in both the EU and United States, as well as US government trade representatives, for lacking a "sound scientific basis" being used inappropriately and "lacking proportionality." In contrast, the European Environmental Agency (EEA) provides a different narrative in their "Late lessons from early warnings" [22] on the use, or rather neglect, of the precautionary principle. This report documents many cases in which societies failed to act in time to prevent serious harm to health and the environment, and contends that over-regulation due to the precautionary principle is the exception, whereas under-regulation tends to be the rule. Increasing globalization and increasingly complex food chains are also likely to lead to (more) food fraud and adulteration. Food fraud and adulteration does not always entail a food safety risk or public health threat, but often involves substituting a cheaper product or component in composite foods. However, a number of food fraud or adulteration incidents, such as melamine in milk in China, have had a clear public health threat. The horsemeat incident illustrates a fraudulent activity that does not bear a public health threat or food safety risk but undermines consumer confidence in food. It also illustrates the concerns of consumers about product contents and increasing complex food chains, and concerns relating to traceability. The legal basis for preventing fraudulent or deceptive practices, the adulteration of food, and any other practices that may mislead the consumer, is established in Article 8 of Regulation 178/2002 (General Food Law, 20).

15.3 PERSISTENT PROBLEMS AND NEW HEALTH THREATS

Another challenge is *persistent problems and new health threats.*

Although globalization and climate change as described earlier will bring changes in vectors of disease and in some cases new diseases, foodborne illness such as salmonellosis and campylobacteriosis are persistent in the world. *Salmonella* and *Campylobacter* are the most frequently reported cause of foodborne outbreaks. Antibiotic-resistant *Salmonella* in particular is increasingly linked to industrial and intensive livestock production systems. Although there has been some success in reducing *Salmonella* and *Campylobacter* in livestock, outbreaks remain a persistent problem.

Further information is available references 23, 24.

Despite changes in food production practices to mitigate risks, these and other foodborne pathogens seem able to evolve quickly, thus contaminating fresh produce and even generating new public health challenges such as antimicrobial resistance [25, 26]

Successful programs for controlling *Salmonella* in poultry and pigs exist. In Denmark, major reductions in the incidence of foodborne human salmonellosis were possible using an integrated approach to control of farms and food processing plants. This has been achieved by monitoring the herds and flocks, eliminating infected animals, and diversifying animals (animals and products are processed differently depending on salmonella status) and animal food products according to the determined risk. The control principles used are applicable to most industrialized countries with modern intensive farming systems. One overall challenge is the generation and maintenance of constructive dialogue and collaboration between public health, veterinary and food safety experts, bringing together multidisciplinary skills and multi-pathogen expertise. Such collaboration is essential to monitor changing trends in well-recognized diseases and detect emerging pathogens. It will also be necessary to understand the multiple interactions these pathogens have with their environments during transmission along the food chain to develop effective programs and solutions. As discussed earlier, microbial pathogens are constantly evolving, which has created new public health problems. Imprudent use of antibiotics in both humans and animal husbandry has led to new challenges relating to antimicrobial resistance. According to WHO, this is one of the major public health challenges of our time "in which common infections and minor injuries which have been treatable for decades can once again kill." Antimicrobial resistance (AMR) presents a substantial challenge to food safety both in terms of impact on public health in general and the capacity of healthcare systems to deal with infections [27, 28].

It is also illustrates the importance of food safety policy that is collaborative across policy areas and sectors. The European Centre for Disease Prevention and Control estimates that AMR results each year in 25,000 deaths and related costs of over EUR 1.5 billion in healthcare expenses and productivity losses [29].

The EU was an early mover in banning antibiotics as growth promoters for livestock. An EU wide ban on the use of antibiotics as growth promoters in animal feed entered into effect in 2006 [30].

The ban is the final step in the phasing out of antibiotics used for non-medicinal purposes as part of the Commission's overall strategy to tackle the emergence of bacteria and other microbes resistant to antibiotics due to their overexploitation or misuse. Banning the use of antibiotics has led to a decrease in resistant bacteria, but the problem persists. AMR is intrinsically related to the way livestock is treated for disease, production methods and animal husbandry practices. Intensive production systems, livestock density and animal husbandry practices increase the dependency on antibiotics

15.4 USE OF CHEMICALS AND RISE OF NEW TECHNOLOGIES

The third challenge is *use of chemicals and rise of new technologies*

Stretching the limits of current regulation, endocrine disrupting chemicals (EDC) are found in a range of product from plastics used for packaging food and drinks to commonly used pesticides [31–33]. EDCs or just EDs (endocrine disruptors) interfere with hormone systems in humans, animals and plants, and cause "adverse health effects in an intact organism, or its progeny, or (sub)populations" according to the position adopted by the WHO's International Program on Chemical Safety [34].

EDs are known or suspected to cause a number of health problems such as learning disabilities, attention deficit disorders and cancer and are increasingly linked to obesity and metabolic disorders such as type II diabetes. Recent research suggests that ED effects can even be transmitted to future generations. In relation to food and food safety, exposure to EDs is mainly related to migration through food and drink packaging, pesticide residues in food and environmental exposure in pesticide application. As part of the revision of its strategy on EDs, the European Commission is currently weighing whether to propose changing EU legislation governing the use of pesticides (Council Regulation (EC) No 1107/2009, 35).

In addition to difficulties related to definition and identification, legislating on ED is challenging because traditional risk-based approaches do not appear suitable to establish appropriate thresholds for exposure: dose is less important compared with exposure and time of exposure in the human life cycle. Scientists have therefore called for hazard-based cut-off criteria for EDCs. Legislation on EDCs provides an illustrative example of the importance of the precautionary principle, providing justification for acting in the face of scientific uncertainty and as a tool for acting on the basis of early warnings. Although support for targeted research is a high priority, the need for further research should not delay necessary policy and regulatory decisions to protect public health. Technologies are no longer presumed safe simply because evidence of risk or adverse effect is unavailable. Precautionary approaches presume that an induced adverse response in animals is a reliable indicator of potential harm in humans, unless informed otherwise by multiple studies. New food chain technologies may increase productivity of the food chain and quality of foods, and can help address a number of societal challenges. However, concerns remain about the safety and acceptability of these technologies in the food chain. Concurrent incremental innovations in conventional technologies can also be anticipated. The use of nanotechnology in the food chain is increasing, but uncertainties over risks remain. Although still at an early stage of development, spending on nanotechnology—technology associated with particles of 1–100 nm in size—is rapidly increasing and the number of nanotech patents is on the rise. Nanotechnologies in the food industry have multiple functions: their first application is in food packaging, where they improve functionality. Other applications of nanotechnology include improving taste, enhancing the bioavailability of certain ingredients, reducing the content of some elements such as sugar and salt, and slowing down microbial activity. In addition, nanotechnology could bring about radical new approaches to assist crop production and storage [36], and disease and pest control. In addition, the unique features of nanomaterials are not fully explored and raise concerns about potential environmental, health and general safety hazards. For example, some new nanomaterials may have the potential to enter the human body through mucous membranes or the skin and migrate via the bloodstream to vital organs, or the brain, interacting with other cells in unpredictable ways, which may have potential cytotoxic or genotoxic effects [37–39]. Nanotechnology use in food illustrates a specific element of novel foods legislation and related challenges. Nanotechnologies are emerging with the capacity to impact both the food industry and consumers (e.g., food processing and packaging, production of agrochemicals and seed). Like other new or modern technologies, nanotechnology can bring significant risks that are hard to assess because of its recent nature. Both animal cloning and nanotechnology are stretching the limits of novel food legislation. More rigorous checks may need to be developed and applied to adequately assess the impact of new food technology on food safety and public health. This also raises the question of whether the current framework can effectively deal with the complexity of issues like nanotechnology, and whether additional specific legislation is required.

15.5 GENETICALLY MODIFIED ORGANISMS

A last challenge is *genetically modified organisms (GMOs).*

GMOs constitute another key theme for food safety authorities: the authorization process of GMOs for import or cultivation remains. In the European Union, no negative environmental or public health impacts of authorized genetically modified (GM) crops are indicated, but public opinion and many Member State governments continue to have concerns about GM crops. Food and feed are generally derived from plants and animals, which have been grown and bred by humans for several thousand years. Plant and animal breeding has developed species and animals selecting desirable characteristics. Biotechnology has made it possible to modify the genetic material of living cells and organisms. Organisms whose genetic material (DNA) has been altered are called GMOs. Food or feed that contains and consists of GMOs or are produced from GMOs are referred to as GM food or feed. Transferring genes from one species to another is particularly problematic for EU citizens. According to a Eurobarometer poll, EU citizens do not see the benefits of horizontal gene transfer, have strong reservations about safety, feel that special labeling of food products is necessary, and do not feel that it should be encouraged; although they see some degree of benefit for vertical gene transfer, they have reservations about impact on the environment and safety aspects of the technology. EU legislation on GMOs has been in place since the early 1990s. GMOs and food products derived from GMOs, which are placed on the market, must also satisfy labeling and traceability conditions. The case of GM food and feed illustrates the importance of consumer confidence and complexity of establishing the burden of scientific proof.

The reader is directed to references 40–42 for further information on GMO foods and food safety.

REFERENCES

[1] Uyttendaele, M., De Boeck, E., & Jacxsens, L. (2016). Challenges in food safety as part of food security: Lessons learnt on food safety in a globalized world. *Procedia Food Science*, *6*, 16–22.

[2] www.itpfoodsafety.ugent.be/

[3] www.europarl.europa.eu/RegData/etudes/IDAN/2014/536287/IPOL_IDA%282014%29536287_EN.pdf

[4] www.europarl.europa.eu/studies

[5] www.cdc.gov/foodsafety/challenges/index.html

[6] www.imf.org/external/datamapper/NGDP_RPCH@WEO/OEMDC/ADVEC/WEOWORLD

[7] Miraglia, M., Marvin, H. J. P., Kleter, G. A., Battilani, P., Brera, C., Coni, E., . . . & Vespermann, A. (2009). Climate change and food safety: An emerging issue with special focus on Europe. *Food and Chemical Toxicology*, *47*(5), 1009–1021.

[8] www.fao.org/documents/card/en?details=cc3017en

[9] Tirado, M. C., Clarke, R., Jaykus, L. A., McQuatters-Gollop, A., & Frank, J. M. (2010). Climate change and food safety: A review. *Food Research International*, *43*(7), 1745–1765.

[10] Duchenne-Moutien, R. A., & Neetoo, H. (2021). Climate change and emerging food safety issues: A review. *Journal of Food Protection*, *84*(11), 1884–1897.

[11] Todirica, I. C., Chiripuci, B. C., & Toderasc, S. A. (2018). Globalisation and food safety implications in developing countries. *International Multidisciplinary Scientific GeoConference: SGEM*, *18*(5.3), 415–422.

[12] Robertson, L. J., Sprong, H., Ortega, Y. R., van der Giessen, J. W., & Fayer, R. (2014). Impacts of globalisation on foodborne parasites. *Trends in Parasitology*, *30*(1), 37–52.

[13] Jacxsens, L., Uyttendaele, M., Holvoet, K., Kierezieva, K., & Luning, P. (2012). The impact of climate change and globalisation on the safety of fresh produce. *International Food Hygiene*, *23*(3), 26–27.

[14] https://eur-lex.europa.eu/legal-content/EN/TXT/HTML/?uri=CELEX:32002R0178

[15] https://food.ec.europa.eu/safety/rasff_en

[16] Menon, J. (2009). Dealing with the proliferation of bilateral free trade agreements. *World Economy*, *32*(10), 1381–1407.

[17] Henson, S., & Humphrey, J. (2009). *The impacts of private food safety standards on food chain and public standard-setting processes*. www.fao.org/3/i1132e/i1132e.pdf

[18] https://ustr.gov/ttip

[19] Anderson, K. (2010). Globalization's effects on world agricultural trade, 1960–2050. *Philosophical Transactions of the Royal Society B: Biological Sciences*, *365*(1554), 3007–3021.

[20] https://food.ec.europa.eu/horizontal-topics/general-food-law_en

[21] www.wto.org/english/res_e/publications_e/sps_agreement_series_e.htm#:~:text=The%20Agreement%20on%20the%20Application,animal%20and%20plant%20health%20regulations

[22] www.eea.europa.eu/publications/late-lessons-2

[23] Thames, H. T., & Theradiyil Sukumaran, A. (2020). A review of Salmonella and Campylobacter in broiler meat: Emerging challenges and food safety measures. *Foods*, *9*(6), 776.

[24] Habib, I., Mohamed, M. Y. I., & Khan, M. (2021). Current state of Salmonella, Campylobacter and Listeria in the food chain across the Arab countries: A descriptive review. *Foods*, *10*(10), 2369.

[25] Bennani, H., Mateus, A., Mays, N., Eastmure, E., Stärk, K. D., & Häsler, B. (2020). Overview of evidence of antimicrobial use and antimicrobial resistance in the food chain. *Antibiotics*, *9*(2), 49.

[26] EFSA Panel on Biological Hazards (BIOHAZ), Koutsoumanis, K., Allende, A., Álvarez-Ordóñez, A., Bolton, D., Bover-Cid, S., . . . & Peixe, L. (2021). Role played by the environment in the emergence and spread of antimicrobial resistance (AMR) through the food chain. *EFSA Journal*, *19*(6), e06651.

[27] Nelson, D. W., Moore, J. E., & Rao, J. R. (2019). Antimicrobial resistance (AMR): Significance to food quality and safety. *Food Quality and Safety*, *3*(1), 15–22.

[28] Freeland, G., Hettiarachchy, N., Atungulu, G. G., Apple, J., & Mukherjee, S. (2023). Strategies to combat antimicrobial resistance from farm to table. *Food Reviews International*, *39*(1), 27–40.

[29] www.ecdc.europa.eu/en/publications-data/ecdcemea-joint-technical-report-bacterial-chal-lenge-time-react

[30] https://eur-lex.europa.eu/legal-content/EN/TXT/?uri=CELEX%3A32003R1831

[31] Kassotis, C. D., Vandenberg, L. N., Demeneix, B. A., Porta, M., Slama, R., & Trasande, L. (2020). Endocrine-disrupting chemicals: Economic, regulatory, and policy implications. *The Lancet Diabetes & Endocrinology*, *8*(8), 719–730.

[32] Duh-Leong, C., Maffini, M. V., Kassotis, C. D., Vandenberg, L. N., & Trasande, L. (2023). The regulation of endocrine-disrupting chemicals to minimize their impact on health. *Nature Reviews Endocrinology*, *19*(10), 600–614.

[33] Yilmaz, B., Terekeci, H., Sandal, S., & Kelestimur, F. (2020). Endocrine disrupting chemicals: Exposure, effects on human health, mechanism of action, models for testing and strategies for prevention. *Reviews in Endocrine and Metabolic Disorders*, *21*, 127–147.

[34] www.who.int/health-topics/chemical-safety#tab=tab_1

[35] https://eur-lex.europa.eu/LexUriServ/LexUriServ.do?uri=OJ:L:2009:309:0001:0050:en:PDF

[36] www.gov.uk/government/publications/government-office-for-science-annual-review-2012-to-2013

[37] Nile, S. H., Baskar, V., Selvaraj, D., Nile, A., Xiao, J., & Kai, G. (2020). Nanotechnologies in food science: Applications, recent trends, and future perspectives. *Nano-Micro Letters*, *12*, 1–34.

[38] Ansari, M. A. (2023). Nanotechnology in food and plant science: Challenges and future prospects. *Plants*, *12*(13), 2565.

[39] He, X., Deng, H., & Hwang, H. M. (2019). The current application of nanotechnology in food and agriculture. *Journal of Food and Drug Analysis*, *27*(1), 1–21.

[40] Teferra, T. F. (2021). Should we still worry about the safety of GMO foods? Why and why not? A review. *Food Science & Nutrition*, *9*(9), 5324–5331.

[41] Gbashi, S., Adebo, O., Adebiyi, J. A., Targuma, S., Tebele, S., Areo, O. M., . . . & Njobeh, P. (2021). Food safety, food security and genetically modified organisms in Africa: A current perspective. *Biotechnology and Genetic Engineering Reviews*, *37*(1), 30–63.

[42] Leonelli, G. C. (2020). GMO risks, food security, climate change and the entrenchment of neo-liberal legal narratives. In *Transnational Food Security* (pp. 128–141). Routledge.

16 Food Products Regulations in the European Union

Varisha Anjum, Vishal Dixit, Pritya Jha, and Irina Potoroko

16.1 INTRODUCTION

Food safety is a major goal of every individual. The United Nations Sustainable Development Goals for 2030 promote an end to hunger and ensuring access by all people—the poor and people in vulnerable situations including infants—to safe, nutritious and sufficient food all year round. Food safety, public health and welfare successfully will be based on medicine events in coming decades. One Health is a holistic or big-picture approach where the tenet is that welfare and well-being is based on human, animal and environmental health and that integration and sharing of information on animal and human health is the key to efficient health systems [1]. The wide growing range of synergistic disciplines includes food safety, public health, health economics, ecosystem health, social science and animal health, for addressing complex health problems [2].

Various zoonoses in Europe affecting human health are foodborne [3], whereas several are also non-zoonotic. Foodborne disease has long symbolised an extensive burden to public health and continues to defy health systems across the globe. Any person can catch a foodborne disease, although susceptible populations such as small children, elderly people, pregnant individuals, those who are immunocompromised, and those living in poverty or who are food insecure are predominantly susceptible. Statistics suggest that foodborne disease are common throughout the world; however, because of the restrictions in the surveillance systems, the actual cases are reported in small proportion. It is presumed that endorsed records on the prevalence of foodborne disease represent only the "iceberg apex." Moreover, very little evidence is available on the burden of foodborne disease that impacts health in terms of mortality, morbidity and disability.

Hence, government should develop and implement food safety policies and strengthen the effectiveness and efficacy of food safety systems, thereby protecting consumers from foodborne disease and their causative agents with more accurate available data. Regulations are needed to manage food safety and to understand the drivers and determinants for the emergence and persistence of human, animal and environmental threats. Without sufficient information about the occurrence and

DOI: 10.1201/9781003296492-18

load of disease allied with specific pathogen/food commodity combinations, prioritisation of foodborne hazards against measured palliation is difficult to put into action.

Statistics on occurrence and disease burden are therefore decisive in evaluating both expenses of control measures and its profits. Moreover, challenges are there in prioritising different public health risks while designing healthcare goals and supporting food safety and public health risk management by measuring pressure of disease and source attribution [4–6]. Technical knowledge about pathogen transmission route is important while designing control strategies against foodborne diseases, for the methods to be more effective, consumer behaviour, food trends, economic incentives, trade and politics need to be considered [7,8]. This review examines food safety aspects focusing on Europe.

16.1.1 Importance of Food Safety in Modernised Food System

Several high-profile food safety events in the previous years have validated the challenges for food safety in modernising food systems. Increased use of certain inputs can result in hazardous residues when such use is unregulated and producers are untrained and intentional adulteration can occur when production cannot be easily traced or monitored. Consumers may demand greater levels of safety with higher incomes and less real or perceived control over food sources at the same time. More rigorous public regulation, upgraded private food supply chain harmonisation and innovative rules for international trade have surfaced in the past two decades to tackle food safety concerns. The developments are the result of various factors, including the growth in trade of perishable and high value products, advances in hazard detection and epidemiology, high-profile health scares, and scientific and regulatory consensus on best approaches to risk management. Thus, food safety is a market access issue for food producers as they seek to meet requirements in modernising global food systems. Furthermore, preventing market interruptions from food safety incidents and assuring consumer confidence is an important part of food market development. Second, food safety risks contribute to the burden of disease in the European Union countries. The World Health Organization (WHO) is engaged in a multi-year process to estimate the global burden of illness from foodborne disease for the year 2015. The purpose of this chapter is to review the international experiences and lessons regarding food safety management, regulation and consumer behaviour, with the goal of identifying how to improve food safety in middle income countries such as Europe. We begin by reviewing the internationally accepted approaches to food safety regulation and management that inform current public and private efforts (Figure 16.1).

Europeans have the right to access safe and nutritious food of the highest standards. In the late 1990s, a few series of food incidents drew awareness to establish universal principles and requirements concerning food and feed law at the EU level. Consequently, a unified approach to food safety "from farm to fork" was established by the European Commission, primarily set out in its White Paper on Food Safety. It protects all segments of the food chain, including feed production, primary production, food processing, storage, transport and retail sale.

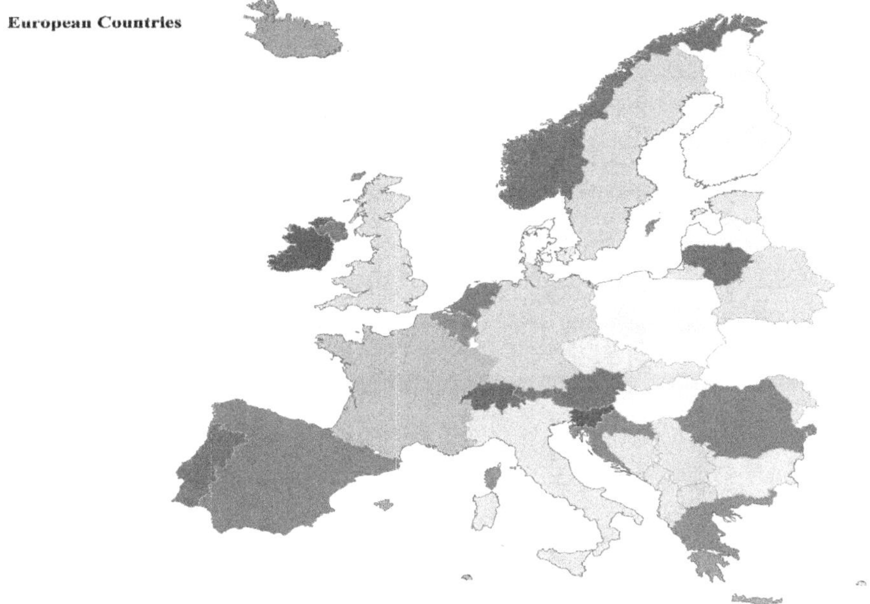

FIGURE 16.1 EU Countries Highlighted in an Outline Map of Europe.

16.1.2 Trends and Sources of Zoonoses, Zoonotic Agents and Foodborne Outbreaks in the EU

In 2015 and 2019, the European Food Safety Authority (EFSA) and the European Centre for Disease Prevention and Control monitored zoonoses activities in 36 European countries (28 Member States (MS) and eight non-MS as four more added after 2015). The first and second most reported zoonoses in humans were campylobacteriosis and salmonellosis, respectively, since 2008 in increasing European Union (EU) movement for confirmed human cases. The EU trend for confirmed human cases of these two diseases was stable (flat) during 2015–2019. In food, the occurrence of *Campylobacter* remained high in broiler meat. The decreasing EU trend for confirmed human salmonellosis cases since 2008 continued, but the proportion of human *Salmonella enteritidis* cases increased since 2008 whereas similar during 2017–2018. The 26 MS met their *Salmonella* reduction targets for poultry with control programmes, whereas 18 met the reduction targets, a further eight failed to meet at least one.

16.1.3 Legal Basis of European Union–Coordinated Zoonoses Monitoring

The monitoring and collection of information for EU system on zoonoses is based on the Zoonoses Directive 2003/99/EC1, which indulges EU Member States (MS)

TABLE 16.1
Summarized Data of Zoonoses Directive 2003/99/ec

S. No.	Article	Chapter	Lists	Annex	Agents	Relevant Information
1.	—	—	A	Annex 1	*Salmonella, Campylobacter, Listeria monocytogenes*, Shiga toxin-producing *Escherichia coli* (STEC), *Mycobacterium bovis, Brucella, Trichinella* and *Echinococcus*	Data on animals, food and feed
2.	—	—	B	Annex 1	i. Viral zoonoses: calicivirus, hepatitis A virus, influenza virus, rabies, viruses transmitted by arthropods	Based on the epidemiological situations in the MS
	—	—	—	—	ii. Bacterial zoonoses: borreliosis, botulism, leptospirosis, psittacosis, tuberculosis due to agents other than *M. bovis*, vibriosis, yersiniosis and their respective agents	—
	—	—	—	—	iii. Parasitic zoonoses: anisakiasis, cryptosporidiosis, cysticercosis, toxoplasmosis and their respective agents	—
	—	—	—	—	iv. Other zoonoses and zoonotic agents such as *Francisella,* Cysticercus and *Sarcocystis*	—
3.	4	II	—	—	—	Monitoring of zoonoses and zoonotic agents of the directive
4.	5 and 6	II	—	—	—	Specific rules for coordinated monitoring programmes and for food business operators
5.	7	III (Antimicrobial resistance)	—	—	—	Specific rules for monitoring of antimicrobial resistance
6.	8	IV (Foodborne outbreak)	—	—	—	Rules for epidemiological investigation of foodborne outbreaks

7.	9	V (Exchange of information)	—	—	—	MS shall assess trends and sources of zoonoses, zoonotic agents and antimicrobial resistance in their territory and each MS shall send their report on trends and sources of zoonoses, zoonotic agents and antimicrobial resistance, covering the data collected under Articles 4, 7 and 8 during the previous year by end of May to the EC
8.	—	—	A–D	Annex IV	—	Monitoring of zoonoses, zoonotic agents and antimicrobial resistance carried out in accordance with Article 4 or 7
9.	—	—	E	Annex IV	—	Regards the monitoring of foodborne outbreaks carried out in accordance with Article 8

TABLE 16.2
Reported Hospitalisations And Case Fatalities Due To Zoonoses In Confirmed Human Cases In The Eu, 2019

Disease	No. of Confirmed Human Cases	Hospitalisation		Death	
		No. of Reporting MS	Reported Hospital Cases	No. of Reporting MS	Reported Deaths
Campylobacteriosis	220,682	16	20,432	17	47
Salmonellosis	87,923	15	16,628	17	140
STEC infections	7775	18	1100	20	10
Yersiniosis	6961	15	648	14	2
Listeriosis	2621	19	1234	20	300
Tularaemia	1280	12	149	13	1
Echinococcosis	739	14	109	14	2
Q fever	950	NA	NA	13	4
West Nile virus infection (a)	443	9	347	11	52
Brucellosis	310	11	98	12	2
Trichinellosis	96	5	6	7	1
Rabies	4	NA	NA	3	3

to collect relevant and comparative statistics on zoonoses, zoonotic agents, antimicrobial resistance and food borne outbreaks. Additionally, MS evaluate trends and sources of outbreaks in their territory and then submit their annual account every year to the European Commission wrapping the data collected. The European Commission later forward these reports to the EFSA.

The task of examining the data and publishing the EU Annual Summary Reports EFSA is assigned. In 2004, the European Commission entrusted EFSA with the task set up the electronic reporting system and database for monitoring zoonoses (EFSA Mandate No. 2004–0178). Data collection on human diseases from MS is conducted in accordance with Decision 1082/2013/EU2 on serious cross-border threats to health. This assessment replaced Decision 2119/98/EC on setting a grid for the epidemiological surveillance and control of communicable diseases in the EU in October 2013. The case definitions were monitored while reporting for infectious diseases to the European Centre for Disease Prevention and Control (ECDC) described in Decision 2018/945/EU3. Initially ECDC used to provided data on zoonotic infections in humans, as well as their analyses, for the EU Summary Reports, subsequently from 2008, reports received via the European Surveillance System (TESSy), maintained by ECDC.

According to List A of the Annex I of the Zoonoses Directive 2003/99/EC data on animals, food and feed must be reported on a mandatory basis. Further reports based on the epidemiological situations in the MS data must be reported on the agents as shown in Table 16.1. Furthermore, MS provided data on certain other microbiological contaminants in foods: histamine, staphylococcal enterotoxins and *Cronobacter sakazakii* for which food safety criteria are set down in the EU legislation.

Severity of the diseases was analysed based on hospitalisation and outcome of the reported cases (Table 16.2).

TABLE 16.3
Yearly Relative Variation (%) Of Foodborne Outbreaks Reporting Rate (Per 100,000 Population) In 2019 Compared With 2018, By Country, In Reporting Eu Ms And Non-Ms

Countries	% Rate	Outbreak Reporting Rate (% variation 2019/2018)
Austria	0.54	–8.0%
Belgium	4.98	44%
Bulgaria	0.23	–11%
Croatia	1.13	92%
Cyprus	0.23	0%
Czechia	0.23	–8.0%
Denmark	0.88	–22%
Estonia	0.98	–13%
Finland	0.98	–27%
France	2.66	10%
Germany	0.48	–3.0%
Greece	0.06	20%
Hungary	0.36	–15%
Ireland	0.51	25%
Italy	0.22	1.0%
Latvia	1.72	0%
Lithuania	1.97	53%
Luxembourg	0	—
Malta	9.12	–4.0%
Netherlands	4.25	–3.0%
Poland	1.17	–15%
Portugal	0.13	18%
Romania	0.04	–76%
Slovakia	—	
Slovenia	0.05	—
Spain	1.08	–19%
Sweden	0.64	–13%
United Kingdom	0.09	16%
EU total	**1.02**	**–12%**
Iceland	0.80	–40%
Montenegro	0.50	–63%
Norway	0.90	5.0%
Rep. of North Macedonia	0.20	5.0%
Serbia	0.50	–39%
Switzerland	0.30	92%

16.1.4 Overview of Countries Reporting Foodborne Outbreaks

During 2019, 27 MS reported 5175 foodborne outbreaks (FBOs), 49,463 cases of illness, 3859 hospitalisations and 60 deaths. In addition, 117 FBOs, 3760 cases of illness and 158 hospitalisations were communicated by six non-MS (Iceland, Montenegro, Norway, Republic of North Macedonia, Serbia, Switzerland). Slovakia did not report data on FBOs.

The total number of outbreaks reported by each MS in 2019 varied importantly, with a small number of MS reporting most of the outbreaks. Altogether, FBOs reported by five countries (Belgium, France, the Netherlands, Poland and Spain) accounted for more than three-quarters of total outbreaks (4042 outbreaks; 78.10% of all outbreaks) and more than two-thirds of total cases observed in the EU in 2019 (32,883 cases; 66.50% of all cases).

The breakdown of FBOs by countries and by strength of evidence is reported in Table 16.3. In this table, the "outbreak reporting rate" (per 100,000 population) describes how frequent was the reporting of FBOs in 2019, in EU/EFTA countries, regardless of the differently sized populations. The range of this value was huge, from 0.04 (Romania) to 9.12 (Malta) outbreaks (per 100,000 population), corresponding to a 253-fold difference.

The "mean outbreak size" (i.e., the mean number of cases per outbreak) and the range of cases per outbreak is shown to characterise the pattern of FBOs reported to EFSA by MS and non-MS. Altogether, these indicators provide evidence of the large variability among MS in the sensitivity of surveillance and the type of FBOs being monitored in each MS. As an example, household outbreaks (i.e., outbreaks in which all the human cases live in one single household) are usually small-sized outbreaks. As not all MS report household outbreaks to EFSA, this may influence the mean outbreak size and the number of outbreaks. Details on the type of FBOs reported to EFSA, by country, are shown in Table 16.3.

16.1.5 Overview of Causative Agents in Foodborne Outbreaks

In 2019 a causative agent was identified in 3101 FBOs (59.90% of total outbreaks) causing 35,969 cases (72.70% of total cases), 3290 hospitalisations (85.30% of total hospitalisations) and 54 deaths (90.0% of total deaths). For a high proportion of outbreaks (40.10%), the causative agent was "unknown" or "unspecified." The Netherlands (693 outbreaks), Belgium (554 outbreaks), France (288 outbreaks) and Spain (229 outbreaks) contributed most to this reporting (1764 outbreaks altogether; 85.10% of outbreaks with an "unknown" or "unspecified" causative agent). Bacteria were reported to have caused most outbreaks ($N = 1364$; 26.40%) followed by bacterial toxins ($N = 997$; 19.30%), viruses ($N = 554$; 10.70%), other causative agents ($N = 155$; 3.0%) and parasites ($N = 31$; 0.60%).

For each pathogen group and single causative agent, the proportion of hospitalisations and deaths among cases and the mean outbreak size facilitate description of the general characteristics of the FBOs and their impact on health. The highest proportion of hospitalisations and deaths were observed for outbreaks caused by bacteria. *Salmonella* was responsible for the highest number of hospitalisations ($N = 1915$)

TABLE 16.4
Foodborne Outbreaks Reported in 2019, by Country and by Unknown/Unspecified Agents Reporting EU MS and Non-MS

Countries	% Rate	Outbreak Reporting Rate (% variation 2019)
Austria	0	—
Belgium	554	46%
Bulgaria	11	
Croatia	6.0	50%
Cyprus	0	—
Czechia	4.0	–20%
Denmark	0	–100%
Estonia	1.0	—
Finland	19	–39%
France	288	6.0%
Germany	35	0%
Greece	2.0	100%
Hungary	5.0	–62%
Ireland	3.0	—
Italy	45	15%
Latvia	0	–100%
Lithuania	2.0	—
Luxembourg	0	—
Malta	21	–5.0%
Netherlands	693	–3.0%
Poland	125	17%
Portugal	6.0	–14%
Romania	0	–100%
Slovakia	—	—
Slovenia	0	—
Spain	229	8.0%
Sweden	19	–27%
United Kingdom	6.0	–33%
MS	2074	7.0%
Iceland	0	—
Montenegro	2.0	–67%
Norway	13	–24%
Rep. of North Macedonia	0	—
Serbia	0	—
Switzerland	19	138%

and *L. monocytogenes* alone caused more than half of the fatal illnesses ($N = 31$) [9]. The number of deaths due to FBOs caused by *L. monocytogenes* doubled, compared with 2018 (10 deaths more than in 2018; 47.60% increase). Fatal cases also increased among outbreak cases caused by *Bacillus cereus* ($N = 7$; 6 cases more than in 2018) mainly due to a single outbreak in France, with five fatal events reported among 17 cases. The monitoring and the reporting of foodborne outbreaks among MS is poorly harmonised, the interpretation of pooled data at the EU level requires caution, as the situation at single MS level may differ importantly.

16.1.6 Outbreaks Caused by Unknown/Unspecified Agents

Several reasons may explain the reporting of unknown/unspecified agents, including late reporting of illness, failure to detect causative agents in patients or in the food, unavailability of clinical or food samples (e.g., leftovers), delay in sample collection and so on. For the same reasons, few outbreaks of unknown aetiology were classified as strong-evidence outbreaks. In 2019, 2074 foodborne outbreaks of unknown aetiology accounted for 40.1% of total outbreaks and 27.30% of illnesses in the EU. At the country level, these proportions varied hugely. Outbreaks with unknown aetiology were mainly reported by Belgium and the Netherlands and these FBOs accounted for 1274 outbreaks (60.10% of all outbreaks caused by unknown agents notified in the EU). They were mainly weak evidence, small-sized (< 10 cases) events that each included fewer than four cases, on average. In Belgium and in the Netherlands, this type of outbreak accounted for the majority of the FBOs (Table 16.4).

These findings suggest that outbreaks caused by unknown agents occurred in confined contexts such as domestic settings or small groups, for which the identification of the link among cases was probably relatively easy. Conversely, 250 outbreaks with unknown aetiology involving each more than ten cases (medium- and large-size outbreak) were reported by 15 MS. Not all MS, however, reported outbreaks of unknown aetiology to EFSA in 2019.

16.2 EUROPEAN UNION REGULATION

The European Parliament and the Council adopted Regulation (EC) No 178/2002 for the general principles and requirements of food law (General Food Law Regulation) in 2002. The General Food Law Regulation is the foundation of food and feed law. It sets out an overarching and coherent framework for the development of food and feed legislation both at Union and National levels. To this end, it lays down general principles, requirements and procedures that underpin decision-making in matters of food and feed safety, covering all stages of food and feed production and distribution. It also sets up an independent agency responsible for scientific advice and support, the European Food Safety Authority (EFSA). Moreover, it creates the main procedures and tools for the management of emergencies and crises, as well as the Rapid Alert System for Food and Feed preceding (RASFF). The General Food Law Regulation ensures a high level of protection of human life and consumers' interests in relation to food while ensuring the effective functioning of the internal market.

16.2.1 Rapid Alert System for Food and Feed (RASFF)

The EU has one of the highest food safety standards in the world, largely thanks to the strong setup of EU legislation in place, which ensures that food is safe for consumers. A key tool to ensure the flow of information to enabling swift reaction when risks to public health are detected in the food chain is RASFF.

Created in 1979, RASFF enables information to be shared efficiently between its members (EU Member State National Food Safety Authorities, Commission, EFSA, ESA, Norway, Liechtenstein, Iceland and Switzerland) and provides round-the-clock service to ensure that urgent notifications are sent, received and responded to collectively and efficiently. Thanks to RASFF, many foods safety risks had been averted before they could have been harmful to European consumers. Vital information exchanged through RASFF can lead to products being recalled from the market. A robust system, which has matured over the years, RASFF continues to show its value to ensure food safety in the EU and beyond. All farms that have been treated by the service treatment company since January 2017 have been immediately blocked by the competent authorities of the concerned Member States, and eggs/chicken meat from these farms can no longer be placed on the EU market nor exported to non-EU countries. The year 2020 was another year of change for the Rapid Alert System for Food and Feed (RASFF).

Regulation (EU) 2019/1715 had entered into force mid-December 2019, implementing the Information Management System for Official Control (IMSOC)1. For RASFF it meant merging the Administrative Assistance and Cooperation (AAC) network with the RASFF network into a whole new entity: the Alert and Cooperation Network (ACN). This integration with AAC allows combining investigations on non-compliances in RASFF notifications or easily escalating non-compliance notifications to RASFF notifications. The fundamental difference between non-compliance and RASFF notifications takes its origin in their different legal basis: Regulation 178/2002 (General Food Law) for RASFF versus Regulation 2017/625 (Official Controls Regulation) for AAC. In 2020, RASFF was in particular confronted with a major food contamination incident in September, when Belgium reported high levels of an unauthorised pesticide, ethylene oxide, in sesame seeds from India, a substance for which a Maximum Residue Limit of 0.05 ppm is set in the legislation for that commodity. It resulted in unprecedented activity in RASFF exchanging information on findings of ethylene oxide, identifying batches of products involved and tracing their distribution.

16.2.2 Integration of the Administrative Assistance and Cooperation Network with the Rapid Alert System for Food and Feed

Although notified within the same electronic system, iRASFF, the AAC non-compliance notifications and RASFF notifications follow two different workflows thanks to a feature specifically developed for this purpose in 2019: the "conversation module." Through the conversation, the notifying country can share its notification with its peers and make requests for assistance. With the rules of the IMSOC Regulation applying from 14 December 2019, the integration between

TABLE 16.5
Summary of the Number of AAS Notifications per Food Product

Food Product	AAS Notification
Fruits and vegetables	362
Dietetic foods, food supplements and fortified foods	294
Meat and meat products (other than poultry)	146
Cereals and bakery products	118
Fish and products thereof	107
Milk and milk products	99
Feed materials	87
Fats and oils	75
Other food products/mixed	71
Prepared dishes and snacks	71
Poultry meat and poultry meat products	69
Food contact materials	59
Cocoa and cocoa preparations, coffee and tea	53
Non-alcoholic beverages	49
Alcoholic beverages	47
Confectionary	47
Bivalve molluscs and product thereof	46
Compounds feeds	41
Herbs and spices	41
Soups broths, sauces and condiments	41
Null	38
Food additives and flavourings	31
Nuts, nut products and seeds	30
Wine	30
Eggs and egg products	21
Feed additives	21
Honey and royal jelly	19
Crustaceans and products thereof	18
Ices and desserts	12
Water for human consumptions (other)	11
Feed premixtures	10
Natural mineral waters	10
Cephalopods and products thereof	6
Pet food	6
Animal by-products	1
Gastropods	1

RASFF and AAC is now complete. In the context of a non-compliance notification, the notifying country can make a request to another country, thereby sharing the notification with only that country and with the Commission. Any participant to the notification can make requests to other countries thereby sharing the notification with these and enlarging the group of countries that cooperate on the notification. A RASFF notification can benefit from the same cooperation mechanism.

16.2.3 AAC Notifications in 2020

The evolution in the number of notifications in RASFF and in AAC between 2017 and 2020 reveals a rapid rise to significance for the non-compliance notifications reported through the AAC. Now that integration into iRASFF (the online platform of the RASFF network) is complete, the AAC network benefits from its new feature (the conversation module) but also from the already long established procedure in iRASFF using follow-up notifications. The use of the system has remained similar in 2020 as in 2019 in terms of the number of non-compliance notifications per notifying country (Table 16.5 and Figure 16.2). Germany has submitted more than three times the number of non-compliances created by Austria, the latter having clearly used the system much more intensively than all other Member States.

16.2.4 Agri-Food Fraud

The free movement of safe and wholesome food is an essential aspect of the internal market and contributes significantly to the health and well-being of citizens and to their social and economic interests. The EU is equipped with a mature and functioning regulatory framework ensuring food safety that deeply relies on enforcement. In that regard, agri-food fraud is an area where the EU is continuously stepping up its efforts. Fraudulent activities are characterised by their intentional nature, aimed at an economic gain, in violation of legal rules and at the expense of the immediate customer or the final consumer. Attempts by some business operators to obtain unfair advantages over competitors by deceiving them (and/or consumers) and the extension of organised groups' crime portfolio to cover food and drink have led to a series of prominent food fraud cases such as the horsemeat scandal. The digital dimension (e-commerce of food) further creates opportunities for deceptive and dishonest practices allowing action from "abroad." The resulting food fraud incidents affect the confidence in the EU food system, with an immediate impact on the functioning of the internal market. The cross-border dimension is often strong as fraudulent operators seek for more profit on the biggest possible scale. Member States can thus not effectively act alone.

The complex nature of our globalised agri-food supply chain and the economic motivation to provide cheaper food products increase the possibility of fraud. Faced with this phenomenon, control authorities losing credibility, companies are losing money and consumers are losing trust in food. This creates a major paradox: "EU food is safer than ever, yet consumer's trust is low." In the wake of the horse meat scandal, the European Parliament's 2013 resolution called on the Commission "to give food fraud the full attention it warrants and to take all necessary steps to make the prevention and combating of food fraud an integral part of EU policy" and "to make the prevention and combating food fraud an integral part of an EU policy." As reaction to the Fipronil incident, the Member States and the Commission agreed on a first set of concrete measures to reinforce the EU's action against food fraud. These measures were presented to the AGRIFISH Council on 9 October 2017. They included a commitment to improved interaction between the rapid alert system (RASFF) and the Administrative Assistance and Cooperation system and to the creation of single

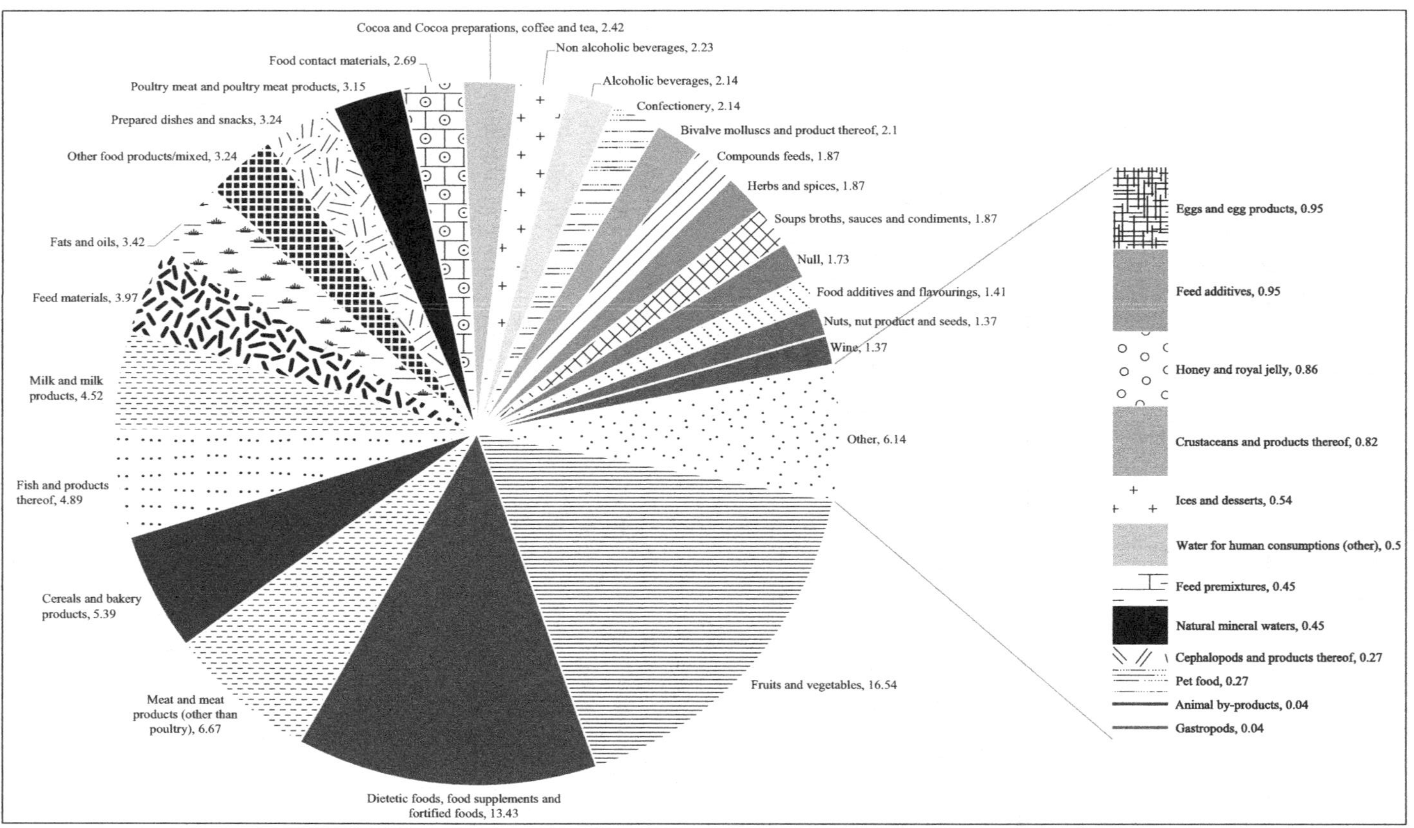

FIGURE 16.2 Summary of the Percent of AAS Notification Per Food Product.

contact points for both systems. The EU re-shaped its agri-food chain official control policies and developed them further with a view to both enhancing citizens' trust and increasing overall efficiency.

On 16 December 2019, the Council of the EU adopted new conclusions on further steps to improve ways of tackling and deterring fraudulent practices in the agri-food chain. In these conclusions, the Council recalled that a high level of protection was an overall objective of EU policies concerning health, safety, environmental protection, and consumer protection, and recognised that the current EU legal framework on tackling food fraud was adequate. The Council nonetheless emphasised the need for continuous and improved cross-sectorial cooperation to fight against food fraud (including not only food and feed control authorities, but also authorities involved in the fight against financial crime and tax, customs, police, prosecution and other law enforcement authorities). The Council called upon the Commission and member states to allocate adequate resources to ensure effective implementation of existing EU legislation by improving the shared understanding of the criteria determining food fraud.

The Council also stressed the need to promote awareness-raising among consumers and to continue to broaden training on countering food fraud.

16.2.5 Regulatory Authority

Name: European Commission (EC)—Directorate General for Health and Consumers

The EC is the European Union's (EU) executive body. Their responsibilities include:

- Proposing and enforcing regulation;
- Representing and upholding the interests of Europe as a whole;
- Drafting proposals for new European laws;
- Managing the day-to-day business of implementing EU policies and allocating EU funds;
- Ensuring that everyone abides by the European treaties and laws.

The responsibilities of the Directorate General for Health and Consumers is to ensure food and consumer goods sold in Europe are safe, that the EU's internal market works for the benefit of consumers, and that Europe helps protect and improve its citizen's health.

16.3 ADVISORY SCIENTIFIC BODY

Name: European Food Safety Authority (EFSA)

It collects information and analyses new scientific developments to identify and assess any potential risks to the food chain. It can carry out scientific assessment on any matter that may have a direct or indirect effect on the safety of the food supply, including matters relating to animal health, animal welfare and plant health.

EFSA also gives scientific advice on non-food and feed genetically modified organisms and on nutrition in relation to EU legislation. It can communicate directly with the public on any issue within its area of responsibility. The five committees that were transferred to EFSA in May 2003 include:

- Scientific Committee on Food (SCF)
- Scientific Committee on Animal Nutrition
- Scientific Committee on Veterinary Measures relating to Public Health
- Scientific Committee on Plants
- Scientific Committee on Animal Health and Animal Welfare.

16.3.1 Role/Responsibility

The Authority shall provide scientific advice and scientific and technical support for the Community's legislation and policies in all fields that have a direct or indirect impact on food and feed safety. It shall provide independent information on all matters within these fields and communicate on risks (178/2002/EC, article 22).

16.3.2 Framework Regulations

178/2002/EC—General principles and requirements of food law, establishing the EFSA and laying down procedures in matters of food safety.

16.3.2.1 Part of an Overarching International Organization

- The EU has been a member of the World Trade Organization since 1995.
- The EU is a member of the Codex Alimentarius Commission.

16.3.2.2 Recent and/or Pending Changes

On 16 December 2008, the regulations of the Package on Food Improvement Agents were adopted. This includes regulations on food additives, food enzymes, and flavourings and food ingredients with flavouring properties, and an additional fourth regulation (Regulation (EC) No. 1331/2008, adopted on 16 December 2010) establishing a common authorisation procedure for additives, enzymes and flavourings.

16.3.3 Regulatory Overview of Specific Food Chemical Groups

Definition of food ingredients

- Any substance, including additives, used in the manufacture or preparation of a foodstuff and still present in the finished product, even if in altered form;
- Where an ingredient of the foodstuff is itself the product of several ingredients, the latter shall be regarded as ingredients of the foodstuff in question;
- The following shall not be regarded as ingredients:

    - The constituents of an ingredient that have been temporarily separated during the manufacturing process and later reintroduced but not in excess of their original proportions;
    - Additives whose presence in each foodstuff is solely because they were contained in one or more ingredients of that foodstuff, if they serve no technological function in the finished product, which are used as processing aids;
    - Substances used in the quantities strictly necessary as solvents or media for additives or flavourings.
- In certain cases, decisions may be taken in accordance with the procedure laid down in Article 20 (2) in Directive 2000/13/EC as to whether the conditions described above are satisfied. Novel foods: Novel foods are foods and food ingredients that have not been used for human consumption to a significant degree within the Community before 15 May 1997.

16.3.4 Regulation

16.3.4.1 Regulation 258/97/EC for Novel Foods

Approval process for a new substance: Foods commercialised in at least one member state before the entry into force of the Regulation on Novel Foods on 15 May 1997, are on the EU market under the "principle of mutual recognition." To ensure the highest level of protection of human health, novel foods must undergo a safety assessment before being placed on the EU market. Only those products considered to be safe for human consumption are authorised for marketing. Companies who want to place a novel food on the EU market need to submit their application in accordance with Commission Recommendation 97/618/EC, which outlines the scientific information and the safety assessment report required. Novel foods or novel food ingredients may follow a simplified procedure, only requiring notifications from the company, when they are considered by a national food assessment body as "substantially equivalent" to existing foods or food ingredients (as regards to their composition, nutritional value, metabolism, intended use and the level of undesirable substances contained therein).

16.3.5 Direct Food Additives

Definition: Food additives are substances that are not normally consumed as food itself but are added to food intentionally for a technological purpose described in Regulation (EC) No. 1333/2008 (e.g., the preservation of food). All food additives should be covered by this Regulation, and therefore in the light of scientific progress and technological development the list of functional classes should be updated (currently there are 26 functional classes listed in the Annex I to Regulation (EC) No. 1333/2008). However, substances should not be considered as food additives when they are used for the purpose of imparting flavour and/or taste or for nutritional purposes, such as salt replacers, vitamins and minerals. Moreover, substances considered as foods that may be used for a technological function, such as sodium chloride or saffron for colouring, and food enzymes also should not fall within the scope of Regulation (EC) No. 1333/2008. However, preparations obtained from foods and other natural source material that are intended to have a technological effect in the final food and that are obtained by selective extraction of constituents (e.g., pigments) relative to the nutritive or aromatic constituents, should be considered additives within the meaning of Regulation (EC) No. 1333/2008.

The new Regulation (EC) No. 1333/2008 does not apply to the following substances unless they are used as food additives:

- Processing aids;
- Substances used for the protection of plants and plant products in conformity with Community rules relating to plant health;
- Substances added to foods as nutrients;
- Substances used for the treatment of water for human consumption falling within the scope of Council Directive 98/83/EC of 3 November 1998 on the quality of water intended for human consumption;
- Flavourings, which fall within the scope of Regulation (EC) No. 1334/2008;
- Regulation (EC) No. 1333/2008 does not apply to food enzymes falling within the scope of Regulation (EC) No. 1332/2008 with effect from the date of adoption of the Community list of food enzymes in accordance with Article 17 of that Regulation.

Regulation: Regulation (EC) No. 1333/2008 includes the Community list of approved food additives for use in foods and conditions of use, and the Community list of food additives approved for use in food additives, food enzymes, food flavourings and nutrients and their condition of use. Before these Community lists apply (1 June 2013) the Annexes to Directives 94/35/EC, 94/36/EC and 95/2/EC are still valid. A food additive may be included in the Community lists only if it meets general conditions: no safety concerns at the level of use proposed; there is a technological need; the consumer is not misled; and there are advantages and benefits for the consumer. Other more specific conditions exist for sweeteners and colours. All authorised food additives have to fulfil purity criteria that are set out in detail in three Commission Directives (EC) No. 10/2009 (food additives other than sweeteners and colours, amending Directive 2008/84/EC), 2008/60/EC (sweeteners), and 2008/128/EC (colours). It should be noted that new regulations on purity criteria were adopted on 9 March 2012 (Regulation (EU) No. 231/2012 on specifications for food additives listed in Annexes II and III) which will repeal the mentioned directives as of 1 December 2012. Food additives must be kept under continuous observation and must be re-evaluated whenever necessary in the light of changing conditions of use and new scientific information.

Therefore, when the EC is informed about new scientific evidence relating to a permitted food additive, it requests EFSA to assess the new data. In addition to this ongoing observation the EC has also asked the EFSA to undertake a re-evaluation of all currently permitted food additives (Regulation (EU) No. 257/2010).

Regulation (EC) No. 1333/2008 on food additives:

- The regulation, except transitional provisions, has been in application since 20 January 2010.
- The regulation strengthens the principle of food safety and consumer information. It allows a more efficient and simplified procedure for authorisation of food additives by comitology. The consolidation of all food additives legislation in one single legal instrument makes legislation user-friendly for citizens and business operators. Comitology is the procedure by which the Commission prepares the draft legislation and member states vote at the Standing Committee on the Food Chain and Animal Health. If a qualified majority is in favour, it is then passed to the European Parliament and the Council, which have 2 months to object. If they do not object, it is published in the Official Journal and then it is EU law.
- In accordance with Article 30 of Regulation (EC) No. 1333/2008, additives that are permitted in food under Directives 94/35/EC, 94/36/EC and 95/2/EC and their conditions of use were entered in the Community list of food additives in Annex II to the regulation. To that end, the compliance with their general and specific conditions of use was reviewed. The new EU lists amending Annexes II and III to Regulation EC 1333/2008 were adopted on 11 November 2011.
- The use of food additives already permitted in Directives 94/35/EC, 94/36/EC and 95/2/EC will continue to be permitted until the application of Annex II as amended by Regulation (EU) No. 1129/2011 (1 June 2013)

Guidance document: The Practical Guidance for Applicants was prepared to provide applicants with information that aims at facilitating the preparation and submission of applications for establishing or updating (adding, removing, or changing conditions, specifications, or restrictions) the Community lists.

Approval process for a new substance: Applicants who wish to introduce new additives into the EU market, or seeking to revise existing provisions regulating individual additives already authorised within the EU, or seeking confirmation that an already approved additive made from a new source or by a new method of production is acceptable, must apply. Beside the Practical Guidance for Applicants there is also the Guidance on Submissions for Food Additive Evaluations by the SCF which provides details on the administrative and technical data required, and the range of toxicological tests generally required for new food additives, and on the format for formal submissions on additives. It must be noted that EFSA is preparing a new guidance document, which will replace the old one. The requirements for the application are also mentioned in Regulation (EU) 234/2011, which implements Regulation (EC) No. 1331/2008. The general requirements consist of:

- Administrative data
- Risk assessment data:
  - Identity of the substance
  - Information on particle size
  - Presence of impurities

  - Microbiological characteristics
  - Proposed chemical and microbiological specifications
  - Manufacturing process
  - Methods of analysis in foods
  - Reaction and fate in food
  - Case of need and proposed uses
  - Exposure
  - Additives produced by microbiological processes
  - Additives produced from genetically modified organisms
  - Information on national authorisations
  - Proposed normal and maximum use levels.
- Toxicological data:
  - General framework for the toxicological evaluation of food additives
  - Study protocols
  - Toxicological section of the dossier (core studies and other studies)
  - Data reporting
  - Review of results and conclusions.
- Risk management data:
  - Function and technological need
  - Investigations on the efficacy
  - Advantages and benefits for the consumer
  - Information why the use would not mislead the consumer
  - Compliance with specific conditions for sweeteners and colours.

16.3.6 Food Contact Substances (Components of Packaging Materials)

Definition: Food contact materials and articles are those that in their finished state are intended to be brought into contact with food, or are already brought into contact with food and intended for that purpose or can reasonably be expected to be brought into contact with food or to transfer their constituents to food under normal and foreseeable conditions of use. This includes packaging materials but also cutlery, dishes, processing machines, containers and so on. The term also includes materials and articles that are in contact with water intended for human consumption but it does not cover fixed public or private water supply equipment.

Regulation: Framework Regulation (EC) No. 1935/2004. Food contact materials should be safe and should not transfer their components into the foodstuff in unacceptable quantities. The transfer of constituents from food contact materials into food is referred to as migration. In the context of the framework Regulation, specific Regulations on plastics (10/2011/EU), Active and intelligent (A&I) FCM substances (450/2009/EC), Recycling of plastics (282/2008/EC), Regenerate cellulose (Directive 2007/42/EC), ceramics (Directive 84/500/EEC) have been published. The specific Regulation on plastic FCM contains a positive list of monomers and additives, which can be used for their manufacture. The EU Food Contact Materials Database lists all approvals and conditions of use from the above Regulations and Directives. To ensure the protection of the health of the consumer and to avoid any contamination of the foodstuff, two types of migration limits have been established for plastic materials:

- An overall migration limit (OML) of 60 mg (of substances) kg^{-1} (of foodstuff or food simulants) that applies to all substances that can migrate from food contact materials to foodstuffs
- A specific migration limit (SML) applies to individual authorised substances and is fixed on the basis of the toxicological evaluation of the substance. The SML is generally established according to the acceptable daily intake (ADI) or the tolerable daily intake (TDI) set by the SCF in the past and by EFSA since 2003. To set the limit, it is assumed that every day throughout his/her lifetime, a person weighing 60 kg eats 1.0 kg of food packed in plastics containing the relevant substance at the maximum permitted quantity.

16.3.6.1 Guidance Document

The guidance document on the submission of a food contact material for evaluation by EFSA by the Panel on Additives, Flavourings, Processing Aids, and Materials in Contact with Food.

16.3.6.2 Approval Process for a New Substance

General requirements include:

- Identity of the substance;
- Physical and chemical properties of the substance;
- Intended use of the substance;
- Authorisation of the substance (authorisation for use of the substance in EU member states and other countries);
- Migration data on the substance;
- Data on the residual content of the substance in the food contact material;
- Microbiological properties of the substance;
- Toxicological data;
- General requirements;
- Core tests (not all types of studies may be applicable for the substance of interest—all tests should be carried out according to EU or OECD guidelines, and including good laboratory practice);
- Three mutagenicity studies in vitro;
- 90-day oral toxicity studies, normally in two species;
- Studies on absorption, distribution, metabolism and excretion;
- Reproduction studies in one species;
- Developmental toxicity studies, normally in two species;
- Long-term toxicity/carcinogenicity, normally in two species;
- Additional studies/special investigations may be required if prior knowledge, or structural considerations indicate that other biological effects such as peroxisomal proliferation, neurotoxicity, immunotoxicity or endocrinological events may occur;

- Dermal or inhalation sensitisation studies, if applicable;
- Depending on the chemical nature of the substance to be used in food contact materials, the list of required tests mentioned above may be modified;
- Additional details available in the guidance document.

16.3.7 Flavouring Agents

Definition: Flavouring substances are defined chemical substances that include flavouring substances obtained by chemical synthesis or isolated using chemical processes, and natural flavouring substances. Flavourings are used to improve or modify the odour and/or taste of foods for the benefit of the consumer. Flavourings and food ingredients with flavouring properties should only be used if they fulfil the criteria specified in Regulation (EC) No. 1334/2008. They must be safe when used, and certain flavourings should therefore undergo a risk assessment before they can be permitted in food.

Regulation: New Regulation (EC) No. 1334 was adopted on 16 December 2008; however, as of 20 January 2011, this new regulation repeals Directives 88/388/EEC and 91/71/EEC. To protect human health, this Regulation should cover flavourings, source materials for flavourings and foods containing flavourings. It should also cover certain food ingredients with flavouring properties that are added to food for the main purpose of adding flavour and that contribute significantly to the presence in food of certain naturally occurring undesirable substances (hereinafter referred to as food ingredients with flavouring properties), their source material and foods containing them. The Regulation sets out flavourings and source materials for which an evaluation and approval is required. The Regulation prohibits the addition of certain substances as such to food and sets maximum levels for certain substances, which are naturally present in flavourings and in food ingredients with flavourings properties, but which may raise concern for human health. As of 20 January 2010, Regulation (EC) No. 1334/2008 on flavouring and certain food ingredients with flavouring properties amended the following: Council Regulation (EEC) No. 1601/91, Regulations (EC) No. 2232/96 and (EC) No. 110/2008, and Directive 2000/13/EC; however, Regulation (EC) No. 2232/96, laying down a community procedure for flavouring substances, will continue to apply until the date of application of the Union list of flavourings and source materials. Smoke flavourings are regulated under Regulation (EC) No. 2065/2003

Approval process for a new substance: After the completion of the evaluation programme but at the latest by 31 December 2010, the EU list of flavouring substances for use in or on foods in the EU shall be adopted [Article 5(1) of Regulation (EC) No. 2232/96]. New substances follow the authorisation procedure laid down in Regulation (EC) No. 1331/2008 on the common authorisation procedure for food additives, food enzymes and food flavourings. Data requirements for flavouring substance application include:

- Manufacturing process;
- Specifications;
- Data on dietary and non-dietary sources;
- Assessment of dietary exposure;

- Assessment of the genotoxic potential of the flavouring substance;
- Examination for structural/metabolic similarity to flavouring substances in an existing flavouring group evaluation (if applicable). Other requirements are specified for other categories of flavouring substances.

16.3.8 Enzymes

Definition: A food enzyme is defined as a product obtained from plants, animals or microorganisms or products thereof including a product obtained by a fermentation process using microorganism containing one or more enzymes capable of catalysing a specific biochemical reaction and added to food for a technological purpose at any stage of the manufacturing, processing, preparation, treatment, packaging, transport or storage of foods. A food enzyme preparation is defined as a formulation consisting of one or more food enzymes in which substances such as food additives and/or other food ingredients are incorporated to facilitate their storage, sale, standardisation, dilution or dissolution. Regulation (EC) No. 1332/2008 does not include food enzymes used in the production of food additives falling within the scope of Regulation (EC) No. 1333/2008 or processing aids. The scope of this Regulation does not extend to enzymes that are not added to food to perform a technological function but are intended for human consumption, such as enzymes for nutritional or digestive purposes.

Regulation: Regulation (EC) No. 1332/2008 on food enzymes amends Council Directive 83/417/EEC, Council Regulation (EC) No. 1493/1999, Directive 2000/13/EC, Council Directive 2001/112/EC and Regulation (EC) No. 258/97. This Regulation harmonises for the first time the rules for food enzymes in the EU. It applies from 20 January 2009, except labelling provisions that apply from 20 January 2010. National provisions concerning the placing on the market and the use of food enzymes and food produced with food enzymes continue to apply in the member states until the adoption of the Union list of enzymes applies.

Approval process for a new substance: Food enzymes shall be subject to safety evaluation by EFSA and approval via an EU list. A 2-year period has been fixed in this Regulation for submission of applications on existing enzymes and new enzymes. This period started on 11 September. The inclusion of a food enzyme in the EU list will be considered by the Commission since Article 6 of Regulation (EC) No. 1332/2008, namely the opinion from EFSA, and also other general criteria such as technological need and consumer aspects. For every food enzyme included in the positive list, specifications including the purity criteria and the origin of the food enzyme shall be laid down. Data required for risk assessment and for risk management of food enzymes are laid down in Regulation (EC) No. 234/2011.

16.3.9 Processing Aids

Definition: According to Article 3.2(b) of Regulation (EC) No. 1333/2088 a processing aid shall mean any substance that is not consumed as a food by itself; is intentionally used in the processing of raw materials, foods or their ingredients, to fulfil a certain technological purpose during treatment or processing; and may result in the unintentional but technically unavoidable presence in the final product of residues of the substance or its derivatives provided they do not present any health risk and do not have any technological effect on the final product.

Regulation: Processing aids are not harmonised at EU level with the exception of food enzymes used as processing aids (see section 16.3.8) and extraction solvents used in the production of foodstuffs and food ingredients (Directive 2009/32/EC). If a processing aid does not meet the criteria outlined in the definition (above), it can be regulated as a food additive, and the applicable Regulation (EC) No. 1333/2008 (regulations for food additive) would be applicable.

16.3.9.1 Approval Process for a New Substance

There is no approval process for processing aids at the EU level.

16.3.10 Nanoscale Materials

Definition: The Commission has adopted a Recommendation for a definition of "nanomaterial" for regulatory purposes that it intends to integrate progressively and where necessary in the EU Food Law [9].

Regulation: Existing legislation covers in principle the potential health, safety and environmental risks in relation to nanomaterials. Recently, specific provisions on the risk assessment of nanomaterials were introduced in EU legislation on food additives and food contact materials (EC 2009). A definition of "engineered nanomaterial" and a mandatory labelling requirement for all food ingredients containing such nanomaterials were introduced in the Regulation on Food Information to consumers. For example, food additives that are prepared through nanotechnology would be considered as new additives. In Article 12 of 1333/2008/EC,

> when a food additive is already included in a Community list and there is a significant change in its production methods or in the starting materials used, or there is a change in particle size, for example through nanotechnology, the food additive prepared by those new methods or materials shall be considered as a different additive and a new entry in the Community lists or a change in the specifications shall be required before it can be placed on the market.

Guidance document: In November 2009, the EC asked EFSA to prepare a guidance document on how to assess potential risks related to certain food-related uses of nanotechnology. Given the knowledge that is currently available, the guidance to be developed will provide practical recommendations on how to assess applications from industry to use engineered nanomaterials in food additives, enzymes, flavourings, food contact materials, novel foods, food supplements, feed additives, and pesticides [9].

Efforts toward developing standards and regulations: The EC has given the Finnish Institute of Occupational Health (FIOH), and Finland as a country, the opportunity to coordinate the EU-funded NanoSafety Cluster, which is a cluster of projects promoting nanomaterial safety:

TABLE 16.6
Top Ten Products That are Most at Risk of Food Fraud

S. No.	Food Product	S. No.	Food Product
1.	Olive oil	6.	Honey and maple syrup
2.	Fish	7.	Coffee and tea
3.	Organic foods	8.	Spices (e.g., saffron and chili powder)
4.	Milk	9.	Wine
5.	Grains	10.	Certain fruit juices

- This project includes all NanoSafety-related areas, such as toxicology, ecotoxicology, exposure assessment, risk management and standardisation;
- The objective of the NanoSafety Cluster is to standardise and harmonise nanotoxicology research and research methods British Standards Institute (BSI);
- National committee NTI/1 on Nanotechnologies Safety of the NanoMaterials Interdisciplinary Research Centre (SnIRC);
- Develop internationally agreed in vivo and in vitro protocols and models for investigating the routes of exposure, bioaccumulation and toxicology of nanoparticles in humans and non-human organisms.

16.3.11 Food Fraud Network

Cooperation between officials with EU agri-food chain knowledge, police and customs officers with investigative powers, and judges and prosecutors' administrations is of the utmost importance either at the national level or at the EU level. The Food Fraud Network, comprises the Commission, the European Union Agency for Law Enforcement Cooperation (Europol), the liaison bodies designated by the Member States, and where relevant, the European Union's Judicial Cooperation Unit (Eurojust). Since 2013, EU Member States and some other European countries (Switzerland, Norway, and Iceland) exchange information and cooperate in matters where they are confronted with violations of the EU agri-food chain legislation of a cross-border nature. It helps the EU Member States and some other European countries to work in accordance with the rules laid down in the Official Controls Regulation [10]. The EU Food Fraud Network allows assisting and coordinating communication between competent authorities and transmitting and receiving requests for assistance. The liaisons bodies are required to exchange information necessary to enable the verification of compliance with EU agri-food chain legislation with their counterparts and, in certain cases, with the Commission, where the results of official controls require action in more than one country (Table 16.6).

16.3.12 Food Fraud: Scope and Definition

1. Deplores the fact that combating food fraud is a relatively new issue on the European agenda, and that in the past it has never been a key priority for legislation and enforcement at EU and national level;

2. Expresses its concern about the potential impact of food fraud on consumer confidence, food safety, the functioning of the food chain and the stability of agricultural prices, and emphasises the importance of quickly restoring European consumers' confidence;
3. Calls, therefore, on the Commission to give food fraud the full attention it warrants and to take all necessary steps to make the prevention and combating of food fraud an integral part of EU policy;
4. Underlines the need to gain further insight into the scale, incidence, and elements of cases of food fraud in the EU; calls on the Commission and the Member States to collect data systematically on fraud cases and to exchange best practices for identifying and combating food fraud;
5. Notes that EU law does not currently provide a definition of food fraud and that Member States adopt different methodologies in the definition thereof; considers a uniform definition to be essential for the development of a European approach to combating food fraud; stresses the need to adopt swiftly a harmonised definition at EU level, based on discussions with Member States, relevant stakeholders and experts, including elements such as non-compliance with food law and/or misleading the consumer (including the omission of product information), intent and potential financial gain and/or competitive advantage;
6. Emphasises the fact that, given the nature of the EU single market, food fraud extends in many cases beyond the borders of Member States and becomes a threat to the health of all European citizens;
7. Notes that recent food fraud cases have exposed different types of food fraud, such as the replacement of key ingredients with cheaper or lower quality alternatives, the incorrect labelling of the animal species used in meat or seafood products, the incorrect labelling of weight, the sale of ordinary foods as organic, the unfair use of quality logos designating origin or animal welfare, the labelling of aquaculture fish as fish caught in the wild or the marketing of an inferior variety of fish under the name of a superior category or a more expensive species, and the counterfeiting and marketing of food past its use-by date;
8. Points out that foods that are often subject to fraudulent activities include olive oil, fish, organic products, grains, honey, coffee, tea, spices, wine, certain fruit juices, milk, and meat;
9. Is concerned about signals indicating that the number of cases is rising and that food fraud is a growing trend reflecting a structural weakness within the food chain [10].

16.3.13 Motion for a European Parliament Resolution

The European Parliament,

- Having regard to the five-point action plan (reference) presented by the Commission in March 2013 after the discovery of a vast network of fraudsters passing off horsemeat as beef;

- Having regard to Regulation (EC) No 882/2004 of the European Parliament and of the Council of 29 April 2004 on official controls performed to ensure the verification of compliance with feed and food law, animal health and animal welfare rules;
- Having regard to Regulation (EC) No 178/2002 of the European Parliament and of the Council of 28 January 2002 laying down the general principles and requirements of food law, establishing the European Food Safety Authority and laying down procedures in matters of food safety;
- Having regard to Regulation (EC) No 1169/2011 of the European Parliament and of the Council of 25 October 2011 on the provision of food information to consumers, amending Regulations (EC) No 1924/2006 and (EC) No 1925/2006 of the European Parliament and of the Council, and repealing Commission Directive 87/250/EEC, Council Directive 90/496/EEC, Commission Directive 1999/10/EC, Directive 2000/13/EC of the European Parliament and of the Council, Commission Directives 2002/67/EC and 2008/5/EC, and Commission Regulation (EC) No 608/2004;
- Having regard to the proposal for a regulation on official controls and other official activities performed to ensure the application of food and feed law, rules on animal health and welfare, plant health, plant reproductive material [and] plant protection products (COM (2013)0265);
- Having regard to the report of the European Court of Auditors of 11 October 2012 on the management of conflicts of interest in four European Union agencies;
- Having regard to Rule 48 of its Rules of Procedure;
- Having regard to the report of the Committee on the Environment, Public Health and Food Safety and the opinions of the Committee on the Internal Market and Consumer Protection and the Committee on Agriculture and Rural Development (A7–0434/2013);
- Whereas the general principles of EU food law, in accordance with Regulation No 178/2002, prohibit the marketing of unsafe food along with fraudulent practices, the adulteration of food, and any other practices that may mislead the consumer;
- Whereas Regulation (EC) No 1924/2006 on nutrition and health claims made on foods and Regulation (EU) No 1169/2011 on the provision of food information to consumers lay down detailed provisions in relation to the ban on misleading advertising and labelling practices;
- Whereas the EU regulatory framework in place for food safety and the food chain has provided a high level of food safety for EU consumers until now; whereas the current legislation is, however, still fragile, and not always reliable, and therefore there is a need for improvements on the ground.

16.3.14 Food-Based Dietary Guidelines (FBDGs)

Food-based dietary guidelines (FBDGs) are important tools for nutrition policies and public health. FBDGs provide guidelines on healthy food consumption and are based on scientific evidence. In the past, disease prevention and nutrient recommendations dominated the process of establishing FBDGs. However, scientific advances and social developments such as changing lifestyles, interest in personalised health and concerns about sustainability require a reorientation of the creation of FBDGs to include a wider range of aspects of dietary behaviour.

FBDGs aim to guide toward recommended food consumption to provide required nutrients and to promote health. They are rooted in scientific evidence [11]. The target groups addressed by FBDGs range from the general public to policy makers. Thus, FBDGs should be easy to understand and easy to follow. It is furthermore crucial for FBDGs to incorporate regions or country-specific food consumption, dietary habits, and burden of diseases. Consequently, they are specific to the population in a region or country [12]. FBDGs reflect a type of "ideal" diet and serve as a basis for the development of nutritional policies that aim to achieve this ideal in members of the general public.

In 1992, the UN Food and Agriculture Organization and the WHO suggested the development of FBDGs and proposed that they should be available for each country of the world [13]. They provided the rationale and gave an overview of the steps that could be taken to develop FBDGs in subsequent publications [11], whereby the reorientation from nutrients to foods in formulating FBDGs was an essential feature. In 2008, the European Food Safety Authority (EFSA) issued a scientific opinion on how to establish FBDGs in Europe. EFSA focused on the process of developing FBDGs and proposed a stepwise approach in which the identification of diet-health relations is the central starting point. EFSA's opinion also considered former reports [11,14,15] which provided guidance for the development, implementation and evaluation of FBDGs. In line with previous reports, EFSA concluded that FBDGs should be established specifically for each country or region because of differences in dietary habits and disease burden.

16.3.15 European FBDGs and Their Derivation

Greece (1999): For establishing the Greek FBDGs, considerations on scientific evidence on diet and health ("key findings" are described without citing references or documented systematic evidence review), as well as nutrient and energy intake in accordance with the nutrient recommendations of the European Scientific Committee for Foods [16] were considered (Dietary guidelines for adults in Greece, 1999). The visual presentation of the FBDGs is an adjusted version of the Mediterranean diet pyramid [17].

Portugal (2003): The derivation of FBDGs in Portugal focused on achieving goals set for energy and nutrient intakes [18,19]. Different Dietary Reference Values (DRVs) for nutrient intake [20] were considered and energy requirements were computed by taking the median of 13 age groups of both sexes [21]. Common usage of food in Portugal was considered in establishing the food groups. The Portuguese Food Wheel reflects the dietary principles of the Mediterranean diet, but evidence on diet-health relations was not considered when deriving the FBDGs.

Slovenia (2007) and Albania (2008): The latest versions of Slovenia's written and graphical models of FBDGs were published in 2007 and 2015, respectively, and the Albanian FBDGs were published in 2008. Both countries adopted the WHO CINDI

(Countrywide Integrated Noncommunicable Diseases Intervention) dietary guide [22] with the WHO food pyramid as the basis of their national food guide. However, detailed information on their approach to establish their FBDGs is not available. The WHO CINDI dietary guide was published by a group of experts from the WHO Regional Office for Europe in 2000. Its aim was to strengthen the capacity of health professionals to help their clients prevent disease and to promote health. The guide includes a summary of the evidence supporting a relation between diet and health. The prevention of noncommunicable chronic diseases (NCDs), such as cardiovascular diseases, certain cancers, hypertension, obesity, and type 2 diabetes. It is stated that the adapted recommendations must cover the nutrient needs of the population and the energy requirements depending on sex, age, body size and physical activity level. Furthermore, it is emphasised that dietary guidelines must consider country-specific dietary patterns and NCD prevalence to make their implementation feasible and effective. The WHO has developed a user-friendly guide in 2012 for the Eastern Mediterranean region on promoting a healthy diet to reduce the risk of major NCDs [23], but it is not yet referred to by the respective countries.

Ireland (2012): The derivation of the FBDGs in Ireland focused on achieving goals set for energy and nutrient intakes [24,25]. Diet-health relations were considered indirectly via nutrient supply (arguments for nutrient goals), but systematic evaluations of the evidence were not performed or used. The food patterns were developed to reflect the typical eating habits of various age and sex groups in Ireland and their affordability was checked (budget pattern).

Germany (2013): In Germany, 2 graphical models were established to implement nutrition recommendations to support health while considering the specific national nutritional situation [26]. The Nutrition Circle implements the DRVs for nutrients at the food level. It is mentioned that the circle is in accordance with the results of evidence-based guidelines and literature reviews by the German Nutrition Society [12,13,27–30] and other professional societies. The Three-Dimensional Food Pyramid combines quantitative and qualitative statements, reflected by ranking of foods because of energy density and nutrient content and other nutritional-physiologic criteria and evidence regarding the prevention of NCDs, in a single model.

Denmark (2013), Finland (2014), Iceland (2014), Norway (2014), and Sweden (2015): The latest versions of the national FBDGs in Denmark, Finland, Iceland, Norway, and Sweden were published between 2013 and 2015. The common Nordic Nutrition Recommendations (NNR) 2012 were used as a basis and adapted according to national requirements. Nordic countries collaborate in setting dietary guidelines through the joint publication of the NNR. The NNR2012 used an evidence-based and transparent approach in assessing associations between nutrients and foods and certain health outcomes. Systematic reviews formed the basis for the recommendations of several nutrients and foods [31,32]. The NNR2012 contains DRVs for nutrients and emphasises the evidence for the role of food and food patterns contributing to the prevention of the major diet-related NCDs. In addition, the NNR2012 contain a chapter on sustainable diets, which explains the interrelations between food, health, and environmental protection [33,34]. It summarises the required changes in food consumption in Nordic countries needed to switch from the current diet to a healthier and more sustainable one. It also highlights the positive and negative effects of the proposed actions [35,36]. For Denmark, Finland, Iceland, and Norway, English-language information on their approach to derive the national FBDGs is not available. The Swedish guidelines [37] are based on the NNR2012 combined with knowledge on the population's dietary habits and on the environmental impact of various food groups. The environmental impacts of individual foods have been analyzed and incorporated into the derivation of the FBDGs. A technical report outlines the evidence that forms the basis for each of the recommendations [38].

Malta (2016): The current FBDGs were published in 2016, in accordance with the Food and Nutrition Policy and Action Plan for Malta (2015–2020) [44]. The process of creating FBDGs appears to have followed the EFSA recommendations and includes a review of the literature on diet-health relations with the use of existing systematic reports (e.g., those from the World Cancer Research Fund, the Centers for Disease Control and Prevention, and WHO). Key recommendations were derived on the information gained from the literature review, based on the principle that nutrient needs are met primarily through consumed foods. They considered local and "traditional" food and food products, as well as today's lifestyle and diet-related health problems. The FBDGs were calculated based on a caloric intake of ~2000 kcal/day, but it is noted that the total amount of food to be consumed depends on the individual's age, sex, height, weight and physical activity [39]. Environmental sustainability was not considered within the derivation of the FBDGs, but reference to the "Green Food Project" is made.

Netherlands (2016): The Dutch FBDGs were updated in 2015–2016. A committee of the Health Council of the Netherlands derived FBDGs described in an advisory report [37] based on a predefined methodology [35], with further background documents in Dutch. Experts systematically evaluated the literature and judged the evidence on nutrients, foods, and food patterns in relation to the risk of the ten most important NCDs in the Netherlands and three causal risk factors. The guidelines were derived based on conclusions that are supported by strong evidence and depending on the actual food consumption pattern [32]. The committee compared their established guidelines with previous findings on ecological aspects of dietary guidelines (Guidelines for a healthy diet: the ecological perspective, 2011) and concluded that complying with a few recommendations would not only result in health gains but also lower the ecological burden. The Netherlands Nutrition Center translated the updated guidelines into public information on healthy eating in 2016 by updating the Wheel of Five. It is mentioned that DRVs were also considered during this process [40], but detailed English information for this step is not available. The Netherlands Nutrition Center refers to a climate balance tool [41] and offers an interactive tool on their website to personalize the food guide by sex and age.

United Kingdom (2016): The Eatwell Guide is the most recent model of the UK FBDGs. Public Health England reviewed healthy eating messages in 2014 considering the conclusion of the Scientific Advisory Committee on Nutrition's Carbohydrate and Health report. Linear programming [14] was used to reshape the guide. This modelling process considered the current intake levels of the most consumed foods in the United Kingdom, applied the revised government dietary recommendations, and modelled the fewest possible changes required to achieve the proposed recommendations. Constraints to shape the Eatwell Guide were energy supply and DRVs for total carbohydrates, free sugars, dietary fiber, total fat, saturated fat, protein and salt. Additional constraints included frequencies or amounts of food items. Checks were made to ensure that requirements for micronutrients, especially in vulnerable age groups, were also met [15].

France (2016, opinion on revision): The French FBDGs are part of the National Nutrition and Health Program (PNNS; Guides nutritions du Programme National Nutrition Santé). The latest edition was published in 2011. In December 2016, an opinion on the revision of the PNNS guidelines was published by the French Agency for Food, Environmental, and Occupational Health and Safety [42]. The work provides the principles and evidence necessary for formulating the FBDGs.

It consists of the following:

- Updating the DRVs (DRVs from international organisations were compared);
- Studying the relations between food consumption and risk of NCDs, worked out in a specific report (French only), using previously conducted work by other organisations such as EFSA, the World Cancer Research Fund, and WHO as a starting point for the literature search;
- The attempt to limit exposure to contaminants [using contamination levels of food from the Total Diet Study (TDS) [11]. A computer tool was developed to identify combinations of foods able to simultaneously cover these three aspects while limiting deviations from the dietary habits observed in France [43].

REFERENCES

[1] Schwabe CW. *Veterinary medicine and human health*. 3rd ed. Baltimore: Williams & Wilkins; 1984.

[2] Xie T, Liu W, Anderson BD, Liu X, Gray GC. A system dynamics approach to understanding the One Health concept. *PLoS ONE*. 2017;12:e0184430.

[3] EFSA (European Food Safety Authority) and ECDC (European Centre for Disease Prevention and Control). The European Union summary report on trends and sources of zoonoses, zoonotic agents and food-borne outbreaks in 2015. *EFSA J*. 2016;14(12):4634, 231 pp.

[4] Mangen MJ, Bouwknegt M, Friesema IH, Haagsma JA, Kortbeek LM, Tariq L, et al. Cost-of-illness and disease burden of food-related pathogens in the Netherlands, 2011. *Int J Food Microbiol*. 2015;196:84–93.

[5] Toljander J, Dovarn A, Andersson Y, Ivarsson S, Lindqvist R. Public health burden due to infections by verocytotoxin-producing Escherichia coli (VTEC) and Campylobacter spp. as estimated by cost of illness and different approaches to model disability-adjusted life years. *Scand J Public Health*. 2012;40:294–302.

[6] Hald T, Vose D, Wegener HC, Koupeev T. A Bayesian approach to quantify the contribution of animal-food sources to human salmonellosis. *Risk Anal*. 2004;24:255–269.

[7] Jurgilevich A, Birge T, Kentala-Lehtonen J, Korhonen-Kurki K, Pietikainen J, Saikku L, Schosler H. Transition towards circular economy in the food system. *Sustainability*. 2016;8:69.

[8] Zinsstag J, Schelling E, Waltner-Toews D, Tanner M. From "one medicine" to "one health" and systemic approaches to health and well-being. *Prev Vet Med.* 2011;101:148–156.

[9] Stamm H, Gibson N, Anklam E. Detection of nanomaterials in food and consumer products: Bridging the gap from legislation to enforcement. *Food Addit Contam Part A.* 2012;29:1175–1182.

[10] Spink J, Moyer DC. Defining the public health threat of food fraud. *J Food Sci.* 2011;75(9):57–63.

[11] Albert J. Global patterns and country experiences with the formulation and implementation of food-based dietary guidelines. *Ann Nutr Metab.* 2007;51:2–7.

[12] Bechthold A. Food energy density and body weight: A scientific statement from the DGE. *Ernahr Umsch.* 2014;61:2–11.

[13] Boeing H, Bechthold A, Bub A, Ellinger S, Haller D, Kroke A, LeschikBonnet E, Müller MJ, Oberritter H, Schulze M, et al. Critical review: Vegetables and fruit in the prevention of chronic diseases. *Eur J Nutr.* 2012;51:637–663.

[14] Buttriss JL, Briend A, Darmon N, Ferguson EL, Maillot M, Lluch A. Diet modelling: How it can inform the development of dietary recommendations and public health policy. *Nutr Bull.* 2014;39:115–125.

[15] Buttriss JL. The Eatwell Guide refreshed. *Nutr Bull.* 2016;41:135–141.

[16] Scientific Committee on Food. *Nutrient and Energy Intakes for the European Community: Reports of the Scientific Committee for Food (Thirty-First Series).* Office for Official Publications of the European Communities, Luxembourg; 1993.

[17] Willett WC, Sacks F, Trichopoulou A, Drescher G, Ferro-Luzzi A, Helsing E, Trichopoulos D. Mediterranean diet pyramid: A cultural model for healthy eating. Am *J Clin Nutr.* 1995;61(1):1402S–1406S.

[18] Pinho I, Franchini B, Rodrigues S. *Guia Alimentar Mediterrânico: Relatório justificativo do seu desenvolvimento.* Academic Press. [Mediterranean diet food guide report]. [Internet] 2016 [cited 2018 Apr 9].

[19] Rodrigues SSP, Franchini B, Graca P, Almeida MDV. A new food guide for the Portuguese population: Development and technical considerations. *J Nutr Educ Behav.* 2006;38:189–195.

[20] WHO. Diet, nutrition, and the prevention of chronic diseases. *World Health Organ Tech Rep Ser.* 1990;797:1–102.

[21] Ferreira FAG. As tabelas portuguesas de necessidades nutrientes. In: Ferreira FAG (ed). *Nutricao Humana.* Lisbon, Portugal: Fundacao Calouste Gulbenkian; 1983, pp. 741–747.

[22] WHO. *CINDI dietary guide.* Copenhagen, Denmark: WHO Regional Office for Europe; 2000.

[23] WHO Regional Office for the Eastern Mediterranean. *Promoting a Healthy Diet for the WHO Eastern Mediterranean Region: Userfriendly Guide.* Academic Press. [Internet] 2012 [cited 2018 Apr 9].

[24] Flynn MAT, O'Brien CM, Faulkner G, Flynn CA, Gajownik M, Burke SJ. Revision of food-based dietary guidelines for Ireland, phase 1: Evaluation of Ireland's food guide. *Public Health Nutr.* 2012a;15:518–526.

[25] Flynn MAT, O'Brien CM, Ross V, Flynn CA, Burke SJ. Revision of food-based dietary guidelines for Ireland, phase 2: Recommendations for healthy eating and affordability. *Public Health Nutr.* 2012b;15:527–537.

[26] Oberritter H, Schäbethal K, Rüsten AV, Boeing H. The DGE nutrition circle—presentation and basis of the food-related recommendations from the German Nutrition Society (DGE). *Ernaehrungs Umschau Int.* 2013;60:24–29.

[27] Hauner H, Bechthold A, Boeing H, Brönstrup A, Buyken A, Leschik Bonnet E, Linseisen J, Schulze M, Strohm D, Wolfram G. Evidence based guideline of the German Nutrition

Society: Carbohydrate intake and prevention of nutrition-related diseases. *Ann Nutr Metab.* 2012;60(1):1–58.
[28] Wolfram G, Bechthold A, Boeing H, Ellinger S, Hauner H, Kroke A, Leschik-Bonnet E, Linseisen J, Lorkowski S, Schulze M, et al. Evidence-based guideline of the German Nutrition Society: Fat intake and prevention of selected nutrition-related diseases. *Ann Nutr Metab.* 2015;67:141–204.
[29] Dinter J, Bechthold A, Boeing H, Ellinger S, Leschik-Bonnet E, Linseisen J, Lorkowski S, Wolfram G. Fish intake and prevention of selected nutrition-related diseases. *Ernaehrungs Umschau Int.* 2016;63:148–154.
[30] Strohm D, Boeing H, Leschik-Bonnet E, Heseker H, Arens-Azevêdo U, Bechthold A, Knorpp L, Kroke A. Salt intake in Germany, health consequences, and resulting recommendations for action. *Ernaehrungs Umschau.* 2016;63:62–70.
[31] Akesson A, Andersen LF, Kristjánsdóttir AG, Roos E, Trolle E, Voutilainen E, Wirfält E. Health effects associated with foods characteristic of the Nordic diet: A systematic literature review. *Food Nutr Res.* 2013;57:227–290.
[32] Fogelholm M, Anderssen S, Gunnarsdottir I, Lahti-Koski M. Dietary macronutrients, and food consumption as determinants of long-term weight change in adult populations: A systematic literature review. *Food Nutr Res.* 2012;56:19103.
[33] Sonestedt E, Overby NC, Laaksonen DE, Birgisdottir BE. Does high sugar consumption exacerbate cardiometabolic risk factors and increase the risk of type 2 diabetes and cardiovascular disease? *Food Nutr Res.* 2012;56:19104.
[34] Domellöf M, Thorsdottir I, Thorstensen K. Health effects of different dietary iron intakes: A systematic literature review for the 5th Nordic Nutrition Recommendations. *Food Nutr Res.* 2013;57:21667.
[35] Forsum E, Brantsaeter AL, Olafsdottir A-S, Olsen SF, Thorsdottir I. Weight loss before conception: A systematic literature review. *Food Nutr Res.* 2013;57:20522.
[36] Hörnell A, Lagström H, Lande B, Thorsdottir I. Breastfeeding, introduction of other foods and effects on health: A systematic literature review for the 5th Nordic Nutrition Recommendations. *Food Nutr Res.* 2013;57:20823.
[37] Livsmedelsverket, National Food Agency. *Find Your Way to Eat Greener, Not Too Much and Be Active.* Springer. [Internet] 2015 [cited 2018 Apr 9].
[38] Konde AB, Bjerselius R, Haglund L, Jansson A, Pearson M, Färnstrand JS, Johansson A-K. *Find Your Way to Eat Greener, Not Too Much and Be Active. Swedish Dietary Guidelines—Risk and Benefit Management Report.* Academic Press. [Internet] 2015 [cited 2018 Apr 30].
[39] Pace L. *Dietary Guidelines for Maltese Adults: Information for Professionals Involved in Nutrition Education. Springer.* [Internet] 2016 [cited 2018 Apr 9].
[40] Kromhout D, Spaaij CJK, Goede J, Weggemans RM. The 2015 Dutch food-based dietary guidelines. *Eur J Clin Nutr.* 2016;70:869–878. Academic Press.
[41] Netherlands Nutrition Center. *The Climate Balance Tool* [Internet] [cited 2018 Apr 9].
[42] French Agency for Food, Environmental and Occupational Health and Safety (47). Springer. *Updating of the PNNA Guidelines: Revision of the Food-Based Dietary Guidelines: ANSES Opinion. Collective Expert Report* [Internet] 2016 [cited 2017 Jun 30].
[43] FAO/WHO. Preparation and use of food-based dietary guidelines: report of a joint FAO/WHO consultation. *World Health Organ Tech Rep Ser.* 1998;880:1–108.

17 Food Products Regulations in Canada

Faraat Ali, Hasan Ali, and Leo M.L. Nollet

17.1 INTRODUCTION

Food quality and safety is an important concern that has an impact on health and commerce across the globe. Low- and middle-income nations suffer more socially and economically as a result of incidents related to food safety (Hoffmann et al., 2019; Tirado-von der Pahlen, 2008; Walia & Sanders, 2019). According to Grace (2017), one of the most important aspects of food security is food safety. Therefore, it can be concluded that diseases caused by foodborne contaminants causing food safety issues are a negative consequence. As a result, it is crucial to ensure that food safety standards are followed by food supply chains across the globe (Nayak & Waterson, 2019). Legislators create regulations, which are then carried out by food safety enforcement and regulatory bodies, these bodies also carry out their effective implementation, enforcement, and communication functions. As a result, it plays a crucial role in the ethical manufacturing and consumption of foods (FAO & WHO, 2019; Wilson et al., 2015). Therefore, the primary goals of food safety regulatory agencies are to enhance ensure the safety of food, support public health, and promote international and domestic trade.

In Canada, industry, local, territorial, and provincial governments, the government of Canada, and consumers all share responsibilities for ensuring the safety of food, similar to many other national food regulatory bodies. The federal government of Canada is responsible for overseeing the food system, however, local, territorial, and provincial governments work together with the federal government to implement policies governing food consumption and manufacturing and within their respective areas of responsibility (Government of Canada, 2009). Additionally, the business sector contributes significantly by recognizing and dealing with risks, working in according to the regulatory policies in place (Bietlot & Kolakowski, 2012). The two federal agencies with the greatest involvement in food risk evaluation and regulation are Health Canada (HC) and the Canadian Food Inspection Agency (CFIA). The group's goals are to assist Canadians to maintain and enhance their health by making sure excellent services and resources are offered also by disseminating pertinent information on diet, health, and risk. These organizations comprise the HC, CFIA, PMRA, and PHAC, in the context of Canada's food system (Cheung-Gertler, 2008; Health Canada, 2011; Ding et al., 2013; Wilson et al., 2017; Verbeke, 2005; James & Marks, 2008).

DOI: 10.1201/9781003296492-19

This chapter fundamentally focuses on the involvement of various national agencies involved in food safety regulation; various laws, acts, and regulations implicated in control and enforcement of rules and regulations in Canadian jurisdiction; and other topics related to food control.

17.2 AGENCIES INVOLVED IN CONTROL AND REGULATION OF FOODS IN CANADA

17.2.1 Health Canada

Many nations have established their own food and drug regulatory agencies and laws, which are in charge of enforcing the laws and issuing directives to control and regulate the development, process, registration, licensing, manufacturing, labeling, and marketing of foods and drugs. For instance, the FDA, MHRA, and TGA are the respective agencies for the United States, the United Kingdom, and Australia (Evans & Day, 2005; Ghosh, 2006). Canada has its own well-established regulatory agency, Health Canada, which is responsible for law enforcement, implementation, and regulation of the food sector and, as a representation of the Canadian government, for the control and regulation of foods and related products.

Health Canada regularly promotes its role in ensuring that the Canadian populace has access to high quality, safe food. Health Canada works to maintain a balance between the risks posed by the food products and the projected health benefits. For the interest of public safety, Health Canada therefore places a high importance on regulating and maintaining the balance between the risk-benefit ratios of food products. To reduce the public's exposure to health-related risk factors while maintaining the enhanced safety nutritional requirements set forth by the regulatory system for these products, Health Canada engages in daily activities related to food regulation that involved manufacturers, industrialists, researchers, and consumers. Additionally, Health Canada works to equip its citizens with the information they need to make better choices and decisions about their well-being. Health Canada is not a manufacturer or distributor of foods and health products (Hajizadeh & Keays, 2023). (For details, see Chapter 6 of this book.)

17.2.2 Food Directorate

The Food Directorate (FD) is the federal agency in charge of overseeing food safety and nutritional value. It also sets norms, standards, laws, and regulations and offers guidance and data on these topics. Territorial, provincial, and federal governments work in concord with the CFIA and PHAC and share accountability for food safety and nutrition to guarantee that the food supply in Canada is healthy and safe. The Food Directorate collaborates extensively with these organizations including industry and health stakeholders. The FD is dedicated to ensuring that Canadian population has access to a reliable supply of healthy food. Additionally, it provides knowledge to assist the Canadian population in choosing safer and better foods to maintain their health and prevent acute and chronic foodborne diseases (Health Canada, 2011). To achieve this goal, FD is authorized to:

- Establish and uphold food standards, norms, guidelines, rules, and regulations that are supported by evidence;
- Perform pre-market safety evaluations of specific food components, food preparation and processing methods, and finished food products;
- Do health risk analyses related to food safety to aid in the oversight of food safety issues;
- Carry out monitoring and surveillance, management, and scientific research to aid in risk assessment and standardization;
- Interact with partners, stakeholders, and the common population.

The FD participates in a global network for nutrition and food safety that organizes standards, broadens knowledge of the threats related to nutrition and food safety of the nutritional qualities of foods, and disseminates early alerts of possible food safety issues. Six bureaus make up the directorate, which is strategically led and steered by the office of the Director General and the Directorate Management Committee (Health Canada, 2011). Three scientific bureaus enforce the core program of FD, related to evaluation of food risk, setting norms, and research and market approval:

- Bureau of Chemical Safety
- Bureau of Nutritional Sciences
- Bureau of Microbial Hazards.

These three bureaus are accountable for integration of operation, science, and policy:

- Bureau of Policy Intergovernmental and International Affairs
- Bureau of Food Surveillance and Science Integration
- Bureau of Business Systems and Operations.

The Bureau of Chemical Safety attempts to make sure that there are no chemicals in food at concentrations that might have a negative impact on the health of the population of Canada. It is in charge of developing regulations, conducting risk analyses, establishing standards, conducting research, and assessing the presence of chemicals in the food of Canadians. The Bureau is divided into four divisions: Food Research, Regulatory Toxicology Research, Scientific Services, and Chemical Health Hazard Assessment. The Bureau of Nutritional Sciences seeks to safeguard Canadians against health risks brought on by inadequate or excessive nutrient intake. This bureau is divided into three sections: Nutrition, Nutrition Research, Nutrition Regulations and Standards, and Pre-market Analysis (Health Canada, 2011).

The Bureau of Microbial Hazards strives to reduce the hazards related to the public's health associated with eating food that has been infected with bacteria, parasite, viruses, prions, or other disease-causing factors. Microbiology Research and Microbiology Evaluation are the two important divisions that make up the Bureau. The Bureau of Policy Intergovernmental and International Affairs provides oversight and guidance on policy at the national and international levels, as well as legislative and regulatory activities for nutrition and food safety. The Bureau maintains close relationships with its various stakeholders, and other bureaus of FD (Health Canada, 2011). Through a bilateral interactions with stakeholders such as the CFIA and PHAC, as well as federal partners like Agriculture and Agri-Food Canada, Global Affairs Canada, and Industry, Science and Economic Development Canada, the Bureau maintains inter-agency interaction and federal position. The Food Surveillance and Science Bureau integrates with other bureaus to cater information, analysis, and advice of experts associated with bioinformatics and biostatistics. The Bureau also offers nutrition and food surveillance service in support of the FD's risk assessments, establishing norms, and market approval (Health Canada, 2011).

With the assistance of three areas of expertise (Biostatistics and Risk Modelling, Bioinformatics High-Capacity Computing, and Food and Nutrition Surveillance), the Bureau collaborates with other related organizations, like federal departments (such as Statistics Canada), international organizations (such as the WHO Collaborating Centre on Food Safety, the International Organization for Standardization for Whole-Genome Sequencing), academia, and territorial and provincial government departments. The Bureau additionally supervises the Submission Management and Information Unit, which acts as a common contact point for pre-market submissions obtained from individual stakeholders and offers administrative assistance and coordination to program the Bureaus (Health Canada, 2011).

17.2.3 Canadian Food Inspection Agency

The Canadian Food Inspection Agency is committed to preserving food, plants, and livestock for the benefit of Canadians' well-being and health, economy, and environment. The President of the CFIA is in charge and accountable to the Minister of Health. In accordance with the CFIA's comprehensive governance framework, every division head is held accountable for a particular assignment that advances one of the agency's objectives. The CFIA has a comprehensive responsibility that covers food safety, animal health, plant health, and access to overseas markets as a science-based regulator. The CFIA's first objective is to reduce the risks to the safety of food, and designing and developing CFIA programs is motivated by the health and safety of Canadians. The CFIA, works in coordination with stakeholders including industry, local, provincial, and federal organizations, and end consumers to make efforts in the direction to protect Canadian population from avoidable health-related hazards associated with health issues derived from foodborne and zoonotic diseases (Health Canada, 2011).

A wholesome and sustainable base of animal and plant resources is necessary for the economic development of Canada's agriculture and forestry industries. As a result, to reduce and manage risks, the CFIA is constantly enhancing the planning and execution of its programs in the areas of plant resources and animal health. The CFIA also does a lot of work to safeguard environmental biodiversity in an effort to safeguard the natural environment from invading animal and plant diseases and plant pests. The objective of the CFIA is to protect food, animals, and plants, which improves the health and well-being of Canadians, the environment, and the country's economy. The CFIA's vision is to thrive as a scientific regulatory body, regarded with confidence and by the population of Canada and the worldwide community (Health

Canada, 2011). Future prosperity depends on CFIA capacity to respond to threats and quick environmental changes. In CFIA, innovative methods of operation are investigated to deliver better, more effective services and programs in the future, eventually ensuring the safety of food, plant, and animal resources for the Canadian population. By expanding information technology infrastructure and giving staff members the resources and equipment they need to transition to a digital way of working, it keeps highlighting digitization efforts. The four upgraded sectors are centered on a state of the future that, at its foundation, represents the agency's reliable alliances and standing as a world leader in protecting Canadians and advancing industry (Health Canada, 2011).

To create a unified and uniform inspection strategy, the CFIA held extensive consultations with front-line inspectors, consumer associations, industry stakeholders, and government stakeholders. The original idea was to first consult on food before developing a model that could be used for all inspection tasks, whether they dealt with the environment or animal, plant, or human health. In response to the Accessible Canada Act, the agency created the CFIA Accessibility Strategy and Plan. The accessibility vision of the CFIA is to create, promote, and preserve a readily available respectful, diverse, and equitable workplace and environment that honors and empowers those with disabilities (Health Canada, 2011).

17.2.4 Public Health Agency of Canada

The federal health ministry includes the PHAC. Its efforts are centered on preventing and controlling diseases, addressing threats to public health, promoting physical and mental well-being, and disseminating knowledge to assist in making informed decisions (Health Canada, 2011). The severe SARS outbreak in Canada led to a number of official queries that led to the creation of the PHAC. Both the Ontario government probe and the National Advisory Committee on SARS and Public Health suggested the establishment of a new organization. It was established in this way by an Order in Council issued by the State Minister for Public Health in Canada in 2004 and later by law that took effect on December 15, 2006. Fundamentally, PHAC is a constituent of the Ministry of Health of the Canadian federal government (Justice Laws Website, 2023).

The president of PHAC is a five-year appointment made by the Governor in Council. Although the Chief Public Health Officer (CPHO), who is required by law to be a scientist, and the President of the PHAC were initially one and the same, the federal government developed to oversee the organization using more flexible civil service, and a split personality with the twin agencies of President and CPHO developed. The top medical authority in Canada is the CPHO. Another role of the CPHO is Governor in Council, whose responsibility is to advise both the Minister of Health and the President of the PHAC. The PHAC Act gives the CPHO the authority to share information on public health issues with other bodies of government, nonprofit groups, the corporate sector, and Canadian population. The Minister of Health is obligated to receive an annual report from the CPHO about the condition of the health system in Canada (Justice Laws Website, 2023). The PHAC include various administrators, namely the Chief Public Health Officer, Senior Assistant

Deputy Minister (Population and Public Health Integration Branch), Assistant Deputy Minister (Infectious Disease and Emergency Preparedness), Deputy CPHO (Health Protection and Chronic Disease Prevention Branch), Chief Science Officer, Executive Director (Corporate Secretariat), Vice-President (Health Security Infrastructure Branch), Vice-President (Strategic Policy and Planning Branch), and Vice-President (Health Promotion and Chronic Disease Prevention Branch) (Justice Laws Website, 2023; Health Canada, 2011).

Because the PHAC's portfolio spans many boundaries, particularly those of jurisdiction, the civil servants have created Special Advisory Committees that consist of territorial, provincial, and federal officials like deputy ministers of health in an effort to guarantee prompt attention and quick response to Canadian population requirements (Health Canada, 2011).

17.2.5 Pest Management Regulatory Agency

In Canada, pesticides are regulated by the PMRA of Health Canada. This division of Health Canada was established in 1995 to combine the duties and resources for regulation for the control of pests. In Canada, pesticides are strictly regulated to ensure that there is no damage to human health or the environment. Health Canada, which is mandated by the Pest Control Products Act, registers and tracks pesticides after a rigorous, scientific assessment that guarantees the hazards are acceptable; it also conducts a 15-year cycle of re-evaluations of pesticides already on the market to make sure that the products continue to meet scientific norms, and it encourages a viable control of pests (Health Canada, 2011). Additionally, Health Canada encourages, confirms, and enforces adherence to the Act, taking appropriate enforcement measures as necessary. Their efforts and programs aim to enhance the regulatory framework and cater Canadian population pest control chemicals and approaches with acceptable risk and value. Health Canada is dedicated to offer an open, clear and participatory course for pesticide control and regulation (Health Canada, 2011).

In Canada, Health Canada collaborates with territory, provincial, and federal agencies to improve and bolster nationwide control and regulation of pesticide. These collaborations guarantee that the various demands of the Canadian population are met at all the tiers of government and that Health Canada's policies fulfil the needs of Canadians. Beyond the borders of Canada, HC collaborates closely with a variety of intergovernmental institutions, such as the Organization for Economic Co-operation and Development and the US Environmental Protection Agency. These intimate links aid in the creation of laws, rules, and regulations (Health Canada, 2011).

Regular publications detailing the pertinent information, such as suggested registration decisions, requests for remarks on suggested decisions or rules and policies, or decisions of pesticide registration, are issued to make sure that stakeholders have knowledge of Health Canada's recommendations and actions regarding pesticides and pesticide control and regulations. The Public Registry serves as a database of non-confidential data regarding registered and intended pesticides, data on pest management, and appropriate application of pesticides (Health Canada, 2011). The Registrants and Applicants section also contains the resources and data required for pesticide producers and applicants, including new applications of pesticide, updates, and reports of incidents. The comments obtained after these meetings consultations are being evaluated by Pest Management Regulatory Agency (PMRA) of HC, which will help to shape the change process and increase its surveillance and protection environment and human health. The PMRA will become more transparent to Canadians as a result of the reform process (Health Canada, 2011).

17.3 LEGISLATION

17.3.1 Food and Drugs Act

All foods, drugs, cosmetics, and medical devices sold and marketed in Canada must comply with quality, safety, and efficacy criteria set by HC. The mandate of the Food and Drugs Act and the Food and Drug Regulations guide the HC in carrying out this task (Health Canada, 2011). The Food and Drug Act is a piece of legislation passed by the Canadian Parliament that regulates the production, export, import, interprovincial transportation, sale, and marketing of food, pharmaceuticals, medical devices, contraceptives, and cosmetics. (See Chapter 6.)

17.3.2 Safe Food for Canadians Act

This is a law concerning food products, including standards for them, registration or authorization of individuals who execute specific related tasks, requirements governing establishments where those operations are carried out, authorization of facilities where those tasks are carried out, and inspections, safety, labeling, and advertising, import, export, and inter-provincial commerce. In an effort to modernize the nation's food safety system, the Canadian government has adopted a new food safety Act. The SFC Act was passed by the federal legislature with the advice and agreement of the Senate and House of Commons of Canada. The Safe Food for Canadians Act went into effect on November 26, 2012. It covers all matters related to food safety. In the past, many Acts such as the Meat Inspection Act, the Consumer Packaging and Labeling Act, the Canada Agricultural Products Act, and the Fish Inspection Act regulated the hygiene and safety of foods in the Canada. (Centre for Science and Environment, 2023; Health Canada, 2011).

The Food Safety and Modernization Act of the United States, which went into effect in January 2011, is reported to have served as an inspiration for the Safe Food for Canadians Act. The Act's main goal is to modernize the entire food safety system to meet the interests of all stakeholders. To ensure industrial compliance, it promises a more advanced and well-equipped inspection system (Health Canada, 2011; Centre for Science and Environment, 2023). The updated legislation will be efficient to handle fraud, dishonest business activities, and tampering with food products. To prevent such acts and protect customers from associated risks, punishments and fines were additionally enhanced. Improved transparency, tracking, and import rules are also promised by the new legislation to further enhance the consumer protection. A food product's manufacturing and distribution history must be recorded to trace it. A product may be tracked downstream to its origin or forward through distribution channels in the event of an epidemic or proof of food contamination, which enables government authorities to take action more rapidly in the event of foodborne disease outbreaks (Centre for Science and Environment, 2023).

The SFC Act will enhance the overall food safety for Canadian populations by

- Safeguarding the Canadian populations from hazards associated with tampered food and frauds. Under the recent legislation, regulators can deal with possible threats to the safety of food more quickly and effectively;
- Outlawing the sale of recalled products and granting the federal government the authority to mandate that the food industry install tracking mechanisms to assist in the swift removal of recalled goods from the market;
- Tightening regulations on food imports into Canada by mandating licenses for importers and banning the entry of hazardous items when risks are identified;
- Setting the rules for the inspection and enforcement processes for every type of food products, including agricultural goods, fish, and meat. By having a single norm, the Canadian population will be safeguarded by the same stringent guidelines (Centre for Science and Environment, 2023; Justice Laws Website, 2023).

17.3.3 Public Health Agency of Canada Act

The Act in question amends numerous laws and relates to the creation of the PHAC. With the help of this Act, the Canadian government has taken steps to improve public health, particularly policies for population health evaluation, disease prevention, health monitoring, and disaster planning and response. Additionally, the Canadian government wants to promote cooperation in the public health sector and to coordinate federal health policy and activities. This law encourages collaboration and consultation with territorial and provincial government authorities, as well as with other stakeholders, intergovernmental agencies, and overseas governments regarding the subject of public health. The Canadian government also believes that the establishment of a public health agency for the country and the selection of a CPHO supports national preparedness for risks to public health and help to recognize and mitigate public health risk factors (Justice Laws Website, 2023). The PHAC was created to support the government of Canada in carrying out its public health-related responsibilities, authorities, and duties. The Minister serves as the president and can depute an officer or employee of the Agency any of the responsibilities, and duties, that the Minister is permitted to carry out or execute under any Act of Parliament or any order, according to any restrictions and conditions that the Minister stipulates, made by the Governor in Council in respect of public health. As per the subsection (1) the Minister is not permitted to assign the authority to create the rules and regulations or to assign a power. A Governor in Council shall by order designate the President of the Agency to a period of up to 5 years, and may be reappointed for another term. The President serves as the Agency's top administrator and has the position of a department's deputy head. According to paragraph 4(2)(h) of the Department of Health Act, the Governor in Council may issue guidelines regarding (a) the gathering, evaluation, interpretation, publication, as well as and distribution of public health information; and (b) the safeguarding of the data if it is secret and confidential, such as private data according to the definition in section 3 of the Privacy Act. Anyone who intentionally owns, uses, or reveals data in violation of a rule imposed under subsection (1) is culpable of an offense and subject to a fine, or a term of prison of up to 6 months, or both, upon summary conviction (Justice Laws Website, 2023).

17.3.4 Canadian Dairy Commission Act

The Canadian Dairy Commission is still in operation as an organization with a Chief Executive Officer, Chairperson. Despite the section 105 of the Financial Administration Act, every member of the Dairy Commission is nominated by the Governor in Council to serve at discretion for such term as the Governor in Council deems suitable. The Health Minister must nominate a chairperson along with eight more members to the Consultative Committee. Every member of the advisory committee must be nominated for a period of not more than 3 years, besides the fact that the first three members appointed will serve for a period of 2 years, three will be appointed for a period of 3 years, and another three members for a duration of 4 years (Justice Laws Website, 2023). The Consultative Committee must convene at such a times as the Commission specifies and will guide the Dairy Commission on any topics pertaining to the manufacturing and sale of milk and dairy products that the Commission refers to it. A rule adopted within the subsection (1) may be broad or specific to a particular dairy product, geographic region, or group or group of people. The Governor in Council can create regulations that require the registration of milk and cream manufacturers as a prerequisite of making any payments under paragraph 9(1)(c) for the sake of those manufactures, as well as prescribing the books and records to be maintained and the data to be provided to the Commission by or on the behalf of those manufacturers. Any individual who fails to comply or violates with any of the provisions of this Act or any rule created under this Act is culpable of a violation and liable (a) on conviction to a fine or to detention for a period not more than 6 months, or to both; or (b) on charges conviction to a fine or to detention for a period not more than 1 year, or to both (Justice Laws Website, 2023).

17.4 DATABASES

17.4.1 Nutrient Data

Two databases published by HC lists the nutritional values of foods available for the Canadian. The Canadian Nutrient File (CNF) is a thorough, computerized multilingual collection of data that provides information about 150 nutrients found in more than 5500 foods. The information in the database, which is updated on a regular basis, may help the Canadians to identify values for substances such as vitamins, minerals, protein, energy, fat, and many more. The CNF provides an accessible web application that enables Canadians to look up the nutritional values of certain foods. The department also publishes the Nutrient Value of Some Common Foods (NVSCF) handbook on a regular basis to give a convenient overview of the most frequently consumed foods in the Canadian market (Health Canada, 2011).

17.4.2 The Canadian Nutrient File

The CNF is an accepted and reference food ingredient database that reports the nutritional content of regularly eaten products by the Canadian population. This database is used as a dietary research tool in a variety of operations at HC, including the development of standards, guidelines, and rules, risk evaluation, and consumption of food studies. Agriculture and Agri-Food Canada (AAFC), Statistics Canada, and the CFIA are among other federal government clients. Furthermore, the CNF is used by a wide range of other users, such as healthcare facilities, educational institutions, food producers, and the general population (Health Canada, 2011). A culmination of growing evidence relating nutrition habits to health and disease, as well as a surge in personal computing technology, has led to a large number of people and groups who are concerned and also using Canadian nutrient data (Health Canada, 2011).

17.4.3 Nutrient Value of Some Common Foods

The NVSCF handbook, published by HC, offers Canadians with a reference that lists nutrients for the most widely consumed foods in Canada. The pamphlet has been in print for many years, with various changes, and it is an invaluable resource for nutritionists and other medical professionals working to assist Canadians better their health. It is crucial to emphasize, however, that although this pamphlet provides nutritional content statistics, it is not meant to counsel Canadians on what constitutes a healthy diet. Canadians should consult the Canada Food Guide for guidance on a healthy eating pattern (Health Canada, 2011).

17.4.4 Nutrition Surveillance Data Tool

The Nutrition Surveillance Data Tool was created by Health Canada's Bureau of Food Surveillance and Science Integration. This data typically portrays calorie, vitamin, and other nutritional element intake based on data from the 2015 Canadian Community Health Survey—Nutrition. It shows where Canadians' intakes lie in relation to Dietary Reference Intakes defined by the National Academies of Science, Engineering, and Institute of Medicine. The purpose is to provide crucial statistics in a dynamic and simple to operate format to supplement the complete typical intake information released in the Government of Canada's Open statistics web page. This tool allows to look at the CCHS—Nutrition normal intake data in three ways: distribution curves, geographic comparison, and data table (Health Canada, 2011).

17.5 SPECIAL FOOD CATEGORIES

17.5.1 Novel Foods Derived from Plants and Microorganisms

Health Canada controls and create the norms, regulations, and guidelines that govern the nutritional quality and safety of foods marketed in Canada. HC regulates the marketing and distribution of novel food products in Canada through a mandated pre-market disclosure procedure outlined in Division 28 of the FDR, called as the Novel Foods Regulation. These instructions help the person filing the petition to prepare a novel food notice and clarify what information is regarded adequate for a safety evaluation. The FD of HC conducts novel food safety evaluations. All novel foods generated from plant or microbial origins, whether whole foods, food items, or food additives, fall under this category. Animal-derived novel food safety standards are being developed. Producers and importers of innovative foods made from animal products should engage with the FD to determine what data is necessary to assess a product safety (Health Canada, 2011).

17.5.2 Supplemented Foods

Supplemented food is a pre-packaged food that have extra minerals, vitamins, amino acids, and/or additional additives like caffeine. These types of foods must fulfill specific criteria to be sold in Canada. Supplemented foods regulations, as well as documents adopted by reference under the FDR, specify the criteria for fortified and supplemented food, covering food ingredients and labeling requirements. The supplemented foods regulations guidance documents are to be obtained upon request to help food makers and dealers in interpreting the supplemented foods regulations (Health Canada, 2011). The guidance document presents information on how to conform with the regulations and discusses:

- Supplemented food is that has a period of transition for meeting the regulation;
- Food that is not allowed to be supplemented;
- Details of food classes that are allowed to be supplemented;
- Knowing the needs linked with employing supplemental composition;
- Labeling description and requirements for supplemented foods, encompassing how to display the compositions on the label;
- Alternative routes to market for items that do not match the standards for approved food categories or additional components;
- Knowing if the product qualifies for supplemented foods regulations;
- How HC created the standards for supplementary ingredients (Health Canada, 2011).

To assist food producers and dealers in interpreting the supplemented foods regulations, HC has created a thorough guide sheet. It presents HC understanding of key standards for supplemented foods. Producers must adhere to strict guidelines to ensure that supplemented foods are safe for consumption. To remain informed of possible dangers, carefully read any warning advice on the package label (Health Canada, 2011). Supplemented foods include additional components that might be harmful to the Canadians health if they (1) consume them in excess or (2) are pregnant, have one or more children, or belong to another group of vulnerable people.

Accountability of food safety, especially supplemented foods, is shared by all territorial, provincial, and federal government—that is, all three levels of government in Canada. HC advises stakeholders to share report any concerns they have concerning a supplemented food (Health Canada, 2011).

17.6 SURVEILLANCE

Food and nutrition policies and programs that boost the population's health and diet need a robust research foundation and the ability to monitor results. To meet these needs, a long-term security food and nutrition monitoring system is critical. The purpose of this framework is to assess and evaluate food and nutrient consumption, food security, nutritional status, nutrition-related health effects, and understanding, beliefs, and behaviors about healthy food and other lifestyle aspects including physical exercise and a healthy environment. This data needs to be connected to information regarding demographics, health indicators, and variables influencing availability of safe, cheap nutritional meals. A food and nutrition monitoring system is a vital tool for detecting nutritional and nutrition-related health issues and to pursue the policy execution for both developmental and emergency programmes (Food and Nutrition Surveillance Systems, World Health Organization [WHO], 2013). A food and nutrition surveillance system is described as the collecting, evaluating, and dissemination of information on nutrition risk factors, nutritional status, and nutrition-related ailments in the Canadian population on a regular and punctual basis. The task is carried out to give information that may be used to encourage, improve, and guide judgments about the necessity of nutritional treatments, as well as the prevalence and distribution of nutrition issues in the community. The goals of nutrition monitoring are (1) to provide an overview of the nutritional status of the general population, with a focus on at-risk subgroups; (2) to explain connections between variables to select preventive actions; (3) to encourage government decisions that will comply with the requirements of both usual national growth and emergency situations; (4) to assemble the key indicators that are associated with food and nutrition and health objectives; (5) to forecast changes in nutritional issues depending on the evaluation of existing trends; and (6) to examine nutrition programs and assess their efficiency (Health Canada, 2011). A balanced diet; the safe availability of nourishing food; and nutritional well-being are all important contributions to a productive and healthy population according to HC. Improving health necessitates monitoring food and nutrient consumption, food safety, nutrient status, and nutrition-related health consequences. It is also critical to track the variables that impact food and nutrient consumption, like social and economic problems, as well as human aspects such as understanding, views, and habits. Food and nutrition surveillance entails collecting information, integration, evaluation, interpretation, and distribution (Health Canada, 2011). It is based on a variety of activities and a wide range of information sources. The Bureau of Food Surveillance and Science Integration in the FD and the Office of Nutrition Policy and Promotion at HC collaborate with territorial and provincial governments and the federal government on a variety of food and nutrition surveillance activities, including:

- Data collection on what the Canadian population eats;
- Determining contamination levels in certain foods;
- Creating methodology, data gathering tools, and guidelines;
- Giving advice on how to evaluate surveillance data;
- Data analysis and interpretation to inform policies and programs (Health Canada, 2011).

17.7 CONCLUSION

Food regulation in Canada comprises the Food and Drugs Act, the Safe Food for Canadians Act, the PHAC Act, and the Canadian Dairy Commission Act, based on the type of food. The Food and Drugs Act is Canada's principal food legislation. The FDA defines regulations concerning food labeling and advertising; food quality and composition criteria, supplementation of foods for particular dietary purposes, food additives, chemical and microbiological hazards, residues of veterinary drugs, pesticides, packaging material, and so on. The Act guarantees that Canadians may make reasonable food choices using reliable data that is not deceptive. As a result, the Act focuses on fair food labeling and forces business to follow laws governing food labeling, advertising, and claims. Moreover, HC, CFIA, PHAC, FD, and PMRA are three important federal government agencies that have supplementary responsibilities in the creation, enforcement, evaluation, and explication of policies and advice based on the Food and Drug Act and its Regulations. Nutritional and health claims must be adequately tested and designed to deliver useful information to the consumer.

REFERENCES

Bietlot, H.P., Kolakowski, B. Risk assessment and risk management at the Canadian Food Inspection Agency (CFIA): A perspective on the monitoring of foods for chemical residues. *Drug Testing and Analysis*, 4 (S1) (2012), pp. 50–58, http://doi.org/10.1002/dta.1352.

Canadian Food Inspection Agency. *About the Canadian Food Inspection Agency* (2015). Academic Press. www.inspection.gc.ca/about-the-cfia/eng/1299008020759/1299008-778654

Centre for Science and Environment (CSE) (2023). www.cseindia.org/canada-adopts-new-food-safety-law-4748

Cheung-Gertler, J.H. *Health Canada* (2008). www.thecanadianencyclopedia.ca/en/article/health-canada

Ding, Y., Veeman, M.M., Adamowicz, W.L. The influence of trust on consumer behavior: An application to recurring food risks in Canada. *Journal of Economic Behavior and Organization*, 92 (2013), pp. 214–223.

FAO & WHO. *Food Control System Assessment Tool: Introduction and Glossary*. Rome (2019).

Ghosh, D., Skinner, M., Ferguson, L.R. The role of the therapeutic goods administration and the medicine and medical devices safety authority in evaluating complementary and alternative medicines in Australia and New Zealand. *Toxicology*, 221 (1) (2006), pp. 88–94.

Government of Canada. *Report of the Independent Investigator into the 2008*. Listeriosis Outbreak (2009).

Grace, D. *Food Safety and the Sustainable Development Goals*. Nairobi, Kenya (2017).

Hajizadeh, M., Keays, D. Ten years after the 2015 Canada Health Transfer reform: A persistent equity concern of insufficient risk-equalization. *Health Policy*, 129 (2023), p. 104711.

Health Canada. *About Mission, Values, Activities* (2011). www.canada.ca/en/health-canada/corporate/about-health-canada/activities-responsibilities/mission-values-activities.html

Hoffmann, V., Moser, C., Saak, A. Food safety in low and middle-income countries: The evidence through an economic lens. *World Development*, 123 (2019), article 104611, http://doi.org/10.1016/j.worlddev.2019.104611.

James, H.S., Marks, L.A. Trust and distrust in biotechnology risk managers: Insights from the United Kingdom, 1996–2002. *AgBioforum*, 11 (2) (2008), pp. 93–105.

Justice Laws Website, Government of Canada (2023). https://laws-lois.justice.gc.ca/eng/

Tirado-von der Pahlen, M. Global food safety and environmental health. *ISEE 20th Annual Conference*, Vol. 19, Epidemiology, Pasadena (2008), pp. S14–S15.

Verbeke, W. Agriculture and the food industry in the information age. *European Review of Agricultural Economics*, 32 (2) (2005), pp. 347–368, http://doi.org/10.1093/eurrag/jbi017

Walia, B., Sanders, S. Curbing food waste: A review of recent policy and action in the USA. *Renewable Agriculture and Food Systems*, 34 (2) (2019), pp. 169–177.

Wilson, A.M., Meyer, S., Webb, T., Henderson, J., Coveney, J., McCullum, D., et al. How food regulators communicate with consumers about food safety. *British Food Journal*, 117 (8) (2015), pp. 2129–2142.

Wilson, A.M., Withall, E., Coveney, J., Meyer, S.B., Henderson, J., McCullum, D., Ward, P.R. A model for (re)building consumer trust in the food system. *Health Promotion International*, 32 (6) (2017), pp. 988–1000, http://doi.org/10.1093/heapro/daw024

18 Food Products Regulations in the United Kingdom

Leo M.L. Nollet

18.1 FOOD LAW ENFORCEMENT AGENCIES

In the United Kingdom, day-to-day responsibility for enforcing food controls is divided between the central and local government.

The central food law enforcement authorities in the United Kingdom are:

- The Food Standards Agency (FSA) in England, Wales and Northern Ireland [1];
- Food Standards Scotland;
- The Department for Environment, Food and Rural Affairs (Defra) and its agencies [28];
- Devolved agriculture and rural affairs departments, including the Department of Agriculture, Environment and Rural Affairs (DAERA) in Northern Ireland [11].

Most food law is enforced by local councils throughout the United Kingdom. The FSA supervises local council enforcement and works with local enforcement officers to make sure food law is applied throughout the food chain.

Food law enforcement in Northern Ireland is done as follows. Local authorities enforce food law for food businesses like cafes, restaurants, food manufacturers and food shops. They are also responsible for enforcement in other food businesses that produce products of animal origin, such as fisheries businesses.

DAERA Agri-food Inspection Branch enforces:

- Food law for primary producers (i.e., farmers and growers);
- Rules for milk and milk products for dairy producers;
- Compliance with hygiene regulations at egg production and egg packing establishments.

The Veterinary Public Health Unit of DAERA enforces meat inspection for meat establishments.

 DOI: 10.1201/9781003296492-20

18.1.1 Food Standards Agency

A strong, scientific, evidence-based approach has been, and will always be, integral to the mission of the Food Standards Agency (FSA) [1] to ensure food is safe, is what it says it is, and to empower consumers to make informed choices in relation to food. FSA uses science and evidence to tackle the challenges of today, to identify and address emerging risks, and to ensure the UK food and feed safety regulation framework is modern, agile and represents consumer interests.

The FSA strategy 2022–2027 [3] states that it bases its decisions on science and evidence, and its produces insights and analysis that inform its own work and the policy and practice of other organizations in the food system. This includes expert advice provided by independent Scientific Advisory Committees [4] and Science Council [5] and making all of the research outputs publicly available, as part of FSA's commitment to being open and transparent.

The issues influencing food and feed safety and standards, and consumers' possible exposure to them, are wide ranging, meaning FSA's Areas of Research Interest (ARI) are broad. FSA's ARI are research questions FSA wants to address to promote and protect public health by ensuring that UK consumers are well informed and have sustainable access to foods that are safe, traceable, and properly labelled.

The FSA first published its ARI in 2017 and a revised set were released in 2020. The 2022 ARI have been updated to align with the FSA Strategy 2022–2027, which will now have a new focus on "food that is healthier and more sustainable," alongside the established pillars of "food is safe" and "food is what it says it is."

Themes presented by FSA form the backbone of its future research ambitions, providing evidence for its policy, advice and operations, highlighting current strategic priorities.

By disseminating, communicating and regularly reviewing the ARI, FSA aims to be better prepared for the future by growing its evidence base and creating opportunities to:

- Build and extend collaborations with other government departments, the devolved administrations, local authorities, industry and consumers (and groups that represent them) to enable a full understanding of the food system and the impact of interventions;
- Develop joint initiatives with UK Research and Innovation (UKRI) [6] and other funders;
- Engage with universities, research institutes and other research providers working at the cutting edge of innovation, by commissioning research, co-designing new projects and supporting fellowships and scholarships to enable them to demonstrate significant impact on the food system and consumer protection;
- Undertake research and development to assure high standards for food safety sampling, including within the Official Control Laboratory system, supported by the UK's Food and Feed National Reference Laboratories [7];
- Contribute to prioritisation activities of partners including those within the UK Food Safety Research Network [8]:
  - Research priority one: Assuring food and feed safety and standards;
  - Research priority two: Understanding consumers and our wider society;

- Research priority three: Adapting to the food and feed system of the future;
- Research priority four: Addressing global grand challenges.

The Food Standards Agency (FSA) issues Food Law Practice guidance [9,10]. This gives advice and practical guidance to enforcement officers on how best to apply the code of practice. The guidance is not legally binding.

The Food Practice guidance covers:

- Administrative matters, such as the qualifications and experience of officers;
- General enforcement matters, including prohibition and improvement notices;
- Guidance on monitoring compliance with food laws and carrying out inspections;
- Guidance relating to establishments dealing with specific products, such as fresh meat or shellfish.

18.2 UK LEGISLATION

The main pieces of UK and European Union (EU) general food legislation are:

- The Food Safety (Northern Ireland) Order, which provides the framework for food legislation in Northern Ireland and creates offences in relation to safety, quality and labelling;
- The General Food Law Regulation (EC), which creates general principles and requirements of food law;
- The Food Hygiene Regulations (Northern Ireland);
- The EU Food Hygiene Regulations;
- The European Communities Act, under which EU food law is transposed into national legislation.

There are also several key Feed Hygiene Regulations that introduce hygiene requirements for those food businesses placing food materials into animal feed, as well as Food Information for Consumers regulations that set out allergen labelling requirements for food manufacturers.

18.2.1 EU References in FSA Guidance Documents

The FSA is updating all EU references to accurately reflect the law now in force, in all new or amended guidance published since the Transition Period ended at the end of 2020. In some circumstances it may not always be practicable to have all EU references updated.

Other than in Northern Ireland, any references to EU Regulations in this guidance should be read as meaning retained EU law. Retained EU law can be attained via the HM Government EU Exit Web Archive [12].

This should be read alongside any EU Exit legislation that was made to ensure retained EU law operates correctly in a UK context. EU Exit legislation is at https://www.legislation.gov.uk [13]. In Northern Ireland, EU law will continue to apply in respect to the majority of food and feed hygiene and safety law, as listed in the Northern Ireland Protocol [14], and retained EU law will not apply to Northern Ireland in these circumstances.

18.2.2 General Food Law

The principal aim of retained EU law Regulation (EC) 178/2002, General Food Law is to protect human health and consumer interest in relation to food [15]. It applies to all stages of production, processing and distribution of food and feed with some exceptions. Food businesses must comply with food and feed safety law.

To place safe food on the market, food businesses must ensure:

- Traceability of food;
- Appropriate presentation of food;
- Suitable food information is provided;
- Prompt withdrawal or recall of unsafe food placed on the market;
- Food and feed imported into, and exported from, the United Kingdom shall comply with food law.

Guidance notes were produced on food safety, traceability, product withdrawal and recall, based on General Food Law.

General Food Law includes principles (Articles 5 to 10) and requirements (Article 14 to 21). The key provisions for food business operators laid down in General Food Law that apply to food business operators are as follows.

18.2.2.1 Safety

Article 14 states that food shall not be placed on the market if it is unsafe. Food is deemed to be unsafe if it is:

- Injurious to health
- Unfit for human consumption.

The article also indicates what factors need to be considered when determining whether food is injurious to health or unfit.

18.2.2.2 Presentation

Article 16 states that labelling, advertising and presentation, including the setting in which the food is displayed, of food shall not mislead consumers.

- Traceability

Article 18 requires food business operators to keep records of the following:

- Food
- Food substances

- Food-producing animals supplied to their business
- Businesses to which their products have been supplied.

In each case, the information shall be made available to competent authorities on demand.

18.2.2.3 Imports

Article 11 requires that food that is imported into the United Kingdom for placing on the market shall comply with the requirements of food law, or if there is a specific agreement between the United Kingdom and the exporting country, then the imported foods must follow agreed requirements.

18.2.2.4 Exported Food

Article 12 requires that food that is exported or re-exported from the United Kingdom must comply with the requirements of food law, unless the authorities of the importing country have requested otherwise, or it complies with the laws, regulations and other legal and administrative procedures of the importing country.

When exporting or re-exporting food, provided the food is not injurious to health or unsafe, the competent authorities of the destination country must have agreed for the food to be exported or re-exported. The competent authorities must confirm this after they have been fully informed as to why the food could not be placed on the market.

Where there is a bilateral agreement between the United Kingdom and another country, food exported from the United Kingdom needs to comply with its provisions.

18.2.2.5 Withdrawal, Recall and Notification

Article 19 requires food business operators to withdraw food that is not compliant with food safety requirements and has left their control. Food business operators must recall the food if it has reached the consumer.

Withdrawal occurs when a food is removed from the market, this includes at point of sale. Recall occurs when customers are asked to return or destroy the product.

Food businesses must also notify the competent authorities (to us and the local authority). Retailers and distributors must help with the withdrawal of unsafe food and pass on information necessary to trace it.

Where food business operators have placed a food on the market that is injurious to health, they must immediately notify the competent authorities. There are also similar provisions for animal feed.

18.3 NATIONAL LEGISLATION

18.3.1 England

In England, the Food Safety and Hygiene (England) Regulations 2013 (as amended) [16] provides for the enforcement of certain provisions of retained EU law Regulation (EC) 178/2002 and for the food hygiene legislation. It also provides national law for bulk transport by sea of liquid oils or fats and raw sugar [17]; the direct supply by the producer of small quantities of meat from poultry or lagomorphs slaughtered on the farm; temperature control in retail establishments; restrictions on the sales and supply of raw drinking milk and derogations relating to low throughput establishments (slaughterhouses).

The General Food Regulations 2004 [18] provide the enforcement of certain provisions of retained EU law Regulation (EC) 178/2002. It also amended the Food Safety Act 1990 to bring it in line with retained EU law Regulation (EC) 178/2002.

18.3.1.1 The Food Safety Act 1990

The main food safety and consumer protection offences created by the Food Safety Act 1990 [19] are:

- Section 7—rendering food injurious to health by:
  - Adding an article or substance to the food;
  - Using an article or substance as an ingredient in the preparation of the food;
  - Abstracting any constituent from the food;
  - Subjecting the food to any process or treatment;
  - With the intention that it shall be sold for human consumption.
- Section 14—selling to the purchaser's prejudice any food that is not of the nature or substance or quality demanded by the purchaser;
- Section 15—falsely describing or presenting food;
- Under section 20, if the commission of an offence is due to the act or default of another person, the other person is guilty of the offence;
- Under section 21 in proceedings for an offence under the provisions of Part 2 of the Act—which includes the offences listed above—it is a defence for a food business operator to prove that they took all reasonable precautions and exercised due diligence to avoid the commission of the offence.

18.3.1.2 Food Hygiene Legislation

Food hygiene legislation is closely related to the legislation on the general requirements and principles of food law but specifically concerns the microbiological safety of food.

The legislation lays down the food hygiene rules for all food businesses, applying effective and proportionate controls throughout the food chain, from primary production to sale or supply to the food consumer.

18.3.1.3 The Food Standards Act 1999

The Food Standards Act gives the Food Standards Agency its functions and powers [20]. The FSA aims to protect public health and consumers' interests. They also aim to ensure food businesses are not burdened by excessive or unclear regulations.

18.3.2 Northern Ireland

18.3.2.1 The Food Safety (Northern Ireland) Order 1991

The Food Safety (Northern Ireland) Order 1991 is an Order to provide with respect to the control of food safety and hygiene in Northern Ireland [21].

18.3.2.2 The Food Hygiene Regulations (Northern Ireland) 2005 and 2006

These regulations, the Food Hygiene Regulations (Northern Ireland) 2005 [23] and 2006 [22], provide for the execution and enforcement in relation to Northern Ireland of certain Community instruments on food hygiene for products of animal origin.

18.3.2.3 Food Law Code of Practice

The Food Law Code of Practice for Northern Ireland [24] sets out how local authorities should enforce food law. It also guides how they should work with food business operators.

Local authorities (usually referred to as district councils in Northern Ireland) must comply with the instructions included in the code of practice when they enforce food law. They must follow and implement all the provisions of the code that apply to them.

The code of practice is revised and updated from time to time to:

- Reduce the paperwork burden on businesses and local councils;
- Update it with changes in legislation;
- Maintain standards of public health and consumer protection.

The latest revision of the Food Law Code of Practice introduced a new model for delivering food standards controls in Northern Ireland. This model aims to help councils take a more risk-based approach to inspection, focusing their time and resources on food businesses that pose the greatest risk to consumers.

The new model is phased in from summer 2023.

18.4 CONCLUSION

As in all countries legislation on food is evolving continuously. For further information the reader is directed to the website of the Food and Drink Federation [25] or https://nibusiness.info.co.uk [26].

A very interesting website is the Foodlaw-Reading website of the University of Reading [27].

REFERENCES

[1] Homepage | Food Standards Agency. www.food.gov.uk/

[2] Food Standards Scotland. www.foodstandards.gov.scot/

[3] Our Strategy | Food Standards Agency. www.food.gov.uk/about-us/our-strategy

[4] Science Advisory Committees | Science Advisory Committees (food.gov.uk). https://sac.food.gov.uk/

[5] Science Council | Science Council (food.gov.uk). https://science-council.food.gov.uk/
[6] UKRI—UK Research and Innovation. www.ukri.org/
[7] National Reference Laboratories (NRLs) | Food Standards Agency. www.food.gov.uk/about-us/national-reference-laboratories-nrls
[8] Food Safety Research Network—Quadram Institute. https://quadram.ac.uk/food-safety-research-network/
[9] Food Law Practice Guidance (October 2015). www.reading.ac.uk/foodlaw/pdf/uk-15020-practice-guidance.pdf
[10] General Food Law | Food Standards Agency. www.food.gov.uk/business-guidance/general-food-law
[11] Home | Department of Agriculture, Environment and Rural Affairs (daera-ni.gov.uk). www.daera-ni.gov.uk/
[12] EU Exit Web Archive—The National Archives. https://webarchive.nationalarchives.gov.uk/eu-exit/
[13] Legislation.gov.uk. www.legislation.gov.uk/
[14] New Protocol on Ireland/Northern Ireland and Political Declaration—GOV.UK (www.gov.uk). www.gov.uk/government/publications/new-protocol-on-irelandnorthern-ireland-and-political-declaration
[15] Regulation (EC) No 178/2002 of the European Parliament and of the Council of 28 January 2002 Laying Down the General Principles and Requirements of Food Law, Establishing the European Food Safety Authority and Laying Down Procedures in Matters of Food Safety (legislation.gov.uk). www.legislation.gov.uk/eur/2002/178/contents
[16] Contents | The Food Safety and Hygiene (England) Regulations 2013 (legislation.gov.uk). www.legislation.gov.uk/uksi/2013/2996/contents/made
[17] Schedule 3 | The Food Safety and Hygiene (England) Regulations 2013 (legislation.gov.uk). www.legislation.gov.uk/uksi/2013/2996/schedule/3/made
[18] The General Food Regulations 2004 (legislation.gov.uk). www.legislation.gov.uk/uksi/2004/3279/made
[19] The Food Safety Act 1990 — A Guide for Businesses. www.food.gov.uk/sites/default/files/media/document/fsactguide.pdf
[20] Food Standards Act 1999 (legislation.gov.uk). www.legislation.gov.uk/ukpga/1999/28/contents
[21] The Food Safety (Northern Ireland) Order 1991 (legislation.gov.uk). www.legislation.gov.uk/nisi/1991/762/contents/made
[22] The Food Hygiene Regulations (Northern Ireland) 2006 (legislation.gov.uk). www.legislation.gov.uk/nisr/2006/3/contents/made
[23] The Food Hygiene Regulations (Northern Ireland) 2005 (legislation.gov.uk). www.legislation.gov.uk/nisr/2005/356/contents/made
[24] Food and Feed Codes of Practice | Food Standards Agency. www.food.gov.uk/about-us/food-and-feed-codes-of-practice#food-law-code-of-practice
[25] Food Regulation | The Food & Drink Federation (fdf.org.uk). www.fdf.org.uk/fdf/what-we-do/food-regulation/
[26] Overview of Food Regulation and Legislation | nibusinessinfo.co.uk. www.nibusinessinfo.co.uk/content/overview-food-regulation-and-legislation
[27] Foodlaw-Reading—University of Reading, UK (rdg.ac.uk). www.foodlaw.rdg.ac.uk/
[28] Department for Environment, Food & Rural Affairs—GOV.UK (www.gov.uk). www.gov.uk/government/organisations/department-for-environment-food-rural-affairs

19 Food Products Regulations in the United States

Leo M.L. Nollet and Faraat Ali

19.1 FOOD SAFETY ORGANIZATIONS IN THE UNITED STATES

All information on food safety in the United States is taken from the websites of the organizations involved in food safety.

FoodSafety.gov [1] is the gateway of the United States to food safety information provided by government agencies.

Several agencies play major roles in carrying out food safety regulatory activities: the Food and Drug Administration (FDA), which is part of the Department of Health and Human Services (DHHS); the Food Safety and Inspection Service (FSIS) of the US Department of Agriculture (USDA); the Environmental Protection Agency (EPA); and the National Marine Fisheries Service (NMFS) of the Department of Commerce. More than 50 interagency agreements have been developed to tie the activities of the various agencies together.

As already said, the United States has federal and governmental organizations that are in control of food safety within its country: FDA [2], FSIS [3], the Centers for Disease Control and Prevention (CDC) [4], state Departments of Public Health [5], and state Departments of Agriculture [6]. These organizations focus on the production and distribution of food, making sure all food distributed to retail stores, restaurants, and consumers is safe, without contamination from foodborne illness. Although there are many other, smaller organizations that participate in the distribution of safe food, these organizations are the most active in regulating food and preventing foodborne illness in the United States.

19.1.1 Food and Drug Agency

19.1.1.1 Core Tasks

FDA has jurisdiction over domestic and imported foods that are marketed in interstate commerce, except for meat and poultry products. FDA's Center for Food Safety and Applied Nutrition (CFSAN) seeks to ensure that these foods are safe, sanitary, nutritious, wholesome, and honestly and adequately labeled [18]. CFSAN exercises jurisdiction over food processing plants and has responsibility

DOI: 10.1201/9781003296492-21

for approval and surveillance of food-animal drugs, feed additives, and all food additives (including coloring agents, preservatives, food packaging, sanitizers, and boiler water additives) that can become part of food. CFSAN enforces tolerances for pesticide residues that are set by EPA and shares with FSIS responsibilities for egg products.

On www.fda.gov/food [7] we find different links:

- Agricultural Biotechnology—Feed your mind [8]

Feed Your Mind is the new education initiative to help consumers better understand genetically engineered foods, commonly called genetically modified organisms (GMOs).

- The New Nutrition Facts Label

The US Food and Drug Administration (FDA) has updated the Nutrition Facts label on packaged foods and drinks [9] (Figure 19.1). FDA is requiring changes to the Nutrition Facts label based on updated scientific information, new nutrition research, and input from the public. The refreshed design and updated information makes it easier to make informed food choices that contribute to lifelong healthy eating habits.

At the What's New with the Nutrition Facts Label we page, one can learn updated information including details on calories, serving sizes, added sugars, and more.

The Nutrition Facts label on packaged foods was updated in 2016 to reflect updated scientific information, including information about the link between diet and chronic diseases, such as obesity and heart disease. The updated label makes it easier for consumers to make better informed food choices. The updated label appears on the majority of food packages. Manufacturers with $10 million or more in annual sales were required to update their labels by January 1, 2020; manufacturers with less than $10 million in annual food sales were required to update their labels by January 1, 2021. The compliance dates are still in place, but the FDA is working cooperatively with manufacturers to meet the new Nutrition Facts label requirements.

- Supplement Your Knowledge

Dietary supplements can help people improve or maintain their overall health, but they may also come with health risks. Whether you're a consumer of dietary supplements or it's your job to inform and educate, it's important to know the facts before deciding to take any dietary supplement [10].

A wide range of downloadable educational resources about dietary supplements, including information about their benefits and risks, and how they are regulated by the US Food and Drug Administration, may be found on this page.

- New Era of Smarter Food Safety

Nutrition Facts	
8 servings per container	
Serving size	**2/3 cup (55g)**
Amount per serving	
Calories	**230**
	% Daily Value*
Total Fat 8g	**10%**
Saturated Fat 1g	**5%**
Trans Fat 0g	
Cholesterol 0mg	**0%**
Sodium 160mg	**7%**
Total Carbohydrate 37g	**13%**
Dietary Fiber 4g	**14%**
Total Sugars 12g	
Includes 10g Added Sugars	**20%**
Protein 3g	
Vitamin D 2mcg	10%
Calcium 260mg	20%
Iron 8mg	45%
Potassium 235mg	6%

* The % Daily Value (DV) tells you how much a nutrient in a serving of food contributes to a daily diet. 2,000 calories a day is used for general nutrition advice.

FIGURE 19.1 Nutrition Facts Label.

FDA is taking a new approach to food safety, leveraging technology and other tools and approaches to create a safer and more digital, traceable food system [11].

- Food Chemical Safety

The FDA protects consumers from harmful exposure to chemicals in food that would have an adverse impact on human health, through a comprehensive, science-driven, and modernized approach [12].

The FDA helps to safeguard the food supply by evaluating the use of chemicals as food ingredients and substances that come into contact with food, such as through food packaging, storage or other handling to ensure these uses are safe. The FDA also monitors the food supply for chemical contaminants and takes action when they find that the level of a contaminant causes a food to be unsafe.

Some chemicals are used because they serve a useful purpose in food or food packaging. Chemicals may be used in food, during food production, and in packaging to preserve quality, add nutritional value, improve texture and appearance, extend shelf life, and protect food from pathogens that can contaminate food and make people sick. These uses of chemicals in food or for food contact must be safe.

Other chemicals may enter the food supply through contamination. For example, environmental contaminants can be present in foods because they are in the soil, water, or air where foods are grown, raised, or processed. Process contaminants, such as undesired chemical by-products, can form during food processing, especially when heating (cooking), drying, or fermenting foods.

Food manufacturers are responsible for marketing safe foods. The food industry has a responsibility to ensure the safety and regulatory status of the chemical substances they use in food or come into contact with food. They are required to implement preventive controls as needed to significantly minimize or prevent exposure to chemicals in foods that are hazardous to human health. The FDA assists the food industry through regulations, guidance documents, and regulatory programs. FDA's work to date has resulted in significant progress in reducing childhood exposure to contaminants from food, and the FDA's Closer to Zero initiative builds on this progress. The agency also helps support innovation to meet demands for foods made using new technologies, ingredients, and food packaging solutions without compromising safety standards. FDA provides factual information about chemicals to help people make the best informed decisions about their food choices. These activities occur both before and after products enter the market.

19.1.1.2 The FDA's Pre-Market Activities

Food additives and color additives must be authorized for their use in food before they enter the market. To obtain this authorization, a manufacturer is required to submit information to the FDA that demonstrates their use meets the safety standard. This submission includes an environmental assessment, unless exempt, for the FDA to review to ensure the use of the additive does not have a significant impact on the environment. The FDA has established several programs to help manufacturers demonstrate with reasonable certainty that a chemical is not harmful when used as proposed. These include:

- *Food additives and color additives*: Food additives and color additives require pre-market review and approval by the FDA. Manufacturers are required to supply the FDA with evidence that establishes each chemical is safe at its intended level of use before it may be added to foods. In the case of food additives and color additives, manufacturers submit data and information to the FDA as a petition requesting approval of the ingredient for a specific intended use. The FDA evaluates the petition, and other existing data and information to determine if the data available demonstrate that the chemical is safe under the proposed conditions of use. If the FDA determines that the intended use of the additive is safe, the FDA publishes a regulation authorizing its use as a food additive or color additive. That authorization can be relied on by any manufacturer for that intended use.

- *Food contact substances*: Food contact substances are substances that come into contact with food, such as through food packaging, processing, storage, or other handling. Companies who wish to use a food contact substance that is a food additive are required to ensure that the food contact substance is authorized by the FDA before marketing the product in the United States. Information about a food contact substance is typically submitted to the FDA through a food contact notification. The FDA reviews information submitted in the food contact notification, and considers other relevant information available to the FDA, to ensure that the intended use is safe. This process includes analyzing testing data that demonstrates the amount of migration of a food contact substance to food because of its intended use, and toxicological data to ensure that the consumer exposure resulting from this migration is safe. If the FDA determines that the intended use of the substance is safe, the use is authorized under an effective food contact notification. Food contact notifications are specific to the company submitting the notification and to the specified intended use of the substance.
- *Generally Recognized as Safe*: The definition of food additive in the Federal Food, Drug, and Cosmetic Act [13] excludes the uses of substances that are Generally Recognized as Safe (GRAS) and therefore do not require premarket review by the FDA. For the use of a substance to be considered GRAS, all data necessary to establish safety must be publicly available and its safe use must be generally recognized by qualified experts. In addition, GRAS uses must meet the same safety standard as for food additives, a reasonable certainty of no harm under the conditions of its intended use and have the same quantity and quality of information that would support the safety of a food additive. The FDA has established a voluntary GRAS notification program [14] to help ensure that these substances are safe under their intended use and to help industry meet its responsibility for ensuring the GRAS status of substances they intend to use in food.

19.1.1.3 The FDA's Post-Market Activities

The FDA is engaged in various post-market activities on an ongoing basis to monitor the food supply for chemical contaminants and help ensure chemicals used as food ingredients and substances that come into contact with food are safe. These include:

- *Continued evaluation of safety information for authorized substances*: The FDA reviews new scientific information on the authorized uses of ingredients and food contact substances to ensure that these uses continue to be safe. The FDA reviews petitions or notifications submitted by industry and other stakeholders that necessitate the reassessment of a previously authorized use. Additionally, FDA scientists proactively reassess a chemical when new information about its safety profile warrants reassessment.

These FDA-initiated reassessments are typically conducted on a case-by-case basis and focus on substances that present the greatest public health concerns.

- *Monitoring the food supply for contaminants*: The FDA monitors the food supply by testing both domestic and imported foods through several different programs. For example, the FDA's Total Diet Study [15] analyzes the food supply for both nutrients and contaminants, and is an essential tool that helps the FDA prioritize food safety and nutrition efforts.
- *Research and method development*: The FDA conducts a variety of research to address chemical contaminants. For example, the FDA researches how process contaminants form and develops measurement methods that allow FDA to survey levels of process contaminants in foods and identify actions to reduce or eliminate any potential harmful exposure. The FDA is also focused on improving testing and methods to better estimate exposure to contaminants and identifying ways to prevent or minimize exposure as much as possible.
- *International scientific activities*: The FDA through collaboration with international regulatory partnerships also limits the allowable amount of a chemical contaminant in specific foods when they are otherwise unavoidable.
- *Oversight activities to address a safety concern*: When FDA identifies new data and information that indicates a chemical is unsafe, steps are taken to protect public health, which can include revoking authorizations or approvals for certain uses, working with industry on voluntary market phase-out agreements and recalls, issuing alerts, and informing consumers.

19.1.1.4 Evaluating Food Chemical Safety

The FDA evaluates the safety of chemicals in food (both intentionally added and contaminants) and that come into contact with food using the scientific and regulatory tools while continually evolving to incorporate new approaches.

- Evaluating the Safety of Chemicals Intentionally Added to Food

When the FDA evaluates if a substance can be safely used in food or come into contact with food, they consider all the relevant information, including:

- Information on the identity of the substance, including its chemical structure and what is known about similar substances;
- The amount of the substance that FDA expects people may be exposed to based on how it will be used and its use level in food;
- Toxicology, safety data, and other information to show that the substance is safe at the calculated exposure levels;
- Evaluating the Safety of Contaminants

The FDA and their state partners regularly monitor the food supply for hundreds of chemical contaminants to help detect when levels in foods may pose a health risk. If a contaminant is detected, to estimate exposure and the potential health risk they consider the level of the contaminant in the food, consumption estimates, vulnerable sub-populations who may be affected, and the most current available toxicological information for that contaminant. If the agency finds that the level of a chemical contaminant in a food poses a potential health risk, they work with the manufacturer to resolve the issue and take action to prevent the product from entering, or remaining in, the US market, as well as informing consumers of the health risks. More information can be found on Chemical Contaminants & Pesticides [16].

19.1.1.5 Modern Methods and Tools

To keep pace with an evolving marketplace, the FDA must be equipped to meet both present and future challenges. These include reviewing an increasing number of submissions from industry and other stakeholders to assess the safety of chemicals added to food or that come into contact with food, which have increased in complexity.

Leveraging modern computational, analytical, toxicology, and research methods and tools will further improve our oversight of chemicals in food. FDA is evaluating how to better incorporate modern methods and tools into our safety assessments to help:

- *Better identify and prioritize the potential risks of chemicals* to ensure the US food supply remains safe, nutritious, and wholesome;
- *Strengthen and update existing approaches and processes* for evaluating and monitoring chemicals in the US food supply.

Modern methods and tools that leverage new and evolving data sources better support pre-market safety evaluations, including reviews of innovative ingredients and food packaging solutions. Modern methods and tools can also help the FDA prioritize our post-market safety review efforts in a science-based, more systematic way that will focus on the chemicals that present the greatest public health concerns.

This approach will also allow the FDA to monitor the food supply for emerging health concerns from chemical exposures. This would enhance how FDA integrates and assesses new science on the safety of chemicals in food and better inform their actions to reduce harmful exposure to chemicals in food.

19.1.1.6 Enhanced Approach

The FDA is enhancing its approach to food chemical safety in three key areas with corresponding objectives that complement the existing food chemical safety monitoring programs. Additional resources will be necessary for the agency to pursue some of these objectives and will help ensure more steady progress toward its goals.

1. Expand tools and methods used when conducting safety reviews and assessments of chemicals in food and substances that come into contact with food to keep pace with scientific advances and technological innovations;
2. Update processes to identify, evaluate, prioritize, and communicate new and evolving information to determine if reassessment of a chemical by the FDA is warranted;
3. Continue to monitor the food supply to ensure that chemicals in food are present at levels that are not a risk to public health.

As FDA continues to enhance its approach toward regulating chemicals in food or that come into contact with food, it will also seek additional scientific and other stakeholder perspectives on the activities, processes, and tools in these key areas and improved transparency.

19.1.1.7 Food Code 2022

The Food Code 2022 is a model for safeguarding public health and ensuring food is unadulterated and honestly presented when offered to the consumer. It represents FDA's best advice for a uniform system of provisions that address the safety and protection of food offered at retail and in food service [17].

19.1.2 Food Safety and Inspection Service—US Department of Agriculture

The Food Safety and Inspection Service of the US Department of Agriculture (FSIS) [19] protects the public's health by ensuring that meat, poultry, and egg products are safe, wholesome and properly labeled.

FSIS shares responsibility with FDA for the safety of intact-shell eggs and processed egg products.

FSIS is part of a science-based national system to ensure food safety and food defense. FSIS ensures food safety through the authorities of the Federal Meat Inspection Act [20], the Poultry Products Inspection Act [21], and the Egg Products Inspection Act [22], as well as humane animal handling through the Humane Methods of Slaughter Act [23].

FSIS has different offices and program areas. Each office plays a key role in protecting America's food supply. Examples include the following:

- Office for Food Safety (OFS)

The Office for Food Safety (OFS) is the USDA mission area that houses the Under Secretary of Agriculture for Food Safety and is charged with carrying out the Administration's food safety priorities.

- Office of Public Health Science (OPHS)

The Office of Public Health Science (OPHS) is responsible for collecting, analyzing, and reporting scientific information. OPHS scientists develop science-based and data-driven advice and recommendations (including risk assessments) for use by Agency decision makers.

19.1.3 Centers for Disease Control and Prevention

The Centers for Disease Control and Prevention (CDC) [4] is the nation's leading science-based, data-driven service organization that protects the public's health. For more than 70 years, the CDC has put science into action to help children stay healthy so they can grow and learn; to help families, businesses, and communities fight disease and stay strong; and to protect the public's health.

The CDC engages in surveillance and investigation of illnesses associated with food consumption in support of the USDA and FDA regulatory missions. The Federal Trade Commission, through regulation of food advertising, plays an indirect role in food safety regulation.

CDC works 24/7 to protect America from health, safety, and security threats, both foreign and domestic. Whether diseases start at home or abroad, are chronic or acute, curable or preventable, and result from human error or deliberate attack, CDC fights disease and supports communities and citizens to do the same.

CDC increases the health security of the nation. As the nation's health protection agency, CDC saves lives and protects people from health threats. To accomplish its mission, CDC conducts critical science and provides health information that protects the nation against expensive and dangerous health threats, and responds when these arise.

The role of the CDC is:

- Detecting and responding to new and emerging health threats;
- Tackling the biggest health problems causing death and disability for Americans;
- Putting science and advanced technology into action to prevent disease;
- Promoting healthy and safe behaviors, communities, and environment;
- Developing leaders and training the public health workforce, including disease detectives;
- Taking the health pulse of the nation.

The four steps to food safety by CDC are: clean, separate, cook and chill [24]:

- Clean: Wash your hands and surfaces often
- Separate: Don't cross-contaminate
- Cook to the right temperature
- Chill: Refrigerate promptly.

19.1.4 Environmental Protection Agency

The Environmental Protection Agency (EPA) [25] licenses all pesticide products distributed in the United States and establishes tolerances for pesticide residues in or on food commodities and animal feed [26]. EPA is responsible for the safe use of pesticides, as well as food plant detergents and sanitizers, to protect people who work with and around them and to protect the general public from exposure through air, water, and home and garden applications, as well as food uses. EPA is also responsible for protecting against other environmental chemical and microbial contaminants in air and water that might threaten the safety of the food.

EPA sets tolerances, which are the maximum amount of a pesticide allowed to remain in or on a food, as part of the process of regulating pesticides. In some countries tolerances are called maximum residue limits (MRLs).

19.1.5 National Oceanic and Atmospheric Administration

The National Oceanic and Atmospheric Administration (NOAA) conducts a voluntary seafood inspection and grading program that is primarily a food quality activity [27]. Seafood is the only major food source that is both "caught in the wild" and raised domestically. Seafood is an international commodity for which quality and safety standards vary widely from country to country. Inspection of processing is a challenge because much of it takes place at sea. Mandatory regulation of seafood processing is under FDA and applies to all seafood related entities in FDA's establishment inventory, including exporters, all foreign processors that export to the United States, and importers. However, fishing vessels, common carriers, and retail establishments are excluded.

NOAA Fisheries, also known as the National Marine Fisheries Service (NMFS) [28], is an office of the National Oceanic and Atmospheric Administration within the Department of Commerce.

19.1.6 US Department of Agriculture

The Agricultural Marketing Service (AMS), Grain Inspection, Packers, and Stockyards Administration (GIPSA), and Animal and Plant Health Inspection Service (APHIS) of the US Department of Agriculture (USDA) [6] oversee the USDA's marketing and regulatory programs. Together they play indirect roles in food safety and more direct roles in marketing, surveillance, data collection, and quality assurance.

19.2 US FOOD LAWS AND REGULATIONS

19.2.1 Laws and Regulations

For an updated list of US food laws see references 29 and 30.

19.2.2 Food Safety Modernization Act (FSMA)

The FDA Food Safety Modernization Act (FSMA) [31,32] is transforming the nation's food safety system by shifting the focus from responding to foodborne illness to preventing it. Congress enacted FSMA in response to dramatic changes in the global food system and in our understanding of foodborne illness and its consequences, including the realization that preventable foodborne illness is both a significant public health problem and a threat to the economic well-being of the food system.

FDA has finalized nine major rules to implement FSMA, recognizing that ensuring the safety of the food supply is a shared responsibility among many different points in the global supply chain for both human and animal foods. The FSMA rules are designed to make clear specific actions that must be taken at each of these points to prevent contamination.

REFERENCES

[1] About FoodSafety.gov | FoodSafety.gov. www.foodsafety.gov/about
[2] U.S. Food and Drug Administration (fda.gov). www.fda.gov/
[3] Home | Food Safety and Inspection Service (usda.gov). www.fsis.usda.gov/
[4] Centers for Disease Control and Prevention (cdc.gov). www.cdc.gov/
[5] State Health Departments | USAGov. www.usa.gov/state-health
[6] USDA. www.usda.gov/
[7] Food | FDA. www.fda.gov/food
[8] Agricultural Biotechnology | FDA. www.fda.gov/food/consumers/agricultural-biotechnology
[9] The Nutrition Facts Label | FDA. www.fda.gov/food/nutrition-education-resources-materials/new-nutrition-facts-label
[10] Supplement Your Knowledge | FDA. www.fda.gov/food/information-consumers-using-dietary-supplements/supplement-your-knowledge
[11] New Era of Smarter Food Safety | FDA. www.fda.gov/food/new-era-smarter-food-safety
[12] Food Chemical Safety | FDA. www.fda.gov/food/food-ingredients-packaging/food-chemical-safety
[13] Federal Food, Drug, and Cosmetic Act (FD&C Act) | FDA. www.fda.gov/regulatory-information/laws-enforced-fda/federal-food-drug-and-cosmetic-act-fdc-act
[14] How U.S. FDA's GRAS Notification Program Works | FDA. www.fda.gov/food/generally-recognized-safe-gras/how-us-fdas-gras-notification-program-works
[15] FDA Total Diet Study (TDS) | FDA. www.fda.gov/food/science-research-food/fda-total-diet-study-tds
[16] 2022–12–31 07:59 | Archive of FDA (pagefreezer.com) https://public4.pagefreezer.com/browse/FDA/31-12-2022T07:59/www.fda.gov/food/food-ingredients-packaging/overview-food-ingredients-additives-colors
[17] Food Code 2022 | FDA. www.fda.gov/food/fda-food-code/food-code-2022
[18] Contact CFSAN | FDA. www.fda.gov/about-fda/center-food-safety-and-applied-nutrition-cfsan/contact-cfsan
[19] About FSIS | Food Safety and Inspection Service (usda.gov). www.fsis.usda.gov/about-fsis
[20] Federal Meat Inspection Act | Food Safety and Inspection Service (usda.gov). www.fsis.usda.gov/policy/food-safety-acts/federal-meat-inspection-act
[21] Poultry Products Inspection Act | Food Safety and Inspection Service (usda.gov). www.fsis.usda.gov/policy/food-safety-acts/poultry-products-inspection-act
[22] Egg Products Inspection Act | Food Safety and Inspection Service (usda.gov). www.fsis.usda.gov/policy/food-safety-acts/egg-products-inspection-act
[23] Humane Methods of Slaughter Act | Food Safety and Inspection Service (usda.gov). www.fsis.usda.gov/policy/food-safety-acts/humane-methods-slaughter-act
[24] Food Safety Home Page | CDC. www.cdc.gov/foodsafety/

[25] U.S. Environmental Protection Agency | US EPA. www.epa.gov/
[26] Regulation of Pesticide Residues on Food | US EPA. www.epa.gov/pesticide-tolerances
[27] National Oceanic and Atmospheric Administration (noaa.gov). www.noaa.gov/
[28] About Us | NOAA Fisheries. www.fisheries.noaa.gov/about-us
[29] Laws—United States Food Law and Regulations—LibGuides at Michigan State University Libraries (msu.edu). https://libguides.lib.msu.edu/c.php?g=212832&p=3135122
[30] Regulations—United States Food Law and Regulations—LibGuides at Michigan State University Libraries (msu.edu). https://libguides.lib.msu.edu/c.php?g=212832&p=3135187
[31] Food Safety Modernization Act (FSMA) | FDA. www.fda.gov/food/guidance-regulation-food-and-dietary-supplements/food-safety-modernization-act-fsma
[32] Full Text of the Food Safety Modernization Act (FSMA) | FDA. www.fda.gov/food/food-safety-modernization-act-fsma/full-text-food-safety-modernization-act-fsma

Index

Note: **Bold** page numbers refer to tables and *italic* page numbers refer to figures.

C

F

G

H

I

J

K

L

M

N

O

P

Q

R

S

T

U

V

W

Y

Z

Printed in the United States
by Baker & Taylor Publisher Services

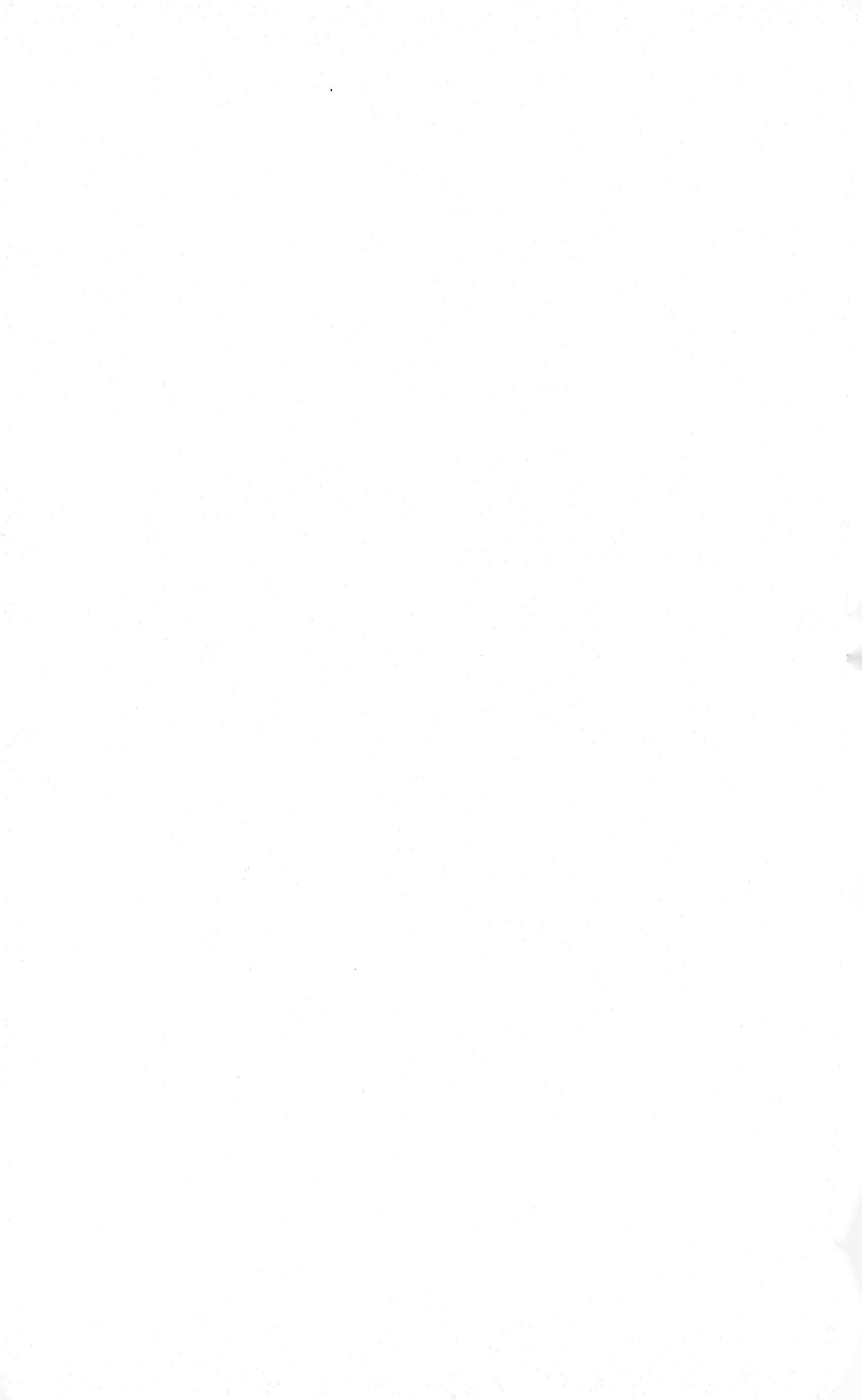